NEURAL TRANSMISSION, LEARNING, AND MEMORY

*International Brain Research Organization
Monograph Series
Volume 10*

INTERNATIONAL BRAIN RESEARCH ORGANIZATION MONOGRAPH SERIES

INTERNATIONAL BRAIN RESEARCH
ORGANIZATION MONOGRAPH SERIES
Volume 10

Neural Transmission, Learning, and Memory

Editors

R. Caputto
Departmento de Quimica Biologica
Facultad de Ciencias Quimicas
Universidad Nacional de Cordoba
Ciudad Universitaria
Cordoba, Argentina

Cosimo Ajmone Marsan, M.D.
Director, IBRO Symposia
Department of Neurology
University of Miami, Medical School
Miami, Florida

Raven Press ■ New York

Raven Press, 1140 Avenue of the Americas, New York, New York 10036

The material contained in this volume was submitted as previously unpublished material, except in the instances in which credit has been given to the source from which some of the illustrative material was derived.

Great care has been taken to maintain the accuracy of the information contained in the volume. However, Raven Press cannot be held responsible for errors or for any consequences arising from the use of the information contained herein.

Library of Congress Cataloging in Publication Data
Main entry under title:

Neural transmission, learning, and memory.

(International Brain Research Organization monograph series ; v. 10)
Includes bibliographical references and indexes.
1. Neural transmission. 2. Learning—Physiological aspects. 3. Memory—Physiological aspects.
I. Caputto, R. II. Ajmone-Marsan, Cosimo. III. Series.
[DNLM: 1. Neural transmission—Congresses. 2. Learning—Physiology—Congresses. 3. Memory—Physiology—Congresses. W1 IN71S v.10 / WL 102.8 N49405]
QP364.5.N47   1983   599'.0188   83-2969
ISBN 0-89004-860-6

Preface

For more than a century, anatomists, physiologists, and pharmacologists have been applying their methods to localize the origin or to measure and to modify activities related to psychological phenomena. Those efforts brought forth impressive progress in our understanding of the problem. The difficulties are such, however, that psychologists sometimes seemed to doubt that those methods would help to solve the problems that interest them most. The term "physiologizing" acquired, at times, a nuance of the meaning of usefulness. The entrance of biochemists into the field is more recent but it was confronted with difficulties not less discouraging than those found by the physiologists. To our knowledge, the term "biochemizing" has not been coined as yet, but its meaning may have come to the minds of many frustrated biochemists confronted with the task of applying very discriminative analytical methods to an intricate mass of anatomical, cellular, and subcellular structures.

The importance of the role played by stimulation in the formation of memory and learning is undeniable. Nonetheless, the span from the molecular aspect of stimulation to those of memory and learning may be too wide to be usefully covered in a symposium. The subject was selected, however, in the hope that a gathering of experts in each aspect of the entire range of the problem may provide more opportunities to show what each of them can offer to help the others. A goal like this in a problem so tremendously complex may have to undergo many failures, but any small success is certainly worth the effort.

The symposium was originally entitled "Molecular Aspects of Nervous Stimulation, Transmission, and Learning Memory" and was held in Cordoba on May 26–29, 1981. Emphasis was on the relationships between neurons, and the presentations were organized to cover the pre- and postsynaptic events related to different neurotransmitters. The transduction of stimulus to a nervous wave or the action of stimulus on procariotic cells were not considered.

R. Caputto

Acknowledgments

Our Academia Nacional de Ciencias Exactas, Físicas y Naturales en Cordoba (Argentina) gratefully acknowledges the following institutions whose generous contributions partially defrayed the costs of organization of the Symposium: Consejo Nacional de Investigaciones Cientificas y Técnicas (Argentina), Sociedad Argentina de Farmacología Experimental, International Brain Research Organization, Roche S.A., Bagó and Medical. The Academy is happy to have organized the assembly of the distinguished group of scientists that attended the meetings and is grateful for the enthusiasm with which they dealt with the different subjects, either as lecturers or discussants.

Contents

The Reactivity of the Neuronal Membrane

Poststimulation Effects on Metabolism

Memory and Learning

Contributors

L. F. Agnati
Department of Human Physiology
University of Modena
41100 Modena, Italy

K. Andersson
Department of Histology
Karolinska Institutet
Box 60400
S-104 01 Stockholm, Sweden

S. Arbilla
Department of Biology
Laboratoires d'Etudes et de
*   Recherches Synthelabo*
58, rue de la Glacière
75013 Paris, France

A. Arce
Departmento de Quimica Biologica
Facultad de Ciencias Quimicas
Universidad Nacional de Cordoba
5000 Cordoba, Argentina

N. G. Bazan
Louisiana State University Eye
*   Center*
136 South Roman Street
New Orleans, Louisiana 70112

D. M. Beltramo
Universidad Nacional de Cordoba
5000 Cordoba, Argentina

F. Benfenati
Department of Human Physiology
University of Modena
41100 Modena, Italy

B. L. Caputto
Departmento de Quimica Biologica
Facultad de Ciencias Quimicas
Universidad Nacional de Cordoba
Ciudad Universitaria
5000 Cordoba, Argentina

R. Caputto
Departmento de Quimica Biologica
Facultad de Ciencias Quimicas
Universidad Nacional de Cordoba
Ciudad Universitaria
5000 Cordoba, Argentina

D. P. Cardinali
CEFAPRIN
V. de Obligado 2490
1428 Buenos Aires, Argentina

M. A. Carrasco
UFRGS
90.000 Porto Alegre
RS, Brazil

B. N. Cemborain
Departmento de Quimica Biologica
Facultad de Ciencias Quimicas
Universidad Nacional de Cordoba
Ciudad Universitaria
5000 Cordoba, Argentina

F. A. Cumar
Departmento de Quimica Biologica
Facultad de Ciencias Quimicas
Universidad Nacional de Cordoba
Ciudad Universitaria
5000 Cordoba, Argentina

E. De Robertis
Instituto de Biologia Celular
Facultad de Ciencias Médicas
Universidad de Buenos Aires
Paraguay 2155
1121 Buenos Aires, Argentina

D. De Souza
Departmento de Bioquimica
Instituto de Biociencias–UFRGS
Rue Sarmento Leite
90.000 Pôrto Alegre
RS, Brazil

R. D. Dias
UFRGS
90.000 Pôrto Alegre
RS, Brazil

H. Dreyfus
Unité 44 de l'INSERM and
Centre de Neurochimie du CNRS
5 Rue Blaise Pascal
67084 Strasbourg Cedex, France

M. Durand
Unité 44 de l'INSERM
5 Rue Blaise Pascal
67084 Strasbourg Cedex, France

K. Fuxe
Department of Histology
Karolinska Institutet
Box 60400
S-104 01 Stockholm, Sweden

E. Giacobini
Laboratory of
 Neuropsychopharmacology
Department of Biobehavioral
 Sciences
University of Connecticut
Storrs, Connecticut 06268

H. Gower
Department of Biochemistry
Institute of Psychiatry
De Crespigny Park
London, SE5 8AF England

S. Harth
CNRS
5 Rue Blaise Pascal
67084 Strasbourg Cedex, France

I. Izquierdo
Departmento de Bioquimica
Instituto de Biociencias
UFRGS (centro)
90.000 Pôrto Alegre
RS, Brazil

S. C. Kivatinitz
Universidad Nacional de Cordoba
5000 Cordoba, Argentina

S. Z. Langer
Department of Biology
Laboratoires d'Etudes et de
 Recherches Synthelabo
58 rue de la Glacière
75013 Paris, France

J. C. Louis
Unité 44 de l'INSERM and
Centre de Neurochimie du CNRS
5 Rue Blaise Pascal
67084 Strasbourg Cedex, France

B. Maggio
Universidad Nacional de Cordoba
Ciudad Universitaria
5000 Cordoba, Argentina

L. Martinez-Millan
CSIC, Patronato "Alfonso el
 Sabio"
Departmento de Anatomia
Zaragoza, Spain

R. Massarelli
CNRS
5 Rue Blaise Pascal
67084 Strasbourg Cedex, France

G. A. Nores
Universidad Nacional de Cordoba
Ciudad Universitaria
5000 Cordoba, Argentina

S-O. Ögren
Astra Pharmaceuticals
S-151 85 Södertälje, Sweden

P. Pasik
Department of Neurology
Mount Sinai School of Medicine of
 the City University of New York
New York, New York 10079

T. Pasik
Department of Neurology
Mount Sinai School of Medicine of
 the City University of New York
New York, New York 10079

A. Pellegrino de Iraldi
Instituto de Biologia Celular
Facultad de Medicina
Universidad Nacional de Buenos
  Aires
Paraguay 2155
1121 Buenos Aires, Argentina

M. L. S. Perry
UFRGS
90.000 Pôrto Alegre
RS, Brasil

J. Prilusky
Laboratorio de Reproduccion y
  Lactancia (LARLAC)
Consejo Nacional de
  Investigaciones Cientificas y
  Tecnicas
Casilla de Correo 855
5500 Mendoza, Argentina

H. Rahmann
Zoological Institute
University of Stuttgart–Hohenheim
7000 Stuttgart 70 (Hohenheim),
  West Germany

M. N. Ritta
CEFAPRIN
V. de Obligado 2490
1428 Buenos Aires, Argentina

R. Rodnight
Department of Biochemistry
Institute of Psychiatry
De Crespigny Park
London SE5 8AF, England

E. B. Rodriquez de Turco
Universidad Nacional del Sur-
  Consejo Nacional de
  Investigaciones Cientificas y
  Tecnicas
Bahia Blanca, Argentina

**G. Rodriguez de Lores
  Arnaiz**
Instituto de Biologia Celular
Facultad de Medicinia
Universidad de Buenos Aires
Paraguay 2155
1121 Buenos Aires, Argentina

P. R. Rose
Brain Research Group
The Open University
Milton Keynes MK7 6AA,
  England

J. Pecci Saavedra
Department of Neurology
Mount Sinai School of Medicine of
  the City University of New York
New York, New York 10079

D. O. Sguza
UFRGS
90.000 Pôrto Alegre
RS, Brazil

G. Toffano
Department of Biochemistry
Fidia Research Laboratories
Via Ponte della Fabbrica 3/A
35031 Abano Terme (PD), Italy

M. I. Vacas
CEFAPRIN
V. de Obligado 2490
1428 Buenos Aires, Argentina

D. A. Vendite
UFRGS
90.000 Pôrto Alegre
RS, Brazil

G. Vincendon
Unité 44 de l'INSERM
5 Rue Blaise Pascal
67084 Strasbourg Cedex, France

T. Y. Wong
Unité 44 de l'INSERM
5 Rue Blaise Pascal
67084 Strasbourg Cedex, France

Neural Transmission, Learning and Memory,
edited by R. Caputto and C. Ajmone Marsan.
Raven Press, New York © 1983.

The Synaptosome. Two Decades of Cell Fractionation of the Brain

E. De Robertis

Instituto de Biología Celular, Facultad de Ciencias Médicas, Universidad de Buenos Aires, Buenos Aires, Argentina

Two decades in science, particularly in neurobiology, represent a very long period, comparable to centuries in other human activities. It is now possible to reflect on the past objectively without the emotions and involvement felt when in 1960 an original observation—the isolation of the synaptosome (13)—started a whole field of research. By that time the application of electron microscopy to the study of the ultrastructure of the central nervous system (CNS) had revealed its great complexity. The synaptic vesicles were discovered in 1954 (12), and many structural details of the synaptic membranes, nerve terminals, perikarya, dendrites, and glial cells had been elucidated. We thought that, to simplify the analysis of the CNS at the structural and biochemical levels, it was essential to develop methods of cell fractionation that could lead to the separation of subcellular fractions as pure and homogeneous as possible. This project involved systematic analysis, by electron microscopy, of the fractions obtained and the use of appropriate biochemical markers (Fig. 1). This work finally led to the separation and identification of the synaptosome. By that time there was some evidence that acetylcholine was associated with a particle generally identified with mitochondria. In 1959, Whittaker (20) presented evidence that this particle could be different from mitochondria. Although the biochemical data suggested that such a particle had about the same gravitational properties as mitochondria, artifacts in the electron microscopy led the author to conclude that he had isolated the synaptic vesicles. The actual explanation was that such a particle (indeed the nerve terminal) had disintegrated as a result of poor fixation and handling of the material.

In May, 1960 we first described the isolation of nerve endings and synaptic vesicles in a paper sent to the *Journal of Biophysical and Biochemical Cytology* (13) that was published in 1961. In the meantime in a short note to *Biochemical Journal*, Gray and Whittaker (17) reached the same conclusion, also describing the presence of isolated nerve endings (later called synaptosomes) in the mitochondrial fraction of the brain.

The investigations carried out independently in Buenos Aires and Cambridge (England) led to the establishment of the foundations for the neurochemical and

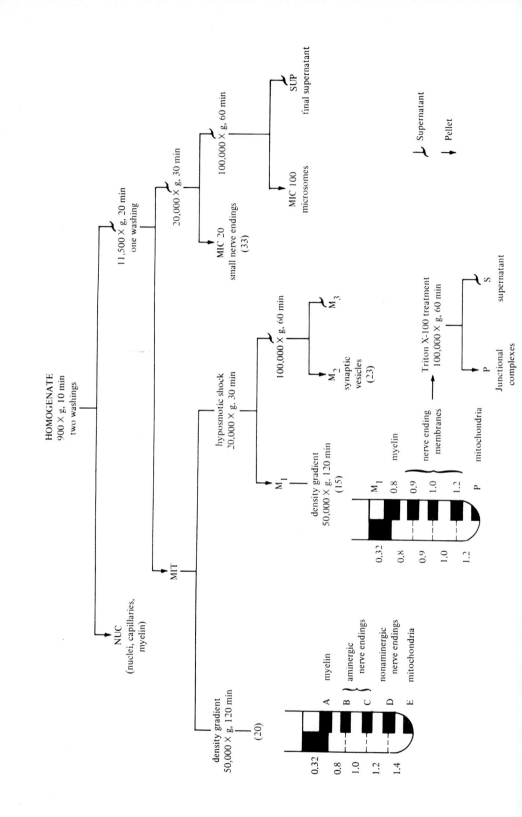

neuropharmacological studies that later developed in many other laboratories throughout the world.

In this chapter I do not intend even to enumerate the many discoveries and insights gained from the isolation of the synaptosome. This information is now dispersed in hundreds of papers. In the past we published a few reviews (14,18,19) and a monograph (8), but today entire symposia and several volumes would be needed to condense the information gathered in these two decades of studies on the synaptosome. In this chapter I wish instead to point out some highlights that could be of interest to neurobiological studies of broad scope.

STRUCTURAL AND BIOCHEMICAL CHARACTERISTICS OF THE SYNAPTOSOME

The isolated synaptosome represents a self-contained particle having all the structural characteristics of the intact synaptic region (8). It comprises not only the presynaptic terminal, with its resealed membrane, but in many cases the postsynaptic membrane also remains attached to the nerve ending. This is a consequence of the fact that it is possible to break up the nerve ending from the axon, together with a portion of the dendrite or the perikaryal membrane and the subsynaptic structures, with the mild shearing forces involved in the homogenization.

The synaptosome is a complex unit of structure and function that represents, in volume, the largest proportion of the gray region of the intact brain (18,19). Studies on the structural and biochemical organization of the synaptosome have demonstrated the presence of at least three subcompartments: soluble axoplasm, synaptic vesicles, and mitochondria. In addition, the synaptosomal membrane, with its pre- and postsynaptic portions, and the postsynaptic density should be considered as integral parts of the synaptosome (Fig. 2). This complex organization may account for the existence of several intrasynaptosomal pools of free amino acids or biogenic amines for the regulation of the rate reactions of the enzyme systems, the availability of substrates, and the permeability of the various membranes limiting such compartments.

The synaptosome is able to carry many of the functions that previously were recognized in brain slices. For example, it produces high-energy compounds through glycolysis and oxidative phosphorylation; it synthesizes lipids, polysaccharides, and a certain amount of protein. Further, it accumulates and extrudes ions and transports different molecules by carrier mechanisms (18).

The early biochemical work was concentrated mainly on the assay of the active substances and the enzymes that are important in chemical transmission (Table 1). It was shown that synaptosomes had a high concentration of acetylcholine, cate-

---

FIG. 1. Diagram showing the various cell fractionation methods developed in our laboratory. These refer to the separation of various types of synaptosomes (nerve endings), synaptosomal (nerve-ending) membranes, synaptic vesicles, junctional complexes, and other fractions from brain.

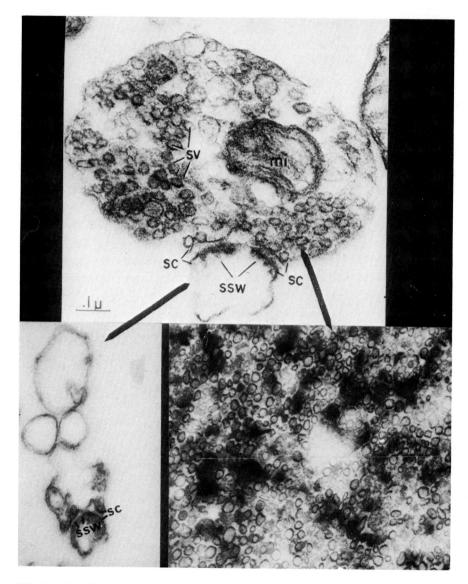

FIG. 2. Top: Electron micrograph of a synaptosome isolated from the rat cerebral cortex. mi, Mitochondria, sc, synaptic cleft, sv, synaptic vesicles, SSW, subsynaptic web or postsynaptic density. **Bottom, left,** synaptosomal membrane after osmotic shock of the synaptosome; **right,** fraction of synaptic vesicles, negatively stained.

cholamines, 5-hydroxytryptamine (5-HT), histamine and substance P (see 8,14,15). The enzymes related to the metabolism of acetylcholine, dopamine, norepinephrine, and 5-HT were also found associated with the synaptosome. An interesting finding was that glutamic acid decarboxylase (GAD), the enzyme that synthesizes GABA,

TABLE 1. *Distribution of biogenic amine and some enzymes in synaptosomes*

	Myelin (A)	Aminergic synaptosomes		Nonaminergic synaptosomes (D)	Mito-chondria (E)
		(B)	(C)		
Amines					
Acetylcholine	0.24	2.02	4.11	0.67	0.27
5-Hydroxytryptamine	0.61	0.78	2.17	0.76	0.48
Norepinephrine	0.32	2.05	1.66	0.77	0.72
Dopamine	0.79	1.85	1.13	0.91	0.71
Histamine	0.72	2.70	1.56	0.44	0.70
Enzymes related to amines					
ChAc	0.10	1.88	0.98	1.00	0.59
AChE	0.15	2.24	2.99	0.94	0.58
5-HTP-D	0.05	1.05	2.05	1.22	0.26
MAO	—	—	0.17	1.16	2.28
Enzymes related to GABA					
GAD	0.02	0.49	1.22	2.00	0.40
GABA-AT	0.15	0.11	0.29	1.10	8.00

Submitochondrial fractions A–E were isolated by gradient centrifugation as described in the legend to Fig. 1. Results are expressed as the relative specific concentration of amine or of enzymatic activity recovered divided by the percentage of protein recovered. (Data from ref. 15).

was concentrated in one of the fractions of synaptosomes (i.e., fraction D, Table 1). This finding led us to interpret the D fraction as representing mainly isolated inhibitory nerve endings (10). This kind of work has expanded, in other laboratories, into numerous investigations, in which different types of synaptosomes were isolated from the striatum, midbrain, cerebellum, hypothalamus, and other regions of the CNS.

As a consequence of the isolation of synaptosomes, several lines of research were initiated in our laboratory. After the injection of convulsant drugs such as methionine sulfoximine, allylglycine, and 6-mercaptopropionate, we found ultrastructural changes in synaptosomes, as well in enzymes related to the amino acid metabolism (see 15). This work has been continued along other lines, into the study of changes in oxygen consumption and protein synthesis in synaptosomes during convulsions.

Another line of work was the production of antibodies against synaptosomes and synaptic membranes (16). In the presence of complement, the antisynaptosomal serum produced lysis of synaptosomes, and, when applied to the cerebral cortex, induced epileptogenic discharges. An antiserum against synaptosomal membranes produced a lytic effect on isolated synaptosomes, and a progressive damage of the membrane of neurons in molluscs. This was observed under the electron microscope, and was also reflected in a progressive deterioration of the bioelectrical properties. This line of work has recently been expanded, in other laboratories, by the use of immunochemical methods applied to purified proteins of the synaptosome. This has led to the biochemical identification of neural types in the intact tissue (see

Pecci Saavendra, *this volume*). The recent use of monoclonal antibodies will certainly produce further advances along these lines. Antimembrane antibodies have been used to produce localized discharges in various regions of the brain, especially the hippocampus. This has provided the opportunity to carry out studies on behavior, memory, and learning.

Because the synaptosome is a self-contained structure, in which the membrane of the nerve ending is totally resealed, it may undergo changes in volume when suspended in media of different osmotic pressures. In 1962 we used this property to disrupt the structure of the synaptosome by osmotic shock and to isolate the above-mentioned subcompartments. If the synaptosome is placed in a hypotonic medium, it swells and eventually the membrane breaks and its content is expelled. By differential and gradient centrifugation it is possible to separate the synaptic vesicles, the mitochondria, the soluble axoplasm, and the synaptosomal membranes (8,14) (Fig. 2). In the vesicular fraction we round the highest concentration of neurotransmitters such as acetylcholine, dopamine, norepinephrine, and histamine, thus demonstrating our previous postulate that the synaptic vesicles were the sites of storage of the neurotransmitters (12).

THE SYNAPTOSOME AND THE LOCALIZATION OF RECEPTORS

In recent years the problem of the localization of synaptic receptors has come to the forefront of neuropharmacological research (see 9). In addition to the postsynaptic receptors that are directly involved in chemical transmission of the nerve impulse, it is now recognized that there are receptors along the entire surface of the neuron, which are particularly concentrated at nerve endings. These presynaptic receptors are involved in the regulation of transmitter release and are found in peripheral, as well as in central synapses (see Langer, *this volume*).

A technique derived from the isolation of the synaptosome and synaptosomal membrane has allowed us to use a direct approach to localize pre- and postsynaptic receptors. In 1967 we found that a mild treatment with 0.1 to 0.2% Triton X-100 produced the preferential dissolution of the presynaptic region of the synaptosomal membrane, leaving intact the postsynaptic membrane with the postsynaptic density (11) (Fig. 3). We also found that the membrane-bound enzymes acetylcholinesterase and Na^+, K^+-ATPase were considerably reduced in the sediment containing the postsynaptic membranes. This suggested a preferential presynaptic localization of these enzymes, the largest proportion of which were found soluble in the supernatant (11).

In experiments in which we studied the binding of [14C]dimethyl-*d*-tubocurarine and [14C]methylhexamethonium we found a different result. Here the radioactivity, expressed per unit of protein mass, instead of decreasing, remained unchanged or increased after the action of Triton X-100. This suggested that the nicotinic receptor is mainly localized postsynaptically in central synapses.

The work on the systemic dissection of the synaptosome has been continued in other laboratories. Cotman and co-workers (6) and Siekevitz and associates (5)

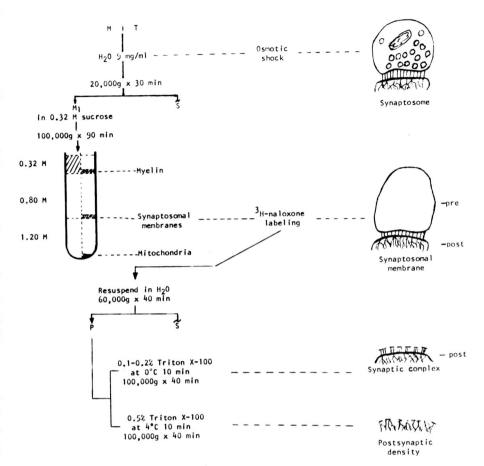

FIG. 3. Diagram showing the cell fractionation techniques used to separate pre- and post-synaptic receptors. On the **right**, morphological representation of the synaptosome and of the Triton X-100 treatment of the synaptosomal membranes. *Pre-, post*, Pre- and postsynaptic membranes; MIT, crude mitochondrial fraction, M_1, crude membrane fraction. (From ref. 7).

found that, by increasing the concentration of detergent and by using a more drastic treatment, it was possible to dissolve also the postsynaptic membrane leaving intact the postsynaptic densities (Fig. 3).

Recently, in collaboration with Aguilar, Criado, Sabato, Gimenez, and others we have started a systematic investigation on the localization of central receptors using this anatomical approach, i.e., by dissecting the synaptosomal membrane into its pre- and postsynaptic portions. Using [^{14}C]dimethyl-d-tubocurarine we confirmed the preferential postsynaptic localization of the nitotinic receptor; however, the muscarinic receptors, labeled with [^{3}H]quinuclidinyl benzylate, behaved differently. With 0.1 to 0.2% Triton X-100 there was a reduction in specific binding per unit mass instead of the increase found with the nicotinic ligand (Fig. 4). This finding

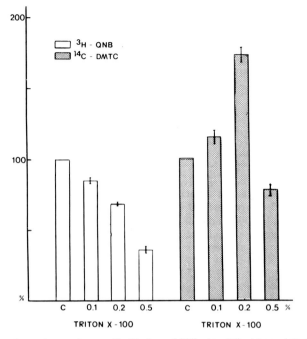

FIG. 4. Percentage change in specific binding of [³H]quinuclidinyl benzylate [³H-QNB] and [¹⁴C]dimethyl-*d*-tubocurarine [¹⁴C-DMTC] in synaptosomal membranes from rat cerebral cortex. (Data From ref. 1). Observe the difference in behavior of nicotinic and muscarinic receptors regarding the action of Triton X-100.

was interpreted as an indication that muscarinic receptors are localized both pre- and postsynaptically.

Similar studies were carried with [³H]dihydroergocriptine to label α-adrenoceptors (3), with [³H]spiroperidol for dopamine receptors, [³H]flunitrazepam for benzodiazepine receptors, and [³H]naloxone for opiate receptors (7). In all cases we found that, with different proportion, there was a pre- and postsynaptic localization of these receptors.

This type of work has had very interesting derivations. For example it has been found that certain central receptors are sensitive to the detergents and can be irreversibly inhibited. However, if a specific ligand is bound prior to the action of the detergent a protection of the receptor is achieved (2). We have also studied the action of local anesthetics, propanolol, and phentolamine on the muscarinic receptor (4) and found that, in the micromolar range, all of them can inhibit the muscarinic receptor by an allosteric type of mechanism.

In conclusion, what are the perspectives for future studies on the synaptosome? As mentioned earlier (18), the time now seems ripe for a breakthrough at the molecular level by the application of some of the powerful methods of immunochemistry and molecular biology. We should follow a more dynamic approach to learn about the synthesis and turnover of the molecular constituents of the synaptosome, including the synaptic vesicles, the nerve ending membranes, and the chemical receptors. However, in this analysis we should not forget that the synapse is a dynamic and self-regulatory unit of the brain endowed with the capacity of transmitting nerve impulses and having other less known functions that are related to the processes of plasticity, memory, and learning. Several chapters of this volume are dedicated to these synaptic functions.

ACKNOWLEDGMENTS

The original work mentioned has been supported by grants from CONICET and SECYT of Argentina.

REFERENCES

1. Aguilar, J. S., Criado, M., and De Robertis, E. (1979): Pre- and postsynaptic localization of central muscarinic receptors. *Eur. J. Pharmacol.*, 57:227–230.
2. Aguilar, J. S., Criado, M., and De Robertis, E. (1980): Protection by atropine of the inhibition caused by Triton X-100 on central muscarinic receptors. *Eur. J. Pharmacol.*, 63:251–257.
3. Aguilar, J. S., Criado, M., and De Robertis, E. (1980): Action of detergents on ^{3}H-dihydroergokriptine binding and localization of α-adrenoceptors in synaptosomal membranes. *Eur. J. Pharmacol.*, 61:47–53.
4. Aguilar, J. S., Criado, M., and De Robertis, E. (1980): Inhibition by local anesthetics, phentolamine and propranolol, of ^{3}H-quinuclidinyl benzilate binding to central muscarinic receptors. *Eur. J. Pharmacol.*, 68:317–326.
5. Cohen, R. S., Blomberg, F., Berzins, K., and Siekevitz, P. (1977): The structure of postsynaptic densities isolated from dog cerebral cortex. *J. Cell. Biol.*, 74:181–203.
6. Cotman, C. W., and Taylor, D. (1972): Isolation and structural studies on synaptic complexes from rat brain. *J. Cell Biol.*, 55:696–711.
7. Criado, M., Aguilar, J. S., and De Robertis, E. (1981): Action of detergents and pre- and postsynaptic localization ^{3}H-naloxone binding in synaptosomal membranes. A structural approach. *J. Neurobiol.*, 12:259–268.
8. De Robertis, E. (1964): *Histophysiology of Synapses and Neurosecretion*. Pergamon Press, Oxford.
9. De Robertis, E. (1975): *Synaptic Receptors. Isolation and Molecular Biology*. Dekker, New York.
10. De Robertis, E. (1968): Isolation of inhibitory nerve endings from brain. In: *Structure and Functions of Inhibitory Neuronal Mechanisms*. Pergamon Press, Oxford, pp. 551–552.
11. De Robertis, E., Azcurra, J. M., and Fiszer, S. (1967): Ultrastructure and cholinergic binding capacity of junctional complexes isolated from rat brain. *Brain Res.*, 5:45–56.
12. De Robertis, E., and Bennett, H. S. (1955): Some features of the submicroscopic morphology of synapses in frog and earthworm. *J. Biophys. Biochem. Cytol.*, 1:47–58.
13. De Robertis, E., Pellegrino de Iraldi, A., Rodríguez de Lores Arnaiz, G., and Gómez, C. J. (1961): On the isolation of nerve endings and synaptic vesicles. *J. Biophys. Biochem. Cytol.*, 9:229–235.
14. De Robertis, E., and Rodríguez de Lores Arnaiz, G. (1969): Structural components of the synaptic region. In: *Handbook of Neurochemistry, Vol. 2*, edited by A. Lajtha, pp. 365–392. Plenum Press, New York.
15. De Robertis, E., Rodríguez de Lores Arnaiz, G., and Alberici, M. (1969): In: *Basic Mechanisms of the Epilepsies*, edited by Jasper, Ward and Pope. Little Brown, New York, pp. 137–165.
16. De Robertis, E., Wald, F., and Lapetina, E. G. (1971): Ultrastructural and bioelectrical effects of antisera against subcellular particles from brain. *Res. Publ. Assoc. Res. Nerv. Ment. Dis.*, 49:8–26.
17. Gray, E. G., and Whittaker, V. P. (1960): The isolation of synaptic vesicles from the CNS. *J. Physiol. (Lond.)*, 153:35P.
18. Rodríguez de Lores Arnaiz, G., and De Robertis, E. (1972): Properties of isolated nerve endings. In: *Current Topics in Membranes Transport, Vol. 3*, pp. 237–272. Academic Press, New York.

19. Rodríguez de Lores Arnaiz, G., and De Robertis, E. (1973): Drugs affecting the synaptic components of the CNS. In: *Fundamentals of Cell Pharmacology*, edited by X. Dikstein, pp. 279–308. Charles C. Thomas, Springfield, Illinois.
20. Whittaker, V. P. (1959): The isolation and characterization of acetylcholine-containing particles from brain. *Biochem. J.*, 72:694–706.

Neural Transmission, Learning and Memory,
edited by R. Caputto and C. Ajmone Marsan.
Raven Press, New York © 1983.

Presynaptic Regulation of Neurotransmitter Release: Physiological and Pharmacological Implications

S. Z. Langer and S. Arbilla

*Department de Biologie, Laboratoires d'Etudes et de Recherches Synthelabo,
Paris, France*

The evidence accumulated during the last 10 years supports the view that several neurotransmitters can modulate their own release through presynaptic inhibitory autoreceptors. Drugs acting as agonists on these presynaptic receptors inhibit, whereas the antagonists facilitate, the stimulated release of neurotransmitters elicited by calcium-dependent mechanisms.

These release modulatory mechanisms have already been described for noradrenaline (33–36,55) dopamine (6,24,30,45,56), acetylcholine (32,51,58), serotonin (13,24,25,44), and γ-aminobutyric acid (GABA) (3). In addition to these presynaptic autoreceptors, there are other presynaptic receptors sensitive to endogenous substances other than the neuron's own neurotransmitter that also play a neuromodulatory role (36,37).

Among all these presynpatic release-modulating mechanisms, the noradrenergic and dopaminergic are at present the most widely studied, and their therapeutic potential is a result of the pharmacological differences existing between presynaptic and postsynaptic receptors for noradrenaline as well as for dopamine.

This chapter deals exclusively with the presynaptic autoreceptors that modulate the release of noradrenaline and dopamine.

CHARACTERISTICS OF THE PRESYNAPTIC AUTOREGULATORY MECHANISMS FOR NORADRENALINE AND DOPAMINE RELEASE

Influence of the Frequency of Nerve Stimulation

The amount of noradrenaline or dopamine released by depolarizing stimuli such as nerve stimulation or exposure to potassium depends either on the frequency of stimulation (34,39,45) or on the concentration of potassium (4,5). The inhibition of the release of noradrenaline obtained in the presence of α_2-adrenoceptor agonists is more pronounced the lower the frequency of nerve stimulation (21,22,39). Similarly, the inhibition of dopamine release by dopamine receptor agonists as apomorphine or pergolide is more pronounced at low frequencies of nerve stimulation (7,45; Kamal, Arbilla and Langer, *unpublished observations*).

On the other hand, a threshold concentration of neurotransmitter in the synaptic cleft appears to be necessary to trigger the disinhibitory effect of receptor antagonists. This has been shown for noradrenaline release on the basis that phenoxybenzamine is unable to facilitate transmitter release by a single pulse or from tissues depleted of noradrenaline by pretreatment with reserpine (18,23,52). Similarly, the electrically evoked release of dopamine from slices of cat caudate nucleus is more efficiently facilitated by the dopamine receptor antagonist sulpiride at 3 or 6 Hz than at 1 Hz (7,45). The fact that dopamine antagonists increase dopamine release suggests that the autoreceptors are activated by endogenously released dopamine and reveal their physiological involvement in modulating transmitter release.

Calcium Dependency of the Negative Feedback Modulation of Transmitter Release Mediated by Presynaptic Receptors

The noradrenergic and dopaminergic autoreceptors also possess the common feature of having the capacity to modulate exclusively the calcium-dependent release of neurotransmitters. The calcium-independent release of noradrenaline elicited by exposure to tyramine is not modified by α-adrenoceptor agonists or antagonists (49,50). Similarly, the release of dopamine elicited by electrical stimulation from the caudate nucleus is modulated through presynaptic dopamine receptors (30,56) whereas, in the same tissue, the calcium-independent release of neurotransmitter elicited by exposure to amphetamine or tyramine is not modified by concentrations of apomorphine that inhibit, or by concentrations of haloperidol that enhance the electrically evoked release of dopamine (30).

Stereoselectivity of α-Adrenoceptors and Dopamine Autoreceptors Modulating Transmitter Release

The pharmacological specificity of these release-modulating receptors has also been confirmed by demonstrating their stereoselectivity. The inhibition of noradrenaline release by noradrenaline itself shows a marked stereoselectivity in favor of the natural enantiomeric form of noradrenaline (57). In the dopaminergic system it is also possible to establish differences in potencies between the two enantiomeric forms of the dopamine receptor antagonists butaclamol and sulpiride at facilitating the release of dopamine elicited by electrical stimulation (6). In addition, only the active enantiomers of butaclamol or sulpiride antagonize the inhibition by apomorphine of dopamine release in the rabbit caudate nucleus (6).

Possible Presynaptic Location of α_2-Adrenoceptors and Dopamine Autoreceptors Modulating Neurotransmitter Release

The presynaptic regulation of noradrenaline release through α_2-adrenoceptors can be demonstrated even in the absence of postsynaptic effector cells. This modulatory mechanism has been shown to be present in recently formed nerve endings in cultured rat cervical ganglion (63), in the rat submaxillary gland after duct ligation (26), and in synaptosomal preparations (19). The modulation by autoreceptors of [³H]dopamine release from the caudate nucleus elicited by potassium stimulation is still present when the possible participation of interneurons is excluded by addition of tetrodotoxin to the perfusion medium (29). In addition, the involvement of transsynaptic mechanisms in the modulation of dopamine release mediated by the dopamine autoreceptor acting through glutamate or acetylcholine were excluded by selective blockade of these receptors (47).

In addition to the presynaptic location of α_2-adrenoceptors (Fig. 1) involved in the regulation of transmitter release, receptor binding studies carried out in the CNS (48,62) indicate that both α_1- and α_2-adrenoceptors are located postsynaptically (Fig. 1). It remains to be clarified if the central postsynaptic α_1-adrenoceptors are preferentially innervated by noradrenergic nerves whereas postsynaptic α_2 adren-

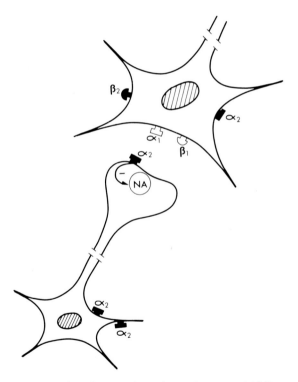

FIG. 1.   Schematic representation of a central noradrenergic neuron. Inhibitory α_2-adrenoceptors involved in the regulation of transmitter release are present in the nerve terminal; in addition, α_2-adrenoceptors with somatodendritic location modulate neuronal firing and their activation would also reduce transmitter release. Postsynaptic α_1-, α_2-, β_1-, and β_2-adrenoceptors are shown schematically. Their presence in the same neuron and the possibility of preferential innervation of α_1- and β_1-adrenoceptors remains to be clarified.

oceptors are predominantly extrasynaptic, as appears to be the case at peripheral neuroeffector junctions in vascular smooth muscle (42,43).

Presynaptic β-adrenoceptors are linked to facilitation of noradrenaline release in peripheral tissues, although the β_1 or β_2 nature of these receptors is not entirely clarified (for review see ref. 36). There is to date no evidence for the existence of facilitatory β-adrenoceptors on the noradrenergic nerve terminals in the CNS. Postsynaptic β_1- and β_2-receptors are present in the CNS (Fig. 1). Again, it is still an open question as to whether there is a preferential intrasynaptic location of one of the receptor subtypes, as shown in the periphery for the β_1-adrenoceptors (9).

Dopamine autoreceptors located in the dopaminergic nerve terminal might be different from those in the postsynaptic neuron (Fig. 2). In support of the view that pharmacological differences exist between presynaptic and postsynaptic dopamine receptors, it was reported that N-chloroethylnorapomorphine is an agonist at the presynaptic dopamine autoreceptor but behaves as an antagonist at the postsynaptic

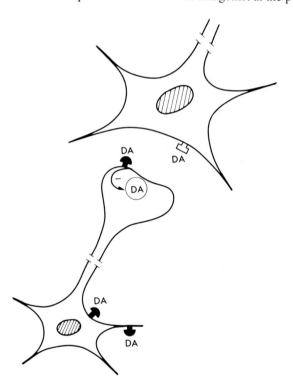

FIG. 2. Schematic representation of a nigro-striatal dopaminergic neuron. Inhibitory dopamine autoreceptors involved in the regulation of transmitter release are present in the nerve terminal. It is possible that a similar presynaptic dopamine autoreceptor is responsible for the regulation of dopamine synthesis. Dopamine autoreceptors with somatodendritic location modulate the firing of the neuron. Postsynaptic dopamine receptors appear to differ from presynaptic receptors in their pharmacological characteristics.

dopamine receptor (46). An additional difference between the dopamine autoreceptor and the postsynaptic receptor is that in the presence of either desipramine or nomifensine the action of agonists on the dopamine autoreceptor is considerably reduced (Arbilla and Langer, *unpublished observations*), while these compounds do not affect the postsynaptic dopamine receptors as shown in behavioral studies and in dopamine receptor binding studies directed toward the identification of postsynaptic dopamine receptors (28; Briley and Langer, *unpublished observations*).

CHANGES IN SENSITIVITY OF PRESYNAPTIC α-ADRENOCEPTORS AND DOPAMINE AUTORECEPTORS

Changes in sensitivity of the presynaptic α-adrenoceptors involved in the regulation of noradrenaline release have been reported in peripheral tissues. Subsensitivity of presynaptic α-adrenoceptors was seen in the cat nictitating membrane after short-term surgical denervation, when postsynaptic changes in sensitivity were not yet developed (40). These changes in sensitivity are probably due to the exposure of presynaptic α-adrenoceptors to the neurotransmitter leaking from the degenerating nerve ending (40). In addition, subsensitivity of presynaptic α-adrenoceptors can also be demonstrated under conditions of exposure to exogenous noradrenaline. In the perfused cat spleen and in the presence of cocaine to inhibit neuronal uptake, presynaptic as well as postsynaptic α-adrenoceptors develop subsensitivity after exposure to noradrenaline (38).

After chronic treatment with tricyclic antidepressant drugs that inhibit neuronal uptake of noradrenaline, increased concentrations of the transmitter in the synaptic cleft result in subsensitivity of the α_2-adrenoceptors modulating noradrenaline release (17,35). Chronic treatment with antidepressants that inhibit neuronal uptake of noradrenaline also produce a functional subsensitivity of presynpatic α-adrenoceptors in the central noradrenergic neurons involved in exploratory behavior in rats (54). Conversely, if α_2-adrenoceptors are blocked chronically they become supersensitive to the presynaptic inhibitory effects of noradrenaline on transmitter release. This effect has been described in brain synaptosomes obtained from rat treated chronically with mianserin, which has α_2-adrenoceptor antagonist properties (14).

The presynaptic dopamine autoreceptors modulating transmitter release undergo changes in sensitivity after chronic treatment with neuroleptics. In slices of the caudate obtained from rabbits chronically treated with haloperidol supersensitivity to the inhibitory effects of apomorphine on dopamine release could be demonstrated (2). After the chronic administration of haloperidol, the dopamine autoreceptors become subsensitive to the effects of the antagonist sulpiride in enhancing dopamine release (Nowak, Arbilla and Langer, *unpublished observations*).

POSSIBLE THERAPEUTIC POTENTIAL OF DOPAMINE AUTORECEPTORS AND α_2-ADRENOCEPTORS AS TARGETS FOR DRUG ACTION

The bradycardic effects of clonidine (11) are likely to be in part due to the peripheral presynaptic effects of this drug at inhibiting noradrenaline release (41). It is also possible that the successful use of clonidine to antagonize the acute opiate withdrawal symptoms in man (27) is due to the stimulation of α_2-adrenoceptors reducing the firing and the release of noradrenaline in the CNS.

Presynaptic α_2-adrenoceptors modulating noradrenaline release are probably implicated in the mechanism of action of tricyclic antidepressants. This effect may be related to the development of subsensitivity of presynaptic α_2-adrenoceptors by the chronic administration of antidepressant drugs. When presynaptic α_2-adrenoceptors are subsensitive, the neuronally mediated release of neurotransmitter will be increased.

There are also some indications suggesting that presynaptic dopamine autoreceptors could be involved in the therapeutic effects of dopamine receptor agonists in schizophrenia, which is probably due to a reduction in dopamine release. In the past, apomorphine was reported to have beneficial effects in schizophrenia, and this drug was recommended by Bleuler as early as in 1911 (8). The activation of presynaptic dopamine autoreceptors can explain the therapeutic effects of low doses of apomorphine in patients with choreiform movements (16,61), in some cases of dyskinesia (10,20,53,59), and in schizophrenia (15,60).

It is also possible that the increase in sensitivity of the dopamine autoreceptors resulting from the long-term administration of neuroleptics will produce a reduction in dopaminergic neurotransmission. The latter would contribute to the antischizophrenic action of neuroleptics. A certain latency period is required after the administration of neuroleptics is started for this change in sensitivity of the dopamine autoreceptor and also for the antipsychotic effects (particularly with regard to the hallucinations, delusions, and thought disturbances) to occur (45).

OTHER AUTORECEPTOR-MEDIATED MECHANISMS CONTROLLING NORADRENERGIC AND DOPAMINERGIC NEUROTRANSMISSION

In addition to the presynaptic negative feedback regulation of transmitter release the somatodendritic autoreceptors contribute to regulate the activity of noradrenergic and dopaminergic neurons. In the locus coeruleus, inhibitory somatodendritic α_2-adrenoceptors reduce the firing of the noradrenergic neurons (12) (Fig. 1). Similarly, somatodendritic dopamine autoreceptors (Fig. 2) are involved in the inhibition of the firing of the nigrostriatal dopaminergic neurons (1).

As discussed throughout this chapter, it appears that the inhibitory autoreceptors in dopaminergic and noradrenergic neurons play a similar role: modulation of the release of the neurotransmitter. There is, however, an important difference between dopaminergic and noradrenergic neurons regarding the involvement of autoreceptors in the regulation of the synthesis of neurotransmitters. Whereas in the dopaminergic neuron the role of dopamine autoreceptors in the regulation of the synthesis of dopamine is well established (31,64), there is no such evidence in support of the involvement of α_2-adrenoceptors in the modulation of the synthesis of noradrenaline.

SUMMARY AND CONCLUSIONS

Presynaptic α_2-adrenoceptors and dopamine inhibitory autoreceptors regulate the release of noradrenaline and dopamine through a negative feedback mechanism where by the neurotransmitter modulates its own release. These presynaptic autoreceptors modulate only the calcium-dependent evoked release of the neurotransmitter, and operate most effectively at intermediate frequencies of nerve stimulation. Like the classic postsynaptic receptors, presynaptic release-modulating receptors are also stereoselective.

Several examples of therapeutic effects of drugs acting on α_2-adrenoceptors and on dopamine autoreceptors suggest that these release-modulating presynaptic receptors represent an important target for the action of drugs.

Both presynaptic autoreceptors for noradrenaline and for dopamine develop changes in sensitivity after chronic activation or blockade by drugs. These changes in sensitivity in presynaptic receptors may have relevance to the therapeutic effects of tricyclic antidepressants and of neuroleptics.

ACKNOWLEDGMENTS

The authors wish to thank Miss Marie-Christine Payen for typing the manuscript.

REFERENCES

1. Aghajanian, G. K., and Bunney, B. S. (1977): Dopamine "autoreceptors": Pharmacological characterization by microiontophoretic single cell recording studies. *Naunyn Schmiedebergs Arch. Pharmacol.*, 297:1–7.
2. Arbilla, S., Galzin, A. M., Langer, S. Z., and Nowak, J. Z. (1981): Supersensitivity of central dopamine autoreceptors following chronic haloperidol treatment in the rabbit. *Br. J. Pharmacol.*, 74:901–902P.
3. Arbilla, S., Kamal, L., and Langer, S. Z. (1979): Presynaptic GABA autoreceptors on gabaergic nerve endings of the rat substantia nigra. *Eur. J. Pharmacol.*, 57:211–217.
4. Arbilla, S., and Langer, S. Z. (1978): Morphine and β-endorphin inhibit release of noradrenaline from cerebral cortex but not of dopamine from rat striatum. *Nature*, 271:559–561.
5. Arbilla, S., and Langer, S. Z. (1979): Facilitation by GABA of the potassium-evoked release of ^{3}H-noradrenaline from the rat occipital cortex. *Naunyn Schmiedebergs Arch. Pharmacol.*, 306:161–168.
6. Arbilla, S., and Langer, S. Z. (1981): Stereoselectivity of presynaptic autoreceptors modulating dopamine release. *Eur. J. Pharmacol.*, 76:345–351.
7. Arbilla, S., Langer, S. Z., and Lehmann, J. (1981): Dopamine autoreceptors inhibiting ^{3}H-dopamine release in the caudate nucleus of the cat: Evidence for a role of endogenously released dopamine. *Br. J. Pharmacol.*, 74:226P.
8. Baldessarini, R. J. (1977): Schizophrenia. *N. Engl. J. Med.*, 18:988–995.
9. Bryan, L. J., Cole, J. J., O'Donnell, S. R., and Anstall, J. C. (1981): A study designed to explore the hypothesis that beta-1 adrenoceptors are "innervated" receptors and beta-2 adrenoceptors are "hormonal" receptors. *J. Pharmacol. Exp. Ther.*, 216:395–400.
10. Carrol, B. J., Curtis, G. C., and Kohmen, E. (1977): Paradoxical response to dopamine agonists in tardive dyskinesia. *Am. J. Psychiatry*, 134:785–789.

11. Cavero, I., and Roach, A. G. (1980): Effects of clonidine on canine cardiac neuroeffector structures controlling heart rate. *Br. J. Pharmacol.*, 70:269–276.
12. Cedarbaum, J. M., and Aghajanian, G. K. (1977): Catecholamine receptors on locus coeruleus neurons: Pharmacological characterization. *Eur. J. Pharmacol.*, 44:375–385.
13. Cerrito, F., and Raiteri, M. (1979): Serotonin release is modulated by presynaptic autoreceptors. *Eur. J. Pharmacol.*, 57:427–430.
14. Cerrito, F., and Raiteri, M. (1981): Supersensitivity of central noradrenergic presynaptic auto-receptors following chronic treatment with the antidepressant mianserin. *Eur. J. Pharmacol.*, 70:425–426.
15. Corsini, G. V., Del Zompo, M., Manconi, S., Cinachetti, G., Manconi, A., and Gessa G. L. (1977): Sedative, hypnotic and antipsychotic effects of low doses of apomorphine in man. *Adv. Biochem. Psychopharmacol.*, 16:645–648.
16. Corsini, G. V., Onali, P., Cianchetti, C., Mangoni, A., and Gessa, G. L. (1978): Apomorphine-hydrocloride induced improvement in Huntington's chorea. *Arch. Neurol.*, 35:27–30.
17. Crews, F. T., and Smith, C. B. (1980): Potentiation of responses to adrenergic nerve stimulation in isolated rat atria during chronic tricyclic antidepressant administration. *J. Pharmacol. Exp. Ther.*, 215:143–149.
18. Cubeddu, L. X., and Weiner, N. (1975): Nerve stimulation-mediated overflow of norepinephrine and dopamine-β-hydroxylase. III. Effects of norepinephrine depletion on the alpha-presynaptic regulation of release. *J. Pharmacol. Exp. Ther.*, 192:1–14.
19. De Langen, C. D. J., Hogenboom, F., and Mulder, A. H. (1979): Presynaptic noradrenergic α-receptors and modulation of ^{3}H-noradrenaline release from rat brain synaptosomes. *Eur. J. Pharmacol.*, 60:79–89.
20. Di Chiara, G., Corsini, G. V., Mereu, G. P., Tissari, A., and Gessa, G. L. (1978): Self-inhibitory dopamine receptors: Their role in the biochemical and behavioral effects of low doses of apo-morphine. *Adv. Biochem. Psychopharmacol.*, 19:275–292.
21. Dubocovich, M. L., and Langer, S. Z. (1974): Negative feed-back regulation of noradrenaline release by nerve stimulation in the perfused cat's spleen. Differences in potency of phenoxyben-zamine in blocking the pre- and post-synaptic adrenergic receptors. *J. Physiol. (Lond.)*, 237:505–519.
22. Dubocovich, M. L., and Langer, S. Z. (1976): Influence of the frequency of nerve stimulation on the metabolism of ^{3}H-norepinephrine released from the perfused cat spleen. Differences observed during and after the period of stimulation. *J. Pharmacol. Exp. Ther.*, 198:83–101.
23. Enero, M. A., and Langer, S. Z. (1973): Influence of reserpine-induced depletion of noradrenaline on the negative feed-back mechanism for transmitter release during nerve stimulation. *Br. J. Pharmacol.*, 49:214–225.
24. Farnebo, L. O., and Hamberger, B. (1971): Drug-induced changes in the release of ^{3}H-monoamines from field stimulated rat brain slices. *Acta Physiol. Scand. (Suppl.)*, 371:35–44.
25. Farnebo, L. O., and Hamberger, B. (1974): Regulation of ^{3}H-5-hydroxytryptamine release from rat brain slices. *J. Pharm. Pharmacol.*, 26:642–644.
26. Filinger, E. J., Langer, S. Z., Perec, C. J., and Stefano, F. J. E. (1978): Evidence for the pre-synaptic location of the alpha-adrenoceptors which regulate noradrenaline release in the rat sub-maxillary gland. *Naunyn Schmiedebergs Arch. Pharmacol.*, 304:21–26.
27. Gold, M. S., Redmond, D. E., and Kleber, H. D. (1978): Clonidine blocks acute opiate-withdrawal symptoms. *Lancet*, 2:599–602.
28. Hall, H., and Ögren, S. O. (1981): Effects of antidepressant drugs òn different receptors in the brain. *Eur. J. Pharmacol.*, 70:393–407.
29. Jackisch, R., Zumstein, A., Hertting, G., and Starke, K. (1980): Interneurons are probably not involved in the presynaptic dopaminergic control of dopamine in rabbit caudate nucleus. *Naunyn Schmiedebergs Arch. Pharmacol.*, 314:129–133.
30. Kamal, L. A., Arbilla, S., and Langer, S. Z. (1981): Presynaptic modulation of the release of dopamine from the rabbit caudate nucleus: Differences between electrical stimulation, amphetamine and tyramine. *J. Pharmacol. Exp. Ther.*, 216:592–598.
31. Kehr, W., Carlsson, A., Lindquist, M., Magnusson, T., and Atack, C. (1972): Evidence for a receptor-mediated feedback control of striatal tyrosine hydroxylase activity. *J. Pharm. Pharmacol.*, 24:744–747.
32. Kilbinger, H., and Wagner, P. (1975): Inhibition by oxotremorine of acetylcholine resting release from guinea pig-ileum longitudinal muscle strips. *Naunyn Schmiedebergs Arch. Pharmacol.*, 287:47–60.

33. Langer, S. Z. (1974): Presynaptic regulation of catecholamine release. *Biochem. Pharmacol.*, 23:1793–1800.
34. Langer, S. Z. (1977): Presynaptic receptors and their role in the regulation of transmitter release. Sixth Gaddum Memorial Lecture. *Br. J. Pharmacol.*, 60:481–497.
35. Langer, S. Z. (1978): Modern concept of adrenergic transmission. In: *Neurotransmitter Systems and Their Clinical Disorders*, edited by N. J. Legg, pp. 29–51. Academic Press, New York.
36. Langer, S. Z. (1980): Presynaptic regulation of the release of catecholamines. *Pharmacol. Rev.*, 32:337–362.
37. Langer, S. Z., and Arbilla, S. (1981): Presynaptic receptors and modulation of the release of noradrenaline, dopamine and GABA. *Postgrad. Med. J.*, 57:18–29.
38. Langer, S. Z., and Dubocovich, M. L. (1977): Subsensitivity of presynaptic α-adrenoceptors after exposure to noradrenaline. *Eur. J. Pharmacol.*, 41:87–88.
39. Langer, S. Z., Dubocovich, M. L., and Celuch, S. M. (1975): Prejunctional regulatory mechanisms for noradrenaline release elicited by nerve stimulation. In: *Chemical Tools in Catecholamine Research II*, edited by O. Almgren, A. Carlsson, and J. Engel, pp. 183–191. Elsevier, North-Holland, Amsterdam.
40. Langer, S. Z., and Luchelli-Fortis, M. A. (1977): Subsensitivity of the presynaptic alpha-adrenoceptors after short term surgical denervation of the cat nictitating membrane. *J. Pharmacol. Exp. Ther.*, 202:610–621.
41. Langer, S. Z., and Massingham, R. (1980): α-Adrenoceptors and the clinical pharmacology of clonidine. In: *Clinical Pharmacology and Therapeutics*, Proceedings of First World Conference, edited by P. Turner, pp. 158–164. Macmillan Publishers, London.
42. Langer, S. Z., Massingham, R., and Shepperson, N. B. (1980): Presence of postsynaptic α_2 adrenoceptors of predominantly extrasynaptic location in the vascular smooth muscle of the dog hind limb. *Clin. Sci.*, 59:225s–228s.
43. Langer, S. Z., Massingham, R., and Shepperson, N. B. (1981): Differential sensitivity to prazosin of blockade of endogenously released and exogenously administered noradrenaline: Possible relationship to the synaptic location of α_1 and the extra synaptic location of α_2 adrenoceptors in dog vascular smooth muscle. *Br. J. Pharmacol.*, 72:123P.
44. Langer, S. Z., and Moret, C. (1982): Citalpram antagonizes the stimulation by LSD of presynaptic inhibitory serotonin autoreceptors in the rat hypothalamus. *J. Pharmac. Exp. Ther.*, 222:220–226.
45. Lehmann, J., and Langer, S. Z. (1982): The pharmacological distinction between central pre- and postsynaptic dopamine receptors: Implications for the pathology and therapy of schizophrenia. In: *Advances in Dopamine Research*, edited by M. Kohsaka, T. Shohmori, Y. Tsukuda, and G. N. Woodruff, pp. 25–39. Pergamon Press, Oxford.
46. Lehmann, J., and Langer, S. Z. (1982): Dopamine autoreceptors differ pharmacologically from postsynaptic dopamine receptors: Effects of $(-)$-N-(2-chloroethyl)-norapomorphine. *Eur. J. Pharmacol.*, 77:85–86.
47. Lehmann, J., and Langer, S. Z. (1982): Muscarinic receptors on dopamine terminals in the cat caudate nucleus: Neuromodulation of ^{3}H-dopamine release *in vitro* by endogenous acetylcholine. *Brain Res.*, 248:61–69.
48. Miach, P. J., Dausse, J. P., and Meyer, P. (1978): Direct biochemical demonstration of two types of α adrenoceptor in rat brain. *Nature*, 274:492–494.
49. Pelayo, F., Dubocovich, M. L., and Langer, S. Z. (1978): Regulation of noradrenaline release from the rat pineal through presynaptic adrenoceptors: Possible involvement of cyclic nucleotides. *Nature*, 274:76–78.
50. Pelayo, F., Dubocovich, M. L., and Langer, S. Z. (1980): Inhibition of neuronal uptake reduces the presynaptic effects of clonidine but not of α-methyl-noradrenaline on the stimulation-evoked release of ^{3}H-noradrenaline from rat occipital cortex slices. *Eur. J. Pharmacol.*, 64:143–155.
51. Polak, R. L. (1971): Stimulating action of atropine on the release of acetylcholine by rat cerebral cortex *in vitro*. *Br. J. Pharmacol.*, 41:600–606.
52. Rand, M. J., Story, D. F., Allen, G. S., Glover, A. B., and McCulloch, M. W. (1973): Pulse-to-pulse modulation of noradrenaline release through a prejunctional receptor auto-inhibitory mechanism. In: *Frontiers in Catecholamine Research*, edited by E. Udsin and S. H. Snyder, pp. 579–581. Pergamon Press, New York.
53. Smith, L. R., Tamminga, C. A., Haraszt, J., Pandey, G. N., and Davis, J. M. (1977): Effects of dopamine agonists in tardive dyskinesia. *Am. J. Psychiatry*, 134:763–768.

54. Spyraki, C., and Fibiger, H. C. (1980): Functional evidence for subsensitivity of noradrenergic α_2-receptors after chronic desipramine treatment. *Life Sci.*, 47:1863–1867.
55. Starke, K. (1977): Regulation of noradrenaline release by presynaptic receptor systems. *Rev. Physiol. Biochem. Pharmacol.*, 77:1–124.
56. Starke, K., Reimann, W., Zumstein, A., and Hertting, G. (1978): Effect of dopamine receptor agonists and antagonists on the release of dopamine in the rabbit caudate nucleus *in vitro*. *Naunyn Schmiedebergs Arch. Pharmacol.*, 305:27–36.
57. Stjarne, L. (1974): Stereoselectivity of presynaptic α-adrenoceptors involved in feedback control of sympathetic neurotransmitter secretion. *Acta Physiol. Scand.*, 90:286–288.
58. Szerb, J. C., and Somogy, I. (1973): Depression of acetylcholine release from cerebral cortex slices by cholinesterase inhibition and by oxotremorine. *Nature (New Biol.)*, 241:121–122.
59. Tamminga, C. A., and Schaffer, M. H. (1979): Antipsychotic and antidyskinetic properties of ergot dopamine agonists. In: *Ergot Alkaloids in Neurologic, Neuropsychiatric and Endocrine Disorders*, edited by M. Goldstein, Raven Press, New York.
60. Tamminga, C. A., Schaffer, M. H., Smith, P. C., and Davis, J. M. (1978): Schizophrenic symptoms improve with apomorphine. *Science*, 200:567–568.
61. Tolosa, E. S., and Sparber, S. B. (1974): Apomorphine in Huntington's Chorea: Clinical observations and theoretical considerations. *Life Sci.*, 15:1371–1380.
62. U'Prichard, D. C., and Snyder, S. H. (1979): Distinct α-noradrenergic receptors differentiated by binding and physiological relationships. *Life Sci.*, 24:79–88.
63. Vogel, S. A., Silberstein, S. D., Berv, K. R., and Kopin, I. J. (1972): Stimulation-induced release of norepinephrine from rat superior cervical ganglion *in vitro*. *Eur. J. Pharmacol.*, 20:308–311.
64. Walters, J. R., and Roth, R. H. (1976): Dopaminergic neurons: An *in vivo* system for measuring drug interactions with presynaptic receptors. *Naunyn Schmiedebergs Arch. Pharmacol.*, 296:5–14.

Neural Transmission, Learning and Memory,
edited by R. Caputto and C. Ajmone Marsan.
Raven Press, New York © 1983.

Role of Sialoglycoconjugates in the Transport of Neurotransmitters

*H. Dreyfus, J. C. Louis, **S. Harth, M. Durand, and
**R. Massarelli

*Unité 44 de l'INSERM and **Centre de Neurochimie du CNRS (Group de
Neurodifférentiation), Strasbourg Cedex, France

The interrelationships between neurotransmitters and neuronal cell membranes are of utmost importance for neurotransmission. This has been well established at the postsynaptic level; its significance might, however, appear rather banal if one does not consider the very dynamic state of the cell membrane which, being in direct contact with the external milieu, adapts, sometimes very rapidly, to any type of change to which it is exposed.

Such changes may come from the extracellular as well as from the intracellular compartments and may lead to important modifications of the membrane conditions. Conversely, it is possible to subject the cell membrane to various procedures and observe the influence of these probable modifications, brought upon the endocellular metabolism, in connection with the exocellular milieu.

The external face of the cell membrane contains a significant amount of sialic acid residues belonging to glycoproteins or glycolipids and conferring an essentially negative charge on the membrane. Ionic bonds have a low energy of association and are dependent upon pH and ionic strength which, especially in the neuron, are subject to rapid changes during nervous conduction and transmission (23). Certain ions, such as quaternary ammonium compounds, which carry one of the most powerful positive charges in the cells, may bind to negatively charged groups that then may have a regulatory role in some basic functions of the nerve cell such as transport or even release mechanisms.

As the validity of such a hypothesis could be tested only by drastic modifications at the membrane level, the membranes of intact cells and of synaptosomes were desialylated. In addition, since from previous studies a correlation was ascertained between transport mechanisms of metabolizable substances and their cellular metabolism (16), the effects of desialylation on the transport of choline and dopamine were studied. Neuraminidase (EC 3.2.1.18; Neuase), which was used to desialylate membranes, is in fact thought not to cross the cell membrane, under normal incubation conditions and after short incubation times.

In a procedure similar to that followed to determine the neurotransmitter characteristics of nerve cell cultures, preliminary experiments were performed to study the basic constituents of the neuronal cell membrane in culture and their analogy with the *in vivo* counterpart.

GANGLIOSIDES

A remarkably similar distribution of polysialogangliosides was found in neuronal cultures when compared with *in ovo* or *in vivo* values. The development of ganglioside accumulation during neuronal maturation indicated the existence of two main periods: a first phase (from 0.25 to 3 days) during which the content of gangliosides increased slightly and correspondingly with the proliferation of the cells and a second phase (from the 3rd day on) characterized by a marked increase in the amount of gangliosides, particularly of polysialogangliosides. During the period of synapse formation (from the 3rd day on when the cultures are derived from an 8-day-old embryo) there was a decrease in GD3 and a high accumulation of GD1a that thereafter remained the major ganglioside species (7).

SYNTHESIS OF SIALIC ACID

When 5-day-old neuronal cultures were incubated with *N*-acetyl-D-[U-^{14}C]mannosamine, the radioactivity was first found in sialic acid residues which thereafter were rapidly incorporated into sialocompounds (Fig. 1). Sialic acid-containing proteins were labeled a few minutes after the addition of the precursor

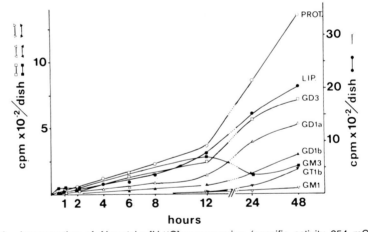

FIG. 1. Incorporation of *N*-acetyl-D-[U-^{14}C]mannosamine (specific activity 254 mCi/mmole, Amersham; 7.5 μCi/dish) into 5-day-old cultured neurons. After incubation for different times at 37°C, cells were intensively washed with 0.147 M NaCl solution and lipids were then extracted and gangliosides purified as previously described (6). Gangliosides were separated by TLC on HPTLC plates (9). Radioactivity contained in total proteins (○——○), total gangliosides (●——●), and individual gangliosides (GM3, ■——■; GM1, ▽——▽; GD3, □——□; GD1a, △——△; GD1b, ▲——▲; and GT1b, ▼——▼) were determined in an Intertechnique scintillation spectrometer using 0.4% Scintimix 3 in toluol as described earlier (6). Proteins were measured according to the method of Lowry et al. (14).

similarly to glycolipids, but in higher amounts. At the beginning of the incubation only hematosides (GM3, GD3) were labeled and, after 4 and 12 hr of incubation, disialo- and trisialogangliosides incorporated the radioactive label.

The different rates of incorporation showed the possibility of a sequential synthesis of gangliosides by the transfer of sugar units to a simple carbohydrate chain.

SYNTHESIS OF GLYCOPROTEINS

Cell homogenates from cultures of different ages (1–7 days) were incubated with GDP-[¹⁴C]mannose and the radioactivity was measured in dolichol monophosphate mannose, dolichol diphosphate oligosaccharides, and in proteins (Fig. 2). The highest capacity of synthesis was found at the 5th day of culture, when the processes of synapse formation are at the highest level (12); the activity decreased afterwards. This transient increase in the synthesis of glycoproteins is a phenomenon that seems to be in fact correlated to synaptogenesis and has been observed during the development of rat cerebellum (26).

GLYCOSYLTRANSFERASE ACTIVITIES

A transient increase in sialyl- and galactosyltransferase activities was observed in homogenates of 5-day-old neuronal cultures while fucosyltransferase activity increased steadily from day 1 to day 7 of culture (Fig. 3), a finding that may indicate a different role of fucosylglycoconjugates in the mechanisms of synaptogenesis. The tests were repeated using intact cells and further demonstrated the presence of glycosyltransferase activities at the surface of the cell membrane. Moreover, the existence of these enzymes at the external surface of the membrane has been confirmed using exogenous acceptors and rigorous experimental conditions (4).

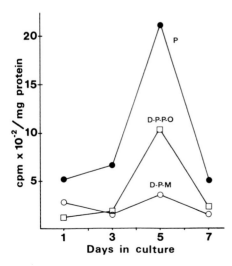

FIG. 2. Incorporation of [¹⁴C]mannose from GDP-[¹⁴C]mannose into lipid and protein acceptors of neuronal cells. Experiments were carried out as described elsewhere (2). Transfer of radioactive mannose was measured into dolichol monophosphate mannose (D-P-M), dolichol diphosphate oligosaccharide (D-P-P-O), and proteins (P).

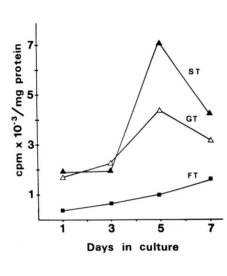

Days in culture

FIG. 3. Sialyltransferase (ST)⁻, galacto-syltransferase (GT)⁻, and fucosyltransferase (FT)⁻ activities during maturation of neuronal cell cultures. Enzymatic assays: for ST, 4 mM MnCl₂, 1 mM NeuAc, 3.5 μM CMP-[¹⁴C]NeuAc (specific activity 304 mCi/mmole, Amersham); for GT, 4 mM MnCl₂, 5 mM GMP, 1 mM galactose, 5 μM UDP-[¹⁴C]galactose (specific activity 254 mCi/mmole, Amersham); for FT, 4 mM MgCl₂, 5 mM UMP, 1 mM fucose, 5 μM GDP-[¹⁴C]fucose (specific activity 118 mCi/mmole, Amersham). 1-, 3-, 5-, and 7-day-old neuronal cultures were homogenized in cold 0.147 M NaCl. For each assay, 50–100 μg of protein were used. Incubations of cell homogenates were performed in a final volume of 1 ml Dulbecco's modified Eagle medium (DMEM) at 37° C during 2 h. Radioactivity linked to the cellular acceptors was determined after precipitation of the cells by 5% phosphotungstic acid (GT, ST), and 10% trichloroacetic acid (FT) (3,10). Radioactivity was measured in a liquid scintillation spectrometer (Intertechnique or Packard-Prias) with Scintimix 3 (Koch and Light) in toluol.

Finally, it should be pointed out that the pattern of these enzymatic activities as a function of the age of the cells was more or less similar to that observed on homogenates.

EFFECTS OF DESIALYLATION ON TRANSPORT MECHANISMS

Cells or synaptosomal fractions from the rat brain were treated with various concentrations of purified Neuase (*Arthrobacter ureafaciens*, Nakarai Chemicals, Japan) preparation at different incubation times. On the basis of its effects and of the lack of proteasic or glycohydrolytic activities, the enzyme used in this study was of the highest purity. The first set of experiments concerned the effects of Neuase treatment on the content and distribution of sialocompounds in the cell membrane.

EFFECTS OF NEURAMINIDASE TREATMENT ON SIALOCOMPOUNDS

Roughly 50% of the liberated sialic is of glycoproteic and 50% of gangliosidic origin. However, after 15 min of incubation with 0.5 U/ml, in synaptosomes, 60% of glycoprotein N-acetylneuraminic acid (= sialic acid; NeuAc) is liberated whereas only 20% of the gangliosidic NeuAc is found in the incubation medium (Table 1). However, the ganglioside pattern is dramatically changed, as polysialogangliosides disappear with a parallel increase in GM1 (Fig. 4).

Similar effects were observed in neurons. It should be pointed out that in each experiment where Neuase action was studied, the release of NeuAc from sialocompounds was measured as a control.

TABLE 1. *NeuAc released after treatment of CSF with neuraminidase*

Treatment	nmoles NeuAc[a] released in the medium/ mg protein	Glycoprotein-NeuAc[b] released in the medium as percent of		Ganglioside-NeuAc[c] released in the medium as percent of	
		Total glycoprotein-NeuAc in CSF	Total NeuAc released in the medium	Total ganglioside-NeuAc in CSF	Total NeuAc released in the medium
1 min without Neuase	1.1	ND	ND	ND	ND
1 min with Neuase (0.5 U/ml)	20.3	61	50	19	50
15 min without Neuase	2.2	ND	ND	ND	ND
15 min with Neuase (0.5 U/ml)	24.3	62	55	25	45

[a]Free NeuAc was measured with the Warren's method after purification, as previously described (5).
[b]Glycoprotein-NeuAc was determined by the Warren's method after lipid extraction (6) and NeuAc acidic hydrolytic release (5).
[c]NeuAc in the ganglioside fractions purified from total lipid extracts (6,11) was measured with the method of Svennerholm (5,21).
Crude synaptosomal fractions (1 mg of protein) were preincubated for 20 min at 37°C with or without (control) 0.5 U/ml of neuraminidase (Neuase, from *Arthrobacter ureafaciens*, Nakarai Chemicals, Japan).
ND, Not detectable. NeuAc, Sialic acid; CSF, Crude synaptosomal fractions.

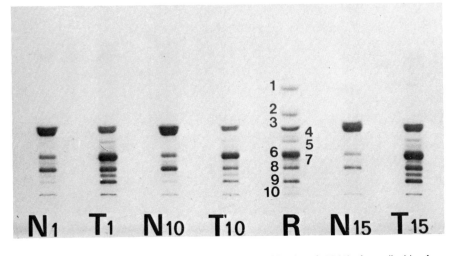

FIG. 4. Thin-layer chromatography on HPTLC plates (Merck, ref. 5641) of gangliosides from a crude synaptosomal fraction of rat brain. Gangliosides were purified as described in the footnote to Table 1 and separated with chloroform-methanol-0.25% aqueous KC1 (60:35:8, by volume) development system. N1, N10, N15: Synaptosomes preincubated 1, 10, or 15 min with 0.5 U/ml neuraminidase. T1, T10, T15: Control synaptosomes preincubated 1, 10, or 15 min in 0.147 M NaCl. R: Reference gangliosides obtained from a mucopolysaccharidosis deceased human brain; 1: GM3; 2: GM2; 3: GM3; 4–5: GD3; 6: GD1a; 7: GX; 8: GD1b; 9: GT1L; 10: GT1b; 11: GQ1b. Svennerholm's nomenclature was used (22) except for GX and GT1L, the structures of which were determined recently (8).

EFFECTS OF NEURAMINIDASE TREATMENT ON DOPAMINE UPTAKE

Treatment of neuronal cultures with 0.5 U/ml of Neuase produced an increase in the uptake of [³H]dopamine. The increase was more pronounced as a function of time (Fig. 5), and is parallel with the release of NeuAc.

EFFECTS OF NEURAMINIDASE TREATMENT ON CHOLINE FLUXES

The effects of Neuase on the uptake of choline in cells and in synaptosomes was quite different when compared with the uptake of dopamine. In fact it was the opposite, as choline influx was severely inhibited in both nerve cells and in synaptosomal fractions. From a kinetic point of view the inhibition actually resulted in the disappearance of the high-affinity K_m value (the lower K_m) (Fig. 6). This might indicate that, possibly, sialocompounds could be implicated in the uptake of choline mediated by the high-affinity mechanism. But before speculating on this hypothesis it was decided to verify whether there was a direct correlation between the high-affinity transport mechanism and the synthesis of acetylcholine. Cells and synaptosomes were preincubated in the presence of Neuase and incubated with [³H]choline. The radioactive distribution of choline in the cell and in the organelles was consequently measured (Table 2). After Neuase treatment an average inhibition of 50% of the radioactive content of the choline pool was observed. However,

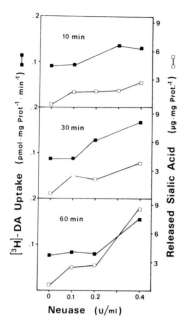

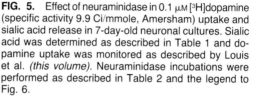

FIG. 5. Effect of neuraminidase in 0.1 μM [³H]dopamine (specific activity 9.9 Ci/mmole, Amersham) uptake and sialic acid release in 7-day-old neuronal cultures. Sialic acid was determined as described in Table 1 and dopamine uptake was monitored as described by Louis et al. *(this volume).* Neuraminidase incubations were performed as described in Table 2 and the legend to Fig. 6.

when the results were expressed as percent of total incorporation no difference was observed in the distribution of the label. Of the total radioactivity, 60% was present in the acetylcholine compartment of synaptosomes with or without Neuase treatment. Further experimental evidence was needed before any tentative explanation could be advanced for these results: the effect of Neuase treatment on the efflux of choline; the answer quickly obtained was that no change could be observed in the outward flux of choline (17).

Finally, a trial was carried out to check whether polysialogangliosides were involved in the uptake of choline. When cells were preincubated with tetanus toxin, no effect was observed on the uptake of choline (Table 3).

DISCUSSION

The significance of the functional role of sialocompounds is still under debate, and although several hypotheses (19,20) have been proposed there is, at present, very little agreement on the significance of the presence of sialocompounds at the cell surface. To approach the study of the possible role of sialocompounds in membrane phenomena it was decided to alter the structure of these molecules by decapping the sialic acid terminals with Neuase under experimental conditions that do not otherwise alter the integrity of the cell membrane.

Recent evidence indicates that the transport of choline might be mediated by a unique mechanism correlated to the endogenous metabolism of the choline pool (16). The ionic and the energy requirement of the influx have shown that this unique mechanism is of the facilitated diffusion type (24,25). The presence of a homoex-

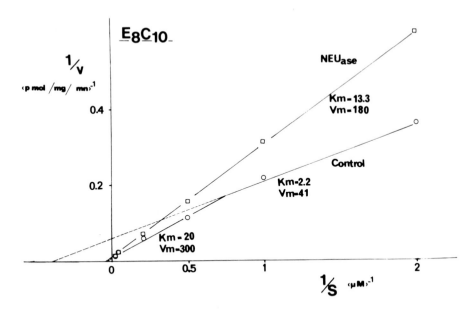

FIG. 6. Effect of neuraminidase on the kinetic parameters of choline uptake in primary mixed nerve cell cultures (E8C10). (□————□), Cells (1.2 mg protein) were pretreated (20 min) with 0.5 ml neuraminidase (0.05 U/ml). (○————○), Controls. Identical effects were observed with crude synaptosomal fractions of rat brain. Uptake of choline was performed as previously described (16).

TABLE 2. *Metabolism of choline after treatment with neuraminidase in primary mixed neural cell cultures[a]*

	10 μM [^{14}C] choline concentration in the medium	
	Control	Neuase-treated
Acetylcholine	1.09 ± 0.4	0.72 ± 0.8
Choline	79.01 ± 0.5	76.02 ± 0.6
Betaine	8.02 ± 0.2	9.80 ± 0.7
Phosphorylcholine	13.09 ± 0.5	13.80 ± 0.8

Separation of choline-containing compounds was accomplished by thin-layer chromatography (on cellulose-coated plates, 100 μm, Merck) with the solvent mixture buthanol-ethanol-acetic acid-water (100:20:17:33, by volume). After visualization with iodine vapors, the compounds were scraped off the plate, added to scintillation vials, and counted with 3 ml water and 10 ml of Instagel. Radioactivity was determined in an Intertechnique scintillation spectrometer.

The values represent means of three experiments ± SD.

[a]Cell cultures (E8C10, 1.2 mg protein) were preincubated for 20 min at 37°C with or without (control) 0.05 U/ml of Neuase and then incubated for 2 min at 37°C with 10 μM [^{14}C] choline (specific activity 30 ci/mmole). Uptake was performed as described elsewhere (17). After neuraminidase treatment the choline uptake was reduced by 30%.

TABLE 3. *Effect of TT on choline uptake in CSF*

Preincubation with TT	Incubation with 10 μM [¹⁴C]choline	pmole choline taken up/mg protein/min $\pm$ SD	
15 min	2 min	$-$TT (control) 3.08 $\pm$ 0.12	(n = 4)
		$+$TT 2.84 $\pm$ 0.18	
20 min	4 min	$-$TT (control) 4.50 $\pm$ 0.44	(n = 6)
		$+$TT 4.74 $\pm$ 0.81	

CSF aliquots (2 mg protein / 200 μl) were preincubated with 2.5 μg TT/ml of Krebs-Ringer phosphate medium at 37°C, then incubated with [¹⁴C]choline. Aliquots of CSF were then filtered on Sartorius filters (SM 11106; 0.45 μm). The excess of radioactivity retained on the filter with the organelles was washed out by 0.147 M NaCl at 4°C. The filters were then transferred into scintillation vials and dissolved in 1 ml dioxane. 10 ml of Scintigel (Roth, Karlsruhe, Germany) scintillation mixture were added and the samples counted. CSF, Crude synaptosomal fraction; TT, tetanus toxin.

change phenomenon adds a further variable to the study of choline fluxes, but to date, no experimental evidence could be shown regarding the nature of the carrier nor of the process responsible for the influx or the efflux (15).

It was previously stated that the study of the movement of choline across the nerve cell membrane is complicated because of three properties of the molecule itself. First, choline is readily metabolized, as observed in synaptosomes and in cells (16); second, the most important metabolites of choline, in any cell, are choline phospholipids, which in nerve cells represent 35 to 45% of all membrane constituents. Third, choline is a very highly charged positive molecule that may form ionic bonds with negatively charged molecules and that may form, and maintain, an electrochemical gradient (in electrophysiological studies choline is the substitute of choice for Na$^+$). As has been demonstrated in our laboratory, all three of these properties may influence and regulate the movements of choline across the cell membrane. A possible fourth point that may be important in the regulation of these movements concerns the dependence of choline fluxes on the electrochemical ionic gradients and consequently nerve activity. However, the response of the cells to the change of ionic gradients seems to be rather slow. In fact, changes in choline fluxes can be observed only after prolonged incubation of cells or synaptosomes in high K$^+$ media (sometimes with very high K$^+$ concentrations) and it is known that after prolonged nervous stimulation the cellular metabolism is deeply affected, especially because of anoxic phenomena. Particularly in the case of choline, Porcellati et al. (18) have shown that under ischemic conditions there is an endocellular accelerated production of choline from phospholipids. Such an increase in the production of choline or of its synthesis from ethanolamine might then represent a further step in the regulation of choline fluxes and, therefore, in the regulation of the synthesis of acetylcholine.

A more thorough discussion on choline fluxes will, however, be presented elsewhere. We now wish to give an interpretation of the evidence herein presented and of the possible role of sialocompounds in the movement of molecules across cell membranes.

The treatment of nerve cells (and of synaptosomes in the case of choline) with Neuase increases the V_{max} of the uptake of dopamine, decreases the V_{max} (we shall discuss of the effects on K_m later) of the uptake of choline, and preliminary results have shown that no effect may be observed on either V_{max} or K_m of the uptake of GABA. The task to reconcile these apparently contradictory results seems to be rather hard and to require a difficult approach. However, a clue to interpretation of these data may be obtained by a careful analysis of these uptake mechanisms.

We have already seen the essential characteristics of choline fluxes. At the moment, for sake of discussion, only the strong positive charge of this molecule should be kept in mind.

The uptake of dopamine presents some important differences when compared with the uptake of choline. It appears in fact to be mediated by a specific carrier and shows no apparent correlation to its endogenous metabolism. Moreover, its affinity for the substrate is established only after the beginning of cell maturation while the V_{max} value, representing the number of binding sites, increases with synaptogenesis (13). On the basis of these characteristics the uptake of dopamine might then be defined as a "simpler" type of transport when compared with the uptake of choline, which appears to be present in all cells, undifferentiated as well as mature, and which is further complicated by the phenomena previously discussed.

The preliminary experimental evidence indicates that the uptake of GABA in nerve cell cultures has many similarities to the uptake of choline and confirms the data obtained in synaptosomes. The study of the uptake of GABA is, however, complicated by the nature of this molecule which, being a neurotransmitter, is bound to release phenomena and consequently is more dependent on ionic gradients and movements.

Treatment with Neuase (under the conditions described) does not alter the status of the cell membrane while it releases sialic acid molecules from sialocompounds. The negative charge of these may play an important role in the transport of choline and of dopamine. The possible binding of choline to gangliosides might suggest that sialic acid terminals that are stretched on the external surface of the cells "attract" and/or "direct" choline molecules toward the carrier situated in the membrane. The capacity of sialocompounds to act as carriers should be excluded at the light of the experiments that showed no effect of Neuase on the efflux of choline, unless influx and efflux movements of choline are not mediated by different carriers. But this seems unlikely considering the presence of an homoexchange phenomenon.

Why does the 10^{-6} MK_m disappear after Neuase treatment? Is it possible that sialocompounds may be relevant for the so-called high-affinity mechanism alone? We think the answer to these questions should be negative. It should be pointed out, in fact, that the inhibition produced by Neuase concerns *both* the high and the low K_m values. At low external concentrations of choline, sialic acid terminals may "capture" these molecules from the milieu (Fig. 7) or may constitute an "umbrella" of charges under which choline molecules are concentrated close to the cell mem-

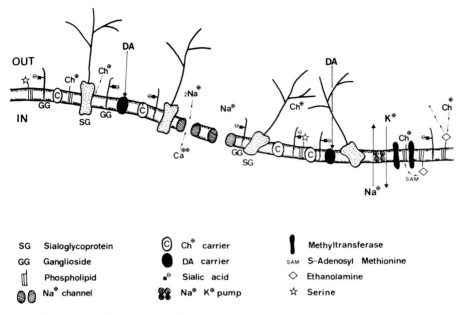

FIG. 7. Hypothesis of involvement of sialoglycoconjugates in choline and dopamine transport in relation to ion fluxes in nerve cell membranes.

brane and to the carrier. The energy for the eventual transfer of choline inside the cell should be provided by the Na^+ gradient.

At high external concentrations of choline, the sialic acid terminals will instead still act as captors for choline molecules and the transport of these will be less dependent upon the Na^+ gradient, as the energy given by the electrochemical gradient created by the choline molecules and maintained by sialocompounds should be enough to drive the same molecules across the membrane (Fig. 7).

Quite differently in the case of dopamine, sialocompounds may actually mask the carrier site, and the desialylation of the membrane unmasks a larger proportion of these. The lack of effect of the K_m on the uptake indicates as well that sialo-compounds should not be considered as possible carriers for dopamine but rather as "regulators" of this transport.

The role of sialocompounds in transport phenomena does not appear, however, to be of general interest, considering the lack of effect on GABA transport after Neuase treatment, but rather limited to some transport systems (1).

Moreover, their role does not seem to be specific (in particular stereospecific) for a certain molecular species but simply a result of their ionized charge. It may then be suggested that some basic cellular phenomena, such as transport for certain nutrients, release of neuromediators, or even cellular recognition, may be regulated by charge distribution and movements (laterally or across the cell membrane) between basic components of the membrane and ionic constituents of the extracellular medium or with basic membrane components of neighbouring cells.

ACKNOWLEDGMENTS

The excellent technical assistance of Mrs. A. Gomez de Gracia is greatly appreciated. We thank Dr. B. Hoflack (Villeneuve d'Ascq) for his kind help in glycosyltransferase activity determination. This work was supported by grants from INSERM (CRL 78.4.017) and the DGRST (aide 80.3.0875).

REFERENCES

1. Balcar, V. J., Borg, J., and Mandel, P. (1977): High affinity uptake of L-glutamate and L-aspartate by glial cells. *J. Neurochem.*, 28:87–93.
2. Cacan, R., Hoflack, B., and Verbert, A. (1980): Metabolism of lipid-linked oligosaccharide intermediates in rat spleen lymphocytes. *Eur. J. Biochem.*, 106:473–479.
3. Cacan, R., Verbert, A., and Montreuil, J. (1976): New evidence for cell surface galactosyltransferase. *FEBS Lett.*, 63:102–106.
4. Dreyfus, H., Harth, S., Massarelli, R., and Louis, J. C. (1981); Mechanisms of differentiation in cultured neurons: Involvement of gangliosides. In: *Gangliosides in Neurological and Neurosurgical Development and Repair*, edited by A. Gorio and M. M. Rapport, Raven Press, New York.
5. Dreyfus, H., Harth, S., Urban, P. F., Mandel, P., Preti, A., and Lombardo, A. (1976): On the presence of a "particle-bound" neuraminidase in retina. A development study. *Life Sci.*, 18:1057–1064.
6. Dreyfus, H., Harth, S., Yusufi, A. N. K., Urban, P. F., and Mandel, P. (1980): Sialyltransferase activities in two neuronal models: Retina and cultures of isolated neurons. In: *Advances in Experimental Medicine and Biology, Vol. 125: Structure and Function of Gangliosides*, edited by L. Svennerholm, P. Mandel, H. Dreyfus, and P. F. Urban, pp. 227–237. Plenum Press, New York.
7. Dreyfus, H., Louis, J. C., Harth, S., and Mandel, P. (1980): Gangliosides in cultured neurons. *Neuroscience*, 5:1647–1655.
8. Ghidoni, R., Sonnino, S., Tettamanti, G., Baumann, N., Reuter, G., and Schauer, R. (1980): Isolation and characterization of a trisialoganglioside from mouse brain containing 9-*O*-acetyl-*N*-acetylneuraminic acid. *J. Biol. Chem.*, 255:6990–6995.
9. Harth, S., Dreyfus, H., Urban, P. F., and Mandel, P. (1978): Direct thin layer chromatography of gangliosides of a total lipid extract. *Anal. Biochem.*, 86:543–551.
10. Hoflack, B., Cacan, R., Montreuil, J., and Verbert, A. (1979): Detection of ectosialyltransferase activity using whole cells. Correction of misleading results due to the release of intracellular CMP-*N*-acetylneuraminic acid. *Biochim. Biophys. Acta*, 568:348–356.
11. Irwin, C. C., and Irwin, I. W. (1979): A simple rapid method for ganglioside isolation from small amounts of tissue. *Anal. Biochem.*, 94:335–339.
12. Louis, J. C., Pettman, B., Courageot, J., Rumigny, J. F., Mandel, P., and Sensenbrenner, M. (1981): Developmental changes in cultured neurons from chick embryo cerebral hemispheres. *Exp. Brain Res.*, 42:63–72.
13. Louis, J. C., Vincendon, G., Massarelli, R., and Dreyfus, H. (1981): Development of dopaminergic properties in cultured neurons from chick embryo cerebral hemispheres. *Biochem. Soc. Trans.*, 9:104–105.
14. Lowry, O. H., Rosebrough, N. J., Farr, A. L., and Randall, R. J. (1951): Protein measurement with the Folin phenol reagent. *J. Biol. Chem.*, 193:265–275.
15. Marchbanks, R. M., and Wonnacot, S. (1979): Relationship of choline uptake to acetylcholine synthesis and release. In: *The Cholinergic Synapse*, edited by S. Tuček, pp. 77–87. Elsevier Scientific Publishing Company, Amsterdam.
16. Massarelli, R., and Wong, T. Y. (1981): Choline uptake in nerve cell cultures and in synaptosomal preparations is regulated by the endogenous pool of choline. In: *Cholinergic Mechanisms*, edited by G. Pepeu and H. Ladinsky, pp. 511–520. Plenum Press, New York.
17. Massarelli, R., Wong, T. Y., Harth, S., Louis, J. C., Freysz, L., and Dreyfus, H. (1982): Possible role of sialocompounds in the uptake of choline into synaptosomes and nerve cell cultures. *Neurochem. Res.*, 7:301–316.

18. Porcellati, G., De Medio, G. E., Fini, C., Floridi, A., Goracci, G., Horrocks, L. A., Lazarewicz, J. W., Palmerini, C. A., Strosznajder, J., and Trovarelli, G. (1978): Phospholipid and its metabolism in ischemia. In: *Proceedings of the European Society for Neurochemistry, Vol. 1*, edited by V. Neuhoff, pp. 285–302. Verlag Chemie, Weinheim, Germany.
19. Rahmann, H., Rösner, H., and Breer, H. (1976): A functional model of sialoglyco-macromolecules in synaptic transmission and memory formation. *J. Theor. Biol.*, 57:231–237.
20. Simonneau, M., Baux, G., and Tauc, L. (1979): Sialic acid containing substrates as intracellular calcium receptors involved in transmitter release. *J. Physiol. (Paris)*, 76:427–433.
21. Svennerholm, L. (1957): Quantitative estimation of sialic acids. II. A colorimetric resorcinol-hydrochloric method. *Biochim. Biophys. Acta*, 24:604–611.
22. Svennerholm, L. (1980): Ganglioside designation. In: *Advances in Experimental Medicine and Biology, Vol. 125: Structure and Function of Gangliosides*, edited by L. Svennerholm, P. Mandel, H. Dreyfus, and P. F. Urban, p. 11. Plenum Press, New York.
23. Weight, F. F. (1974): Physiological mechanisms of synaptic modulation. In: *The Neurosciences: Third Study Program*, edited by F. O. Schmitt and F. G. Worden, pp. 929–941. MIT Press, Cambridge, Massachusetts.
24. Wong, T. Y., Dreyfus, H., and Massarelli, R. (1981): Transport and metabolism of choline in synaptosomes: Ionic requirement. *Biochem. Soc. Trans.*, 9:84–85.
25. Wong, T. Y., Louis, J. C., Vincendon, G., and Massarelli, M. (1981): Transport and metabolism of choline in synaptosomes: Energy requirement. *Biochem. Soc. Trans.*, 9:83–84.
26. Zanetta, J. P., Roussel, G., Gandhour, M. S., Vincendon, G., and Gombos, G. (1978): Postnatal development of rat cerebellum: Massive and transient accumulation of concanavalin A binding glycoprotein in parallel fiber axolemma. *Brain Res.*, 142:301–319.

Neural Transmission, Learning and Memory,
edited by R. Caputto and C. Ajmone Marsan.
Raven Press, New York © 1983.

Effect of Gangliosides and Other Fusogenic Agents on the Neurotransmitter Movements in Nerve Endings. Importance of the Membrane Interfacial Potential

F. A. Cumar, B. Maggio, and R. Caputto

Departmento de Química Biológica, Facultad de Ciencias Químicas, Universidad Nacional de Córdoba, Ciudad Universitaria, Córdoba, Argentina

An important step in interneuronal transmission is the release of chemical substances at the nerve endings. A proposed mechanism for this process involves a Ca^{2+}-mediated exocytosis in which the synaptic vesicle fuses with the synaptosomal plasma membrane (7,11,18,21). Since membrane-membrane interactions must take place in this phenomenon it is generally agreed that changes in the molecular organization of these membranes are occurring. However, a perusal of the literature reveals that most of the mechanisms proposed to explain this process usually consider isolated or very specific molecular mechanisms that are seldom integrated within the general dynamic metastable state of the membrane. On the other hand, considerable experimental evidence has been accumulated during the last decade showing that in processes involving membrane fusion in general, *several* transient modifications of the molecular organization of both the lipid and protein components, with concomitant changes of the membrane permeability, must occur simultaneously; usually, if only one of the requirements is not fulfilled the end result is not obtained (cf. 33,39).

On this basis, the problem of neurotransmitter release is just another example regarding changes of the overall membrane metastable state with several features in common with many other general processes of exocytosis. Obviously, there must exist in the membrane system or its surroundings natural compounds that, according to the interactions established with other membrane components, can lead to and regulate the final event.

As a result of previous experiments on glycosphingolipids in our laboratory (cf. 8,39) we have been interested in investigating whether gangliosides can be involved in neurotransmitter movements. As described below, these lipids, which are enriched in the synaptosomal plasma membranes, share several interfacial properties with many other natural and synthetic compounds involving changes of intermolecular organization and electrical field at the membrane interface that can lead to permeability changes and membrane fusion (39).

INTERFACIAL PROPERTIES OF GLYCOSPHINGOLIPIDS

The chemical structure of a complex glycosphingolipid such as a trisialoganglioside is shown in Fig. 1. For most of the glycosphingolipids the hydrophobic (ceramide) portion is, on average, very similar and the oligosaccharide chain may contain several neutral carbohydrates and, in the case of gangliosides, a variable number of sialosyl residues.

When glycosphingolipids are oriented at interfaces, the complexity of the oligosaccharide chain and dipolar properties of individual carbohydrate residues has a profound influence on the surface behaviour. The liquid character of the interface and molecular area of these lipids increases according to the number of negatively charged sialosyl residues as a consequence of electrostatic repulsions (37). From studies performed with lipid monolayers on subphases at different pH values it was suggested that the oligosaccharide chain can dynamically move from an approximately perpendicular orientation with respect to the interface at a close molecular packing to an angle displaced as much as 80 degrees at loose packing (37–39). These movements of the polar head group extending to variable degrees into the aqueous phase according to changes of molecular packing (e.g., as due to isothermal phase changes and interactions) in the membrane plane may constitute information transducers that can regulate membrane-ligand interactions (cf. 46).

The constraints imposed on the conformation of the oligosaccharide chain by the glycosidic linkages and its anchoring to the interface through the ceramide moiety determine the orientation of the dipole moment vector of each carbohydrate residue (Fig. 2), and this is revealed by measurements of the interfacial potential (37). Neutral carbohydrate residues seem to contribute with an electrical field in a direction opposite to that of the hydrocarbon chains; in view of the fact that sialosyl residues are chemically indistinguishable a rather unexpected finding was that their dipolar properties depended on how they are located along the oligosaccharide chain. This is probably related to the relative position that, according to the linkages involved, the carboxylate group is forced to adopt with respect to both the interface and the rest of each of the sialosyl moieties (Fig. 2) (38).

The above studies indicated that, on the basis of the orientation of dipole moment vectors of the different carbohydrate residues in the oligosaccharide chain, two

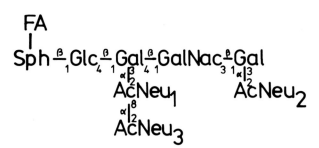

FIG. 1. Chemical structure of a trisialoganglioside. Sph, sphingoid; FA, fatty acid; G1c, glucose; Gal, galactose; ga1Nac, *N*-acetylgalactosamine; AcNeu, *N*-acetylneuraminic (sialic) acid.

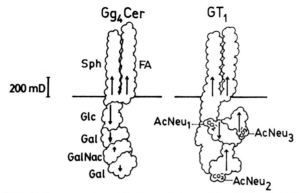

FIG. 2. Resultant dipole moment contributions of glycosphingolipids at pH 5.6. Outline projections of Corey-Pauling-Koltun molecular models are given with indicated vertical dipole moment contibutions from each moiety. For more detailed explanation of the configuration of molecular models see legend to Fig. 5. (From ref. 39, with permission.)

groups of glycosphingolipids can be distinguished: neutral glycosphingolipids and monosialogangliosides that contain only dipolar components oriented opposite to those of the hydrocarbon portion of the molecule, and polysialogangliosides that contain in the polar head group dipolar components oriented in the same direction as those of the ceramide moiety. These different dipolar properties strongly influenced the interactions that the two groups of glycosphingolipids can establish with membrane phospholipids in interfaces (36).

The different glycosphingolipids showed interactions with phospholipids that are independent of the type of hydrophobic chains of the phospholipid. Conversely, the molecular organization adopted by the glycolipid-phospholipid interface depended on the type of polar head group of both lipids as shown in Fig. 3. A definite change in the tendency of the interactions with all the phospholipids, in both molecular packing and surface potential, can be seen for di- and trisialogangliosides, compared with monosialogangliosides and neutral glycosphingolipids (36).

Energetic considerations indicated that the interactions between phosphatidyl-choline and polysialogangliosides are thermodynamically favored, as shown by the negative value of the excess free energy for these mixtures (Fig. 4) (36,39). This suggested that, in absence of other constraints, polysialogangliosides would spontaneously associate with phosphatidylcholine preferably to other phospholipids in a complex lipid interface such as a natural membrane. The polysialoganglioside-phosphatidylcholine interactions occur with a closer than expected molecular packing and a reduced interfacial potential (Fig. 3) with respect to a noninteracting state. Molecular details of the interactions were obtained from studies with lipid monolayers on subphases at different pH values and using compounds that contain only one of the two charged groups present in phosphatidylcholine. These studies revealed that to obtain thermodynamically stable ganglioside-phospholipid interactions with reductions in molecular packing and surface potential it seems necessary that the lipid interface may establish certain dipolar interactions that lead to its stabilization;

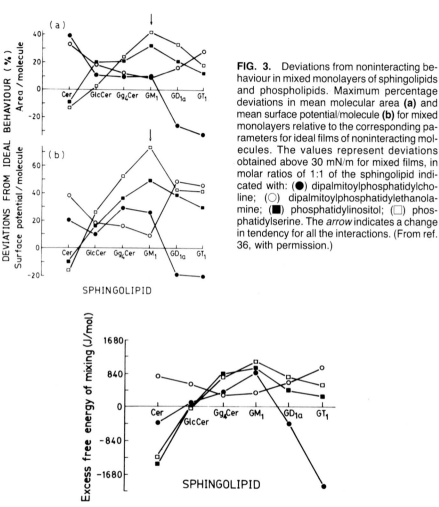

FIG. 3. Deviations from noninteracting behaviour in mixed monolayers of sphingolipids and phospholipids. Maximum percentage deviations in mean molecular area **(a)** and mean surface potential/molecule **(b)** for mixed monolayers relative to the corresponding parameters for ideal films of noninteracting molecules. The values represent deviations obtained above 30 mN/m for mixed films, in molar ratios of 1:1 of the sphingolipid indicated with: (●) dipalmitoylphosphatidylcholine; (○) dipalmitoylphosphatidylethanolamine; (■) phosphatidylinositol; (□) phosphatidylserine. The *arrow* indicates a change in tendency for all the interactions. (From ref. 36, with permission.)

FIG. 4. Excess free energy of mixing for mixed monolayers of sphingolipids and phospholipids. The excess free energy of mixing values were obtained by calculation of the area under the pressure-area isotherm up to a surface pressure of 30 mN/m by Simpson's rule. The values are given for mixed films in molar ratios 1:1, of the sphingolipids indicated with: (●) dipalmitoylphosphatidylcholine; (○) dipalmitoylphosphatidylethanolamine; (■) phosphatidylinositol; (□) phosphatidylserine. (From ref. 36, with permission.)

for this, the participating groups need not even be present on the same molecule to the same extent as they are present in the interface as a whole (38).

In summary, the decreased molecular packing and reduced surface potential obtained in mixed monolayers of polysialogangliosides with phosphatidylcholine can be explained by a partial matching and neutralization of two oppositely oriented dipole moment vectors, one in the zwitterionic phospholipid and the other in one of the sialosyl residues (AcNeu$_2$ or AcNeu$_3$) (Fig. 5). These arrangements can account for reductions in molecular packing through both an increase of polar head group and hydrocarbon chain interactions accompanied by a "molecular cavity" effect (38).

MEMBRANE FUSION AND NEUROTRANSMITTER MOVEMENTS IN NERVE ENDINGS

Another evidence that the type of interactions referred to above were not exclusive of only one type of molecule (e.g., polysialogangliosides) but were due to more general interfacial effects is that the reductions in molecular packing and decreased surface potential observed for the interactions of polysialogangliosides with phosphatidylcholine resembled those exhibited by more than 15 lipid- or water-soluble compounds that in natural membrane preparations are able to induce membrane fusion (cf. 33,39). On this basis, it was possible to anticipate that gangliosides GD$_{1a}$, GD$_3$, and GT$_1$, but not GM$_3$, GM$_1$, or the neutral glycosphingolipids Cer, GlcCer, and Gg$_4$Cer could induce fusion of chicken erythrocytes (35) in an experimental system similar to that described by Ahkong et al. (1).[1] The morphological changes observed in chicken erythrocytes incubated in the presence of polysialogangliosides involved cell rounding and the formation of multinucleated cells. In the case of ganglioside GD$_3$, the process of fusion also showed the formation of vesicles pinched off the membrane of a same cell besides the more usual intercellular fusion (Fig. 6). As in the case of fusogenic agents (cf. 33), it was found that free Ca^{2+} is required for the ganglioside-induced fusion.

In view of the possible participation of a membrane fusion process for the release of neurotransmitter, our next attempt was to investigate the effect of the compounds described above on neurotransmitter release when incubated with a synaptosomal preparation.

Release of [^{3}H]dopamine from synaptosomes ranging from 60 to 80% was observed for all the compounds able to decrease the surface potential of phosphatidylcholine interfaces and to induce membrane fusion in chicken erythrocytes (14,15). As for membrane fusion processes in general (cf. 33), induction of dopamine release did not occur if Ca^{2+} was omitted from the incubation medium. On the other hand, compounds chemically related to the effective fusogenic agents but that have a different behavior with phosphatidylcholine in monolayers and that did not induce

---

[1]*Abbreviations used*: Cer, ceramide (*N*-acylsphingoid); GlcCer, Glcβ1→1Cer; LacCer, Galβ1 → 4Glcβ1 → 1Cer; Gg$_3$Cer, GalNAcβ1 → 4Galβ1 → 4Glcβ1 → 1Cer; Gg$_4$Cer, Galβ1 → 3GalNAcβ1 → 4Galβ1 → 4Glcβ1 → 1Cer; GM$_3$, NeuGcα2 → 3Galβ1 → 4Glcβ1 → 1Cer; GD$_3$, NeuAcα2 → 8NeuAcα2 → 3Galβ1→ 4Glcβ1 → 1Cer; GM$_1$, Galβ1 → 3GalNAcβ1 → 4Gal (3 ← 2αNeuAc)β1 → 4Glcβ1 → 1Cer; GD$_{1a}$, NeuAcα2 → 3Galβ1 → 3GalNAcβ1 → 4Gal (3 ← 2αNeuAc)β1 → 4Glβ1 → 1Cer; GT$_1$, NeuAcα2 → 3Galβ1 → 3GalNAcβ1 →4Gal(3 ← 2α(NeuAc8 ← 2αNeuAc)β1 → 4Glcβ1 →1 Cer. Abbreviations are those recommended by IUPAC-IUB (cf. 25) for neutral glycosphingolipids and by Svennerholm (54) for gangliosides.

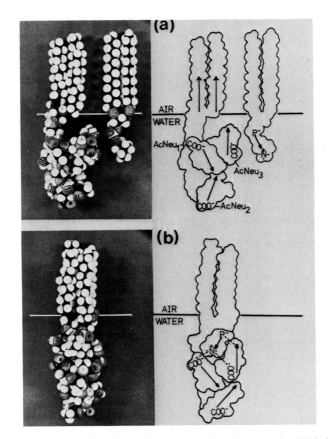

FIG. 5. Molecular models of trisialoganglioside and dipalmitoylphosphatidylcholine. Space-filling Corey-Pauling-Koltun molecular models illustrating some possible conformations and interactions of ganglioside GT_1 and dipalmitoylphosphatidylcholine. Outline projections of the models are also shown to illustrate relevant moieties and interactions. The molecules are considered to be in a closely packed state (i.e., above a surface pressure of 30 mN/m). The position of the air–water interface should be considered an example only. An equimolar mixture of ganglioside GT_1 and dipalmitoylphosphatidylcholine exhibiting noninteracting behaviour is shown in **(a)**; **(b)** shows a possible arrangement showing intermolecular interactions. In **(a)** the phospholipid is represented with the acyl chains in all-*trans*configuration and its polar head group in an average position according to the work of Phillips et al. (49) and Gally et al. (20). For ganglioside GT_1, the conformation of the ceramide moiety is represented essentially according to the work of Pascher (48) and with three cooperative rotational isomers of the type "2gl kink" (51,56) in each hydrophobic chain. The position of the oligosaccharide chain is represented as deduced from monolayer studies (37). The vectors in the outline projections represent dipole-moment contributions (positive toward the arrow; cf. ref. 19). In **(b)** the phospholipid acyl chains are represented exhibiting rotational isomers occurring co-operatively with those of ganglioside GT_1 so that the phosphocholine moiety fits in the "pocket" circumscribed by $AcNeu_3$, with the quaternary nitrogen atom pointing toward the observer. Broken lines joining particular groups in the outline projections represent possible electrostatic interactions between corresponding charged groups (see the text). (From ref. 38, with permission.)

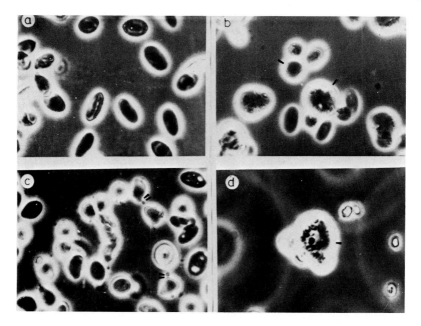

FIG. 6. Morphological changes during ganglioside- and monooleoylglycerol-induced fusion of chicken erythrocytes. Erythrocytes were incubated at 37° C as described by Ahkong et al. (1) **(a)** in absence of added lipids; in presence of 100 μg/ml of: (b) monooleoylglycerol; (c) GD₃; (d) GT₁. Phase contrast microscopy, ×600. Single arrows show bi- or multinucleated cells; *double arrows* indicate membrane pinching off. (From ref. 35, with permission.)

erythrocyte fusion were not effective in inducing release of neurotransmitter (Table 1; Fig. 7). Substances able to reduce the interfacial potential but not their ineffective chemical analogs were also found to inhibit by about 70 to 90% the high-affinity Na$^+$-dependent uptake of neurotransmitter (15) (Table 1).

MOLECULAR MECHANISMS OF FUSION-MEDIATED
NEUROTRANSMITTER RELEASE

The above results indicated that the possible molecular mode of action of the compounds studied were not related to a common chemical feature but seemed a consequence of a more general physicochemical property related to combined intermolecular interactions concerning the whole system (39). It has been proposed that a fusogenic lipid may initially interact with choline-containing phospholipids so that a new and more stable arrangement of molecular dipoles is produced that, in turn, allows a closer packing and reduced surface potential (36,40,41). Besides altering the polar head group properties, the presence of the low-melting fusogenic lipid might cooperatively increase the number of rotational isomers of the hydrophobic chains in the membrane interior, giving a bilayer containing hydrocarbon chains individually more disordered but that can still be packed intermolecularly

TABLE 1. *Dopamine movements induced by different effectors*

	Effector (μM)	Dopamine retained (%)	Effector (μM)	Dopamine uptake (%)	Membrane fusion in chicken erythrocytes	Surface potential and packing in lecithin monolayers
No effector (control)	—	69	—	100	Negative	—
Monooleoylglycerol	280	23	280	32	Positive	Decreased
Oleic acid	280	12	280	14	Positive	Decreased
Palmitoleic acid	280	12	—	—	Positive	Decreased
Sulphatide	280	20	280	18	Positive	Decreased
GD_3	210	32	—	—	Positive	Decreased
GD_{1a}	210	23	280	28	Positive	Decreased
GT_1	140	23	—	—	Positive	Decreased
Myelin basic protein	8	14	8	36	Positive	—
Dimethylsulphoxide	3.9×10^6	8	—	—	Positive	Decreased
Sucrose	9.0×10^5	13	9.0×10^5	8	Positive	Decreased
Monostearoylglycerol	280	109	280	84	Negative	No change or increased
Stearic acid	280	82	280	105	Negative	No change or increased
Palmitic acid	280	81	—	—	Negative	No change or increased
Galcer	280	76	160	82	Negative	No change or increased
Gg_4Cer	260	88	—	—	Negative	No change or increased
GM_1	260	88	280	123	Negative	No change or increased
Albumin	8	94	8	92	Negative	—

The dopamine retained represents the [³H]dopamine in a synaptosomal preparation, previously loaded with this compound, after 15 min of incubation with an effector and 1.5 mM $CaCl_2$ with respect to zero time. For uptake the values represent the [³H]dopamine accumulated after 2.5 min of incubation with an effector, compared with control. (From ref. 15, with permission.)

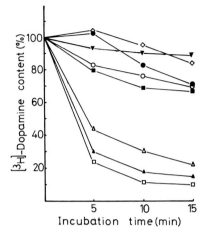

FIG. 7. Time dependence of dopamine release in synaptosomal preparations induced by different effectors. The preparation contained: (○) no effector; (□) 3.9 M dimethylsulphoxide; (▲) 14 μM myelin basic protein; (△) 160 μM GD_{1a}; (▼) 160 μM GM_1; (●) 160 μM GD_{1a} plus 8 μM myelin basic protein; (■) 3.9 M dimethylsulphoxide without $CaCl_2$; (◇) 160 μM GD_{1a} without $CaCl_2$. (From ref. 15, with permission.)

in a fairly ordered manner (36,41,44,51). These changes may produce lateral segregation of different lipid domains (12) as well as induce nonbilayer phases (13,23) and a concomitant increase of the membrane permeability. In lipid bilayers the increase of membrane permeability has been related to the presence of intermolecular "defects" brought about by the establishment of dissimilar interactions between molecules in different mesomorphic states (31,45,47). This situation can lead to the appearance of ionic channels, fluctuating in time (4) and occurring in a voltage-dependent manner, probably due to a voltage-dependent enhancement of occurrence of rotational isomers present in hydrophobic chains involved in mesomorphic transitions (53). The effect of water-soluble compounds in membrane fusion is thought to occur by changes of the long-range water structure of the bulk phase which affects the interactions taking place among the phospholipid polar head groups (34,42) that can modify the phase behaviour and surface potential of the phospholipid interface (2,5,42,55). Thus, the intermolecular interactions induced by either lipids or water-soluble substances can produce conditions leading to a new overall organizational metastable state of the membrane system, allowing an increased permeability and the intermixing of components in closely adjacent membranes (cf. 33,39).

As a result of the presence of considerable concentration gradients for Na^+, K^+, and Ca^{2+} an increased permeability produced in nerve endings by fusogens will allow these ions to move "downhill" across the membrane, causing depolarization and further permeability increases as an amplified response. An increase in the concentration of cytoplasmic Ca^{2+} is generally required for the fusion of membranes (cf. 33) or for release of neurotransmitter mediated by exocytosis (43,50) and it has been shown that fusogenic substances lead to an increased entry of Ca^{2+} into the cell (6). Uptake of transmitters by Na^+-coupled cotransport requires a proper maintenance of low membrane permeability to Na^+ so that the energy stored in the transmembrane Na^+ gradient can be utilized for the transmitter transport process.

An enhanced permeability of the nerve ending membrane brought about by a fusogenic agent will reduce the Na^+ gradient through an increased Na^+ influx and thus decrease the uptake of neurotransmitter. This conclusion was supported by experiments using water-soluble fusogenic agents and ouabain (15).

PHYSIOLOGICAL REGULATION OF TRANSIENT MEMBRANE INSTABILITY PROCESSES

The amount of components with fusogenic properties in the membrane might be regulated by several mechanisms. A naturally present "nonactive" fusogenic substance may be "activated" in the membrane plane by dissociation of constraining interactions (cf. 46). Once interactions are modified either by normal fluctuations, in the time order of about 10^{-6} sec (28), of the dynamic steady state of the membrane or as a consequence of perturbations induced by an effector or "physiological" stimulus, a fusogenic component would be able to exert its function through the establishment of new energetically favored interactions (cf. 39). In this connection, it has been shown that the unstabilizing action of sulphatides and gangliosides on membranes can be inhibited by certain proteins (Fig. 7) (15,44), probably because of favored and thermodynamically more stable interactions occurring between them in which the individual molecular properties of both the lipids and the proteins are modified (16, Fidelio et al., in preparation). In the case of gangliosides this type of effect could be of functional importance, as it has been reported that tetanus and botulinum toxins, which bind to complex gangliosides, inhibit the release of neurotransmitter (26,30).

Alternative mechanisms would be the metabolic formation in the membrane of fusogenic compounds such as unsaturated diacylglycerol (1,3), which has been implicated in processes of vesicle exocytosis and membrane recycling in nerve endings (24) or lysolecithin (cf. 33), for which an increased production occurs in mast cells concomitantly with Ca^{2+} entry and histamine release by exocytosis following antigenic stimulation (22). The formation of lysolecithin and unsaturated fatty acids in nerve endings was achieved by exogenously added phospholipase A_2 and this was accompanied by a modification of the membrane potential as evidenced by cyanine dyes together with an increased release and depressed uptake of neurotransmitter (52,57). A similar mechanism of action can be applied to the effects of β-bungarotoxin at presynaptic levels, as this preparation contains an associated phospholipase A_2 activity (32,52). In living cells, disialoganglioside GD_{1a} has been implicated in membrane fusion processes as its concentration transiently increases just before the fusion of myoblasts in cultures and mutant myoblasts, unable to fuse into myotubes, do not synthesize GD_{1a} while still producing monosialogangliosides (58). In the central nervous system (CNS) gangliosides are synthesized in the neuronal perikarya and reach the synaptosomal plasma membrane, presumably through the process of axonal transport (17,29). In this respect, it has been reported that the transport of gangliosides from retina to the optic tectum in chicken exposed to light was increased with respect to animals kept in the dark (see Caputto et al.

this volume). This could represent an increased flux of gangliosides to the nerve endings required by a greater activity (including release of neurotransmitter) under conditions of visual stimulation (9,10).

The functional behaviour described for natural membrane preparations shows a good correlation with the interfacial properties of the compounds studied and a key step for triggering the final process seems related to the possibility of obtaining a decrease of the surface potential of phosphatidylcholine interfaces, However, it should not be disregarded that membrane fusion processes related to exocytosis and neurotransmitter release and uptake are final events dependent on transmembrane potential, not in every case requiring necessarily the direct involvement of a fusogenic membrane component. The transmembrane potential is a complex parameter arising not only from the dipolar contributions from molecules or their dynamic associations at the interface but also from electrogenic pump potentials and large ionic diffusion potentials. Therefore, changes of the steady-state conditions that could affect the overall transmembrane potential such as transient changes in local ionic concentrations, chemically or electrically induced depolarizations (including action potentials), receptor-ligand associations, leading to modified intermolecular interactions both in the short and long range in the whole membrane system that can involve an increased ionic permeability, in cases through specific ionic channels (27), would result in the same end effect.

ACKNOWLEDGMENTS

Work from this laboratory was supported in part by the Organización de los Estados Americanos, SECYT and CONICET, Argentina. The authors are Career Investigators of the latter institution. We thank the Departamento de Medios Audiovisuales, Universidad Nacional de Córdoba for Assistance in preparing the illustrations.

REFERENCES

1. Ahkong, Q. F., Fisher, D., Tampion, W., and Lucy, J. A. (1973): The fusion of erythrocytes by fatty acids, esters, retinol and α-tocopherol. *Biochem. J.*, 136:147–155.
2. Ahkong, Q. F., Tampion, W., and Lucy, J. A. (1975): Promotion of cell fusion by divalent cation ionophores. *Nature*, 256:208–209.
3. Allan, D., Low, M. G., Finean, J. B., and Michell, R. H. (1975): Changes in lipid metabolism and cell morphology following attack by phospholipase C *(Clostridium perfringens)* on red cells or lymphocytes. *Biochim. Biophys. Acta*, 413:308–316.
4. Antonov, V. F., and Petrov, U. V., Molnar, A. A., Prednoitelev, D. A., and Ivanov, A. S. (1980): The appearance of single-ion channels in unmodified lipid bilayer membranes at the phase transition temperature. *Nature*, 283:585–586.
5. Blow, A. M. J., Botham, G. M., Fisher, D., Goodall, A. H., Tilcock, C. P. S., and Lucy, J. A. (1978): Water and calcium ions in cell fusion induced by poly(ethylene glycol). *FEBS Lett.*, 94:305–310.
6. Blow, A. M. J., Botham, G. M., and Lucy, J. A. (1979): Calcium ions and cell fusion. Effects of chemical fusogens on the permeability of erythrocytes to calcium and other ions. *Biochem. J.*, 182:555–563.
7. Boyne, A. F. (1978): Neurosecretion: Integration of recent findings into the vesicle hypothesis. *Life Sci.*, 22:2057–2066.

8. Caputto, R., Maccioni, H. J. F., Arce, A., and Cumar, F. A. (1976): Biosynthesis of brain gangliosides. *Adv. Exp. Med. Biol.*, 71:27–44.
9. Caputto, B. L., Maccioni, A. H. R., Landa, C. A., and Caputto, R. (1979): Effects of light on the labelling of optic tectum gangliosides after an intraocular injection of *N*-[³H]acetylmannosamine. *Biochem. Biophys. Res. Commun.*, 86:849–854.
10. Caputto, R., Maccioni, A. H. R., Maccioni, H. J. F., Caputto, B. L., and Landa, C. A. (1980): The gangliosides of the chicken retina and optic tectum. The influence of light on their labelling after an injection of labelled precursors. *Neurochemistry*, 1:43–57.
11. Ceccarelli, B., and Hurlbut, W. P. (1980): Vesicle hypothesis of the release of quanta of acetylcholine. *Physiol. Rev.*, 60:396–441.
12. Chapman, D. (1976): Physicochemical studies of cellular membranes. In: *Mammalian Cell Membranes, Vol. 1*, edited by G. A. Jamieson and D. M. Robinson, pp. 97–137. Butterworths, London.
13. Cullis, P. R., and de Kruijff, B. (1979): Lipid polymorphism and the functional roles of lipids in biological membranes. *Biochim. Biophys. Acta*, 559:399–420.
14. Cumar, F. A., Maggio, B., and Caputto, R. (1978): Dopamine release from nerve endings induced by polysialogangliosides. *Biochem. Biophys. Res. Commun.*, 84:65–69.
15. Cumar, F. A., Maggio, B., and Caputto, R. (1980): Neurotransmitter movements in nerve endings. Influence of substances that modify the interfacial potential. *Biochim. Biophys. Acta*, 597:174–182.
16. Fidelio, G. D., Maggio, B., Cumar, F. A., and Caputto, R. (1981): Interaction of glycosphingolipids with melittin and myelin basic protein in monolayers. *Biochem. J.*, 193:643–646.
17. Forman, D. S., and Ledeen, R. W. (1972): Axonal transport of gangliosides in the goldfish optic nerve. *Science*, 177:630–633.
18. Fried, R. C., and Blaustein, M. P. (1978): Retrieval and recycling of synaptic vesicle membrane in pinched-off nerve terminals (synaptosomes). *J. Cell. Biol.*, 78:685–700.
19. Gaines, G. L. (1966): Insoluble monolayers at liquid-gas interfaces. In: *Interscience Monographs on Physical Chemistry*, edited by I. Prigogine, pp. 136–207. Interscience, New York.
20. Gally, H. U., Niederberger, W., and Seelig, J. (1975): Conformation and motion of the choline head group in bilayers of dipalmitoyl-3-*sn*-phosphatidylcholine. *Biochemistry*, 14:3647–3652.
21. Heuser, J. E., Reese, T. S., Dennis, M. J., Jan, L., and Evans, L. (1979): Synaptic vesicle exocytosis captured by quick freezing and correlated with quantal transmitter release. *J. Cell Biol.*, 81:275–300.
22. Hirata, F., and Axelrod, J. (1980): Phospholipid methylation and biological signal transmission. *Science*, 209:1082–1090.
23. Hope, M. J., and Cullis, P. R. (1981): The role of non bilayer lipid structures in the fusion of human erythrocytes induced by lipid fusogens. *Biochim. Biophys. Acta*, 640:82–90.
24. Hawthorne, J. N., and Pickard, M. R. (1979): Phospholipids in synaptic function. *J. Neurochem.*, 32:5–14.
25. IUPAC-IUB (1977): Commission on biochemical nomenclature. The nomenclature of lipids. Recommendations (1976) *Lipids*, 12:455–468.
26. Kelly, R. B., Deutsch, J. W., Carlson, S. S., and Wagner, J. A. (1979): Biochemistry of neurotransmitter release. *Annu. Rev. Neurosci.*, 2:399–446.
27. Keynes, R. D. (1976): Organization of the sodium channels in excitable membranes. In: *The Structural Basis of Membrane Function*, edited by Y. Hatefi and L. Djavadi-Ohaniance, pp. 331–338. Academic Press, New York.
28. Knowles, P. F., Watts, A., and Marsh, D. (1979): Spin-label studies of lipid immobilization in dimyristoylphosphatidylcholine-substituted cytochrome oxidase. *Biochemistry*, 18:4480–4487.
29. Landa, C. A., Maccioni, H. J. F., and Caputto, R. (1979): The site of synthesis of gangliosides in the chick optic system. *J. Neurochem.*, 33:825–838.
30. Ledeen, R. W., and Mellanby, J. (1977): Gangliosides as receptors for bacterial toxins. In: *Perspectives in Toxinology*, edited by A. W. Bernheimer, pp. 15–42. Wiley, New York.
31. Lee, A. G. (1977): Analysis of the defect structure of gel-phase lipid. *Biochemistry*, 16:835–841.
32. Livengood, D. R., Manalis, R. S., Donlon, M. A., Masukawa, L. M., Tobias, G. S., and Shain, W. (1978): Blockade of neuromuscular transmission by enzymatically active and inactive β-bungarotoxin. *Proc. Natl. Acad. Sci. USA*, 75:1029–1033.
33. Lucy, J. A. (1978): Mechanisms of chemically induced cell fusion. In: *Membrane Fusion*, edited by G. Poste and G. L. Nicolson, pp. 267–304. Elsevier/North Holland, The Netherlands.
34. Maggio, B., Ahkong, Q. F., and Lucy, J. A. (1976): Poly(ethylene glycol), surface potential and cell fusion. *Biochem. J.*, 158:647–650.

35. Maggio, B., Cumar, F. A., and Caputto, R. (1978): Induction of membrane fusion by polysialo-gangliosides. *FEBS Lett.*, 90:149–152.
36. Maggio, B., Cumar, F. A., and Caputto, R. (1978): Interactions of gangliosides with phospholipids and glycosphingolipids in mixed monolayers. *Biochem. J.*, 175:1113–1118.
37. Maggio, B., Cumar, F. A., and Caputto, R. (1978): Surface behaviour of gangliosides and related glycosphingolipids. *Biochem. J.*, 171:559–565.
38. Maggio, B., Cumar, F. A., and Caputto, R. (1980): Configuration and interactions of the polar head group in gangliosides. *Biochem. J.*, 189:435–440.
39. Maggio, B., Cumar, F. A., and Caputto, R. (1981): Molecular behaviour of glycosphingolipids in interfaces. Possible participation in some properties of nerve membranes. *Biochim. Biophys. Acta*, 650:69–87.
40. Maggio, B., and Lucy, J. A. (1975): Studies on mixed monolayers of phospholipids and fusogenic lipids. *Biochem. J.*, 149:597–608.
41. Maggio, B., and Lucy, J. A. (1976): Polar-group behaviour in mixed monolayers of phospholipids and fusogenic lipids. *Biochem. J.*, 155:353–364.
42. Maggio, B., and Lucy, J. A. (1978): Interactions of water-soluble fusogens with phospholipids in monolayers. *FEBS Lett.*, 94:301–304.
43. Miledi, R. (1973): Transmitter release induced by injection of calcium ions into nerve terminals. *Proc. R. Soc. Lond. (Biol.)*, 183:421–425.
44. Monferrán, C. G., Maggio, B., Roth, G. A., Cumar, F. A., and Caputto, R. (1979): Membrane instability induced by purified myelin components. Its possible relevance to experimental allergic encephalomyelitis. *Biochim. Biophys. Acta*, 553:417–423.
45. Nagle, J. K., and Scott, H. L. (1978): Lateral compressibility of lipid mono- and bilayers. Theory of membrane permeability. *Biochim. Biophys. Acta*, 513:236–243.
46. Nicolson, G. L. (1976): Transmembrane control of the receptors on normal and tumor cells. I. Cytoplasmic influence over cell surface components. *Biochim. Biophys. Acta*, 457:57–108.
47. Papahadjopoulos, D., Jacobson, K., Nir, S., and Isac, T. (1973): Phase transitions in phospholipid vesicles. Fluorescence polarization and permeability measurements concerning the effect of temperature and cholesterol. *Biochim. Biophys. Acta*, 311:330–348.
48. Pascher, I. (1976): Molecular arrangements in sphingolipids. Conformation and hydrogen bonding of ceramide and their implication on membrane stability and permeability. *Biochim. Biophys. Acta*, 455:433–451.
49. Phillips, M. C., Finer, E. G., and Hauser, H. (1972): Differences between conformations of lecithin and phosphatidylethanolamine polar head groups and their effects on interactions of phospholipid bilayer membranes. *Biochim. Biophys. Acta*, 290:397–402.
50. Rahamimoff, R., Meir, H., Erulkar, S. D., and Barenholz, Y. (1978): Changes in transmitter release induced by ion-containing liposomes. *Proc. Natl. Acad. Sci. USA*, 75:5214–5216.
51. Seelig, A., and Seelig, J (1974): The dynamic structure of fatty acyl chains in a phospholipid bilayer measured by deuterium magnetic resonance. *Biochemistry*, 13:4839–4845.
52. Sen, I., and Cooper, J. R. (1978): Similarities of β-bungarotoxin and phospholipase A_2 and their mechanism of action. *J. Neurochem.*, 30:1369–1375.
53. Sujar, I. P. (1979): A theory of the electric field-induced phase transition of phospholipid bilayers. *Biochim. Biophys. Acta*, 556:72–85.
54. Svennerholm, L. (1963): Chromatographic separation of human brain gangliosides. *J. Neurochem.*, 10:613–623.
55. Tilcock, C. P. S., and Fisher, D. (1979): Interaction of phospholipid membranes with poly(ethylene glycol)s. *Biochim. Biophys. Acta*, 557:53–61.
56. Trauble, H., and Haynes, D. H. (1971): The volume change in lipid bilayer lamellae at the crystalline-liquid crystalline phase transition. *Chem. Phys. Lipids*, 7:324–335.
57. Wernicke, J. F., Vanker, A. D., and Howard, B. D. (1975): The mechanism of action of β-bungarotoxin. *J. Neurochem.*, 25:483–496.
58. Whatley, R., Ng, S. K.-C., Rogers, J., McMurray, W. C., and Sanwal, B. D. (1976): Developmental changes in gangliosides during myogenesis of rat myoblast cell line and its drug resistant variants. *Biochim. Biophys. Res. Commun.*, 70:180–185.

Neural Transmission, Learning and Memory,
edited by R. Caputto and C. Ajmone Marsan.
Raven Press, New York © 1983.

Uptake, Transport, and Metabolism of Neurotransmitters in Pure Neuronal Cultures

J. C. Louis, H. Dreyfus, T. Y. Wong,
G. Vincendon, and R. Massarelli

Unité 44 de l'INSERM and Centre de Neurochimie du CNRS (Group de Neurodifférentiation), Strasbourg Cedex, France

The only general widespread point of agreement among neuroscientists at present is the recognition of the difficulties inherent to the study of the nervous system, essentially because of its great complexity. It has thus become a common lieu to seek models that may be utilized as simplified approaches to the study of the nervous system.

In this respect synaptosomal preparations have been a tool offering the possibility of determining certain basic mechanisms intrinsic to the metabolic function of the neuron and related to its most important function, communication.

Nerve cell cultures have, as well, been used as simple models of the nervous system. The first type of culture that has undergone thorough studies has been the neuroblastoma C1300 of the mouse (1,20). The possibility of cloning these tumoral cells and obtaining cell cultures uniquely capable of synthesizing acetylcholine or catecholamines has for the first time overcome the multicellular complexity of the nervous system.

Neuroblastoma cells, however, being of tumoral origin, possess a severe drawback as a consequence of their nature: they can mutate rapidly, and consequently, rapidly lose those properties that had made them biochemically useful as models or acquire new ones.

A safer approach in the search for a simple model of the nervous system is given by the use of primary nerve cell cultures that are usually prepared from embryonic tissues (for review see refs. 17,21). Dissociated nerve cells from chick embryo cerebral hemispheres grow, differentiate, and establish cell-to-cell contacts and functional synapses. Recently, it has been possible to obtain primary cultures of exclusively neuronal cells (8,18). This new tool provides the opportunity to study the metabolism of neurotransmitters and its relationship with basic constituents of the neuronal membrane in well-differentiated neurons grown in the absence of supportive cells.

Primary nerve cell cultures have been used in the study of catecholamines and choline metabolism and the results obtained in the course of this work will be herein reviewed.

The basic steps of the metabolism of catecholamines are well known and the interest of approaching this study in pure neuronal cultures resides in the fact that, as it will be shown later on, these cultures express predominantly dopaminergic characteristics and thus represent an ideal subject for the metabolic analysis of dopamine.

In the case of the metabolism of acetylcholine, present knowledge is not very much different from what was known 20 or 30 years ago. The mechanism of regulation of the synthesis of acetylcholine is still unknown, although in recent years several hypotheses have been forwarded with various success. One of the most recent hypotheses concerns the regulation of the neurotransmitter through the supply of the precursors as, apparently, the enzyme of synthesis (choline acetyl-transferase, EC 2.3.1.6) should not be rate-limiting in the synthesis of acetylcholine. The supply of choline, particularly, has been (and still is) widely used as a possible tool in regulating acetylcholine synthesis. The hypothesis was based on two prem-ises: that choline is not synthesized in the nervous system and that a certain type of transport of choline, which then should be the only method of bringing this precursor to the site of acetylcholine synthesis, is specific for cholinergic neurons and for acetylcholine metabolism.

The study of these neurotransmitter systems has been approached by using neu-ronal cultures. However, before discussing these metabolic pathways, certain basic characteristics of neurons in culture will be shown and elucidated.

PRIMARY NERVE CELL CULTURES

Mechanically dissociated nerve cells from 8-day-old chick embryo cerebral hem-ispheres (E8) when put in culture for 8 to 10 days (C8–10) will give a uniform layer of glia cells on top of which neurons will grow and differentiate (mixed nerve cells) (2). If older embryos are used (E12–14) glia cells will develop while neurons whose differentiation *in vivo* starts from the 10th day of embryonic life, will rapidly degenerate. In these conditions, pure glial cell cultures will be obtained (2). If plastic Petri dishes are precoated with poly-L-lysine, dissociated E8 neurons attach to this substrate preferentially and develop whereas supporting cells do not (18).

Morphology

The morphology of mixed nerve cell and of pure glia cultures has been shown in several reports (see, e.g., ref. 2). Figure 1 shows the appearance of a pure neuronal culture after 6 days *in vitro*. When kept in culture neurons will grow and develop cell-to-cell contacts starting from C3. From this time to C7–9 the number of synaptic contacts will increase, and electron microscopy has revealed the presence of synaptic thickenings and of synaptic vesicles (of clear and dense-cored nature) (Fig. 1B). The purity of the cultures has been established by using three different histochemical approaches (8,18). Acetylcholinesterase staining showed a heavy labeling of all cells. The second criterion used was the histofluorescence of cate-cholamines. By means of this technique a large percentage (95%) of cells was

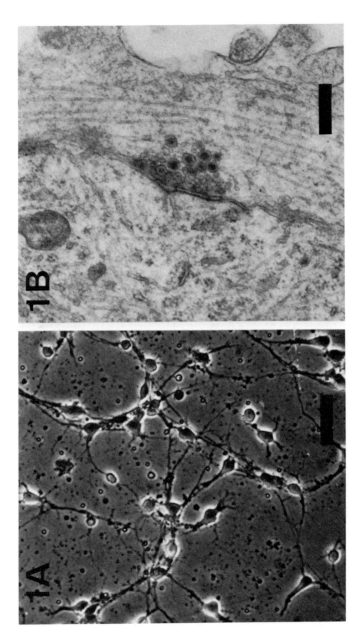

FIG. 1. Morphological aspect of cultures from 8-day-old chick embryo cerebral hemispheres. **A:** Phase-contrast micrograph of a 6-day-old culture. Scale: 50 μm. **B:** Electron micrograph of a characteristic axo–somatic synapse in a 6-day-old culture. The presynaptic element is filled with many dense-cored, as well as clear, vesicles. Scale: 0.4 μm.

found to react positively to glioxilate treatment, suggesting a predominance of catecholaminergic cells. This result was confirmed by the biochemical studies, as shown in the next section.

The most clear-cut evidence showing the purity of these cultures has been the immunohistochemical labeling of cell membranes with tetanus toxin. With this approach the purity of the cultures was established as at least 98%.

Presence of Neurotransmitters

To detect the presence of neurotransmitters the activities of some enzyme markers have been analyzed. Figure 2 shows that tyrosine hydroxylase (EC 1.14.16.2), glutamic acid decarboxylase (EC 4.1.1.15), and choline acetyltransferase (EC 2.3.1.6) activities were detectable, while no activity of dopamine-β-hydroxylase (EC 1.14.17.1) activity was measurable (8).

The results indicated that these cells, during their maturation, express predominantly dopaminergic and GABAergic properties while the cholinergic characteristics do not develop in this system.

TRANSPORT OF NEUROTRANSMITTERS AND THEIR PRECURSORS

To approach the study of the metabolism of neurotransmitters it was necessary to examine the mechanism of transfer of their precursors, especially in the case of choline where the presence of a high- and a low-affinity uptake systems had provided the opportunity to introduce new hypotheses in the regulation of acetylcholine metabolism, as discussed in a later section.

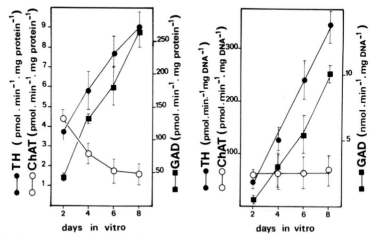

FIG. 2. Development of tyrosine hydroxylase (TH ●———●), glutamate decarboxylase (GAD ■———■), and choline acetyltransferase (ChAT ○———○) activities with time in culture. The enzyme activities are expressed as pmole·min^{-1}·mg protein^{-1} **(left panel)** and as pmole·min^{-1}·mg DNA^{-1} **(right panel)**. Enzymatic assays have been performed as described elsewhere (8).

Tyrosine

When neurons were incubated (2 min) in the presence of various concentrations of [^{3}H]tyrosine the uptake was saturable as a function of substrate and the kinetic parameters were measured according to Michaelis-Menten kinetics (Table 1). It should be pointed out that during maturation of the cells the K_m of tyrosine uptake did not change significantly ($\sim$ 45 μM) while V_{max} values increased twice (when expressed on a DNA basis), a finding that might suggest an increase in the number of carrier sites in the neuronal membrane as a function of increasing cellular maturation. Tyrosine can then be taken up in neurons through a saturable mechanism that, however, on the basis of experiments performed with metabolic inhibitors and ouabain appeared to be of a facilitated diffusion type (Table 2).

TABLE 1. *Development of kinetic parameters of tyrosine transport with time in culture*

Days in culture	K_m (μM)	V_{max} nmole·min^{-1} ·mg Prot^{-1}	V_{max} nmole·min^{-1} ·mg DNA^{-1}	k_{DIFF} pmole·min^{-1} ·mg Prot^{-1}·μM^{-1}
3	49.3 ± 9.7	8.33 ± 0.35	122.6 ± 5.2	4.7
5	42.8 ± 6.8	8.80 ± 0.38	236.5 ± 8.8	4.9

The kinetic parameters (K_m and V_{max}) were determined by the statistical analysis of Cleland (3) from the 2-min points of the uptake experiments. Cultures were preincubated (10 min) with a Krebs-Ringer-HEPES solution, pH 7.3 and incubated (2 min) with Krebs-Ringer-HEPES solution containing various concentrations (from 10^{-5} M to $2 \cdot 10^{-3}$M) of L − [3,5 − ^{3}H] tyrosine (Amersham, specific activity 50 Ci/mmole). K_{DIFF}, Diffusion coefficient.

TABLE 2. *Energy dependence, ionic dependence, and specificity of tyrosine and dopamine uptakes*

	Tyrosine uptake (% of control)	Dopamine uptake (% of control)
Control	100	100
+2°C	36.9 ± 14.3	23.4 ± 4.4
KCN (1 mM)	87.9 ± 12.9	44.3 ± 3.4
2,4-Dinitrophenol (1 mM)	98.6 ± 4.5	57.8 ± 6.8
Ouabain (1 mM)	87.7 ± 13.6	53.2 ± 4.4
Low Na$^+$ (25 mM)	—	45.0 ± 5.2
D-Amphetamine (10^{-7}M)	—	42.2 ± 7.8
Nomifensine (10^{-7}M)	—	28.2 ± 5.6
Desipramine (10^{-7}M)	—	82.6 ± 9.3

The 2-min incorporation of [^{3}H]tyrosine or [^{3}H]dopamine was measured after 30 min of preincubation of 7-day-old cultures in Krebs-Ringer-HEPES solution kept in the cold (2°C) or containing the metabolic inhibitors KCN (1 mM), 2,4-dinitrophenol (1 mM) or ouabain (1 mM).

Dopamine uptake was measured after a 10-min preincubation in Krebs-Ringer-HEPES medium containing D-amphetamine (10^{-7}M), nomifensine maleate acid (10^{-7}M), or desipramine (10^{-7}M).

Uptake in low Na$^+$ conditions was performed by replacing Na$^+$ with isomolar choline chloride.

Dopamine

It is widely accepted that the reuptake of dopamine following its presynaptic release is an efficient mechanism for the termination of its postsynaptic effects. Neurons can transport dopamine via a mechanism that becomes saturable starting from the 3rd day in culture (Table 3). In the case of dopamine, similarly to what was observed for the uptake of tyrosine, the affinity of the uptake did not change with time in culture while V_{max} values increased, from day 3 to day 7 of culture, of 22-fold, suggesting an increase in the number of carrier sites with cell maturation. The uptake of dopamine appeared to be specific for this substrate, as it was highly inhibited by nomifensin and, to a minor extent, by amphetamine while only a very small inhibitory effect could be observed with desipramine, a strong inhibitor of noradrenaline uptake (Table 2). Reserpine (10^{-5} M) had no inhibitory effect on the accumulation of dopamine before 3 days in vitro. After the 3rd day in culture reserpine produced progressively greater inhibition with time (30% of inhibition of the 30-min accumulation of [^{3}H]dopamine at day 3, 55% at day 5, and 60% at day 7). Figure 3 shows the effect of reserpine on the accumulation of dopamine after 1 and 5 days in culture. Since reserpine is known to inhibit the uptake of catecholamines into the synaptic vesicles (10), these findings may suggest an increasing storage capacity corresponding with the maturation of the cells.

In this respect, it should be considered that noradrenaline enters these neurons only via a nonsaturable uptake (9), a finding that should be correlated to the absence of the expression of noradrenergic characteristics.

The uptake of dopamine was highly inhibited by metabolic agents and ouabain (Table 2). Further proof of the specificity of the carrier system for dopamine stems from the observation that after changing the substrate concentration range the K_m value remained unchanged (~ 1 μM), in contrast with observations on the uptake of GABA and choline (see next two sections).

TABLE 3. *Development of kinetic parameters of dopamine uptake with time in culture*

Days in culture	K_m (μM)	V_{max} pmole·min^{-1} ·mg Protein^{-1}	V_{max} pmole·min^{-1} · mg DNA^{-1}	K_{DIFF} pmole·min^{-1} ·mg Protein^{-1} ·μM^{-1}
1	Nonsaturable	—	—	—
3	0.91 ± 0.17	4.2 ± 0.5	61.3 ± 7.2	3.3
4	1.12 ± 0.52	20.2 ± 3.7	457.5 ± 73.2	3.4
7	1.11 ± 0.38	37.9 ± 4.8	1353.6 ± 178.0	4.2

The kinetic parameters (K_m and V_{max}) were determined as described in Table 1 with various concentrations of [^{3}H]dopamine -0.05 to 20 μM$-$ (Amersham, specific activity 9.9 Ci/mmole). The incubation medium contained pargyline (1 mM) to inhibit monoamine oxidase (EC 1.4.3.4) activity.
K_{DIFF}, Diffusion coefficient.

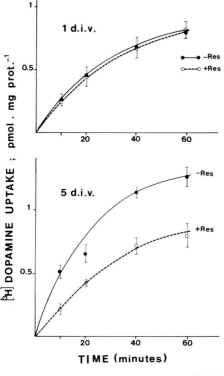

FIG. 3. Effect of reserpine on the accumulation of [³H]dopamine after 1 and 5 days in culture. Cultures were preincubated for 30 min in a solution of Krebs-Ringer-HEPES containing 1 mM pargyline in the absence (− Res ●———●) or in the presence (+ Res ○---○) of 10⁻⁵ M reserpine. After removal of the incubation medium, the accumulation of [³H]dopamine (present at a concentration of 0.1 μM in the incubation medium) was determined at different times of incubation. d.i.v., Days *in vitro*.

GABA

Neuronal cell cultures possess an uptake mechanism for GABA that is saturated with increasing concentrations of the substrate. The endogenous compartment of GABA was saturated as well, within a few minutes, with 10 or 20 μM exogenous GABA (Fig. 4A and B).

The uptake of GABA into the presynaptic terminals represents the only possible inactivation step following the release of the neurotransmitter. Several authors have observed the presence of a high-affinity mechanism for GABA transport and have suggested that this might be an efficient mechanism to stop the action of the neurotransmitter (13). However, the studies by the groups of Levi and Raiteri (7) have suggested the provocative conclusion that GABA may enter the presynaptic terminal by homoexchange through the mediation of a carrier-mediated diffusion-like process. A result that may corroborate their suggestion stems from the analysis of the kinetic parameters of GABA uptake into neurons when the concentration range of the substrate was changed (Table 4). Using a concentration range of 0.1 to 20 μM the K_m was 3.6 μM; with a 10-fold diluted range the K_m was 0.33 μM. A carrier-mediated transport process should not change in affinity with changing the substrate concentration range (in fact this does not happen in dopamine or in serotonin uptakes), unless the transport mechanism is strictly correlated to its endocellular metabolism as it was shown in choline transport (6), and as it may happen for GABA.

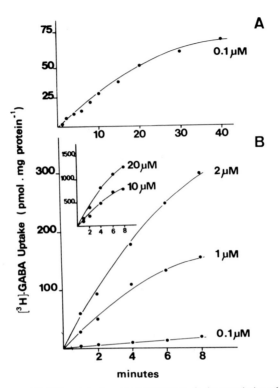

FIG. 4. Time course of GABA uptake in cultured neurons. **A:** Accumulation of [³H]GABA during incubation with 0.1 μM GABA. **B:** Relationship between GABA concentrations in the incubation medium and GABA uptake, as a function of time. Uptake is expressed as nmoles of [³H]GABA taken up/mg protein. Experiments were performed on 8-day-old cultures in a HEPES-buffered Krebs-Ringer medium, pH 7.3. Each point represents the mean of five or six cultures.

TABLE 4. *Kinetic parameters of GABA uptake at different concentration ranges of substrate*

	Concentration range (μM)	K_m (μM)	V_{max} pmole·min^{-1}·mg Protein^{-1}
GABA uptake	0.01→2.0	0.33 ± 0.07	7.6 ± 0.7
	0.1→20	3.6 ± 1.6	789 ± 124

Kinetic parameters were determined as described in Table 1 by statistical analysis (3) of the values obtained with two different ranges of concentrations of GABA.

Choline

The uptake of choline is rather peculiar and its peculiarity depends essentially on the fact that choline is not only a rapidly metabolized substance in synaptosomes and in nerve cells (15), but it is as well a basic constituent of phospholipids that themselves represent the structural backbone of cell membranes. The study of the transport of choline across cell membranes should be approached carefully also because of the presence of the base exchange mechanisms and of the enzymes related to it that were found to be present on the outer cell membrane (19).

Two different affinities were found for the uptake of choline into synaptosomes (for review see ref. 5). The values of these K_m's could, however, vary in changing the substrate concentration ranges (5,14). The K_m with higher affinity has been considered as specific for cholinergic neurons, and possibly rate-limiting in the synthesis of acetylcholine (6). However, its presence in noncholinergic neurons, glia, and even in nonnervous cells (14) limits its usefulness as a cholinergic marker and raises some doubts regarding its role in the regulation of acetylcholine metabolism.

It was found that in nerve cells the free choline compartment may rapidly change in relation to the presence or absence of exogenous choline (14,15). This observation led to the study of the uptake of choline in nerve cells whose endogenous pool of choline was kept in steady-state or in non-steady-state conditions. The results showed (Table 5) that two apparent affinities of choline uptake were found only when the endocellular pool of choline was in non-steady-state conditions. When the physiological concentrations[1] were preserved only one K_m was detected with a value

TABLE 5. *Kinetics of choline uptake in nonsteady-state and in steady-state conditions of the endocellular free choline levels*

	Choline (μM)	Affinity mechanism	K_m (μM)	V_{max} pmole·mg Protein^{-1}·2 min^{-1}
E8C10	0	High	0.8	44.8
	0	Low	14.3	333.3
	50		14.2	545.5
E8CN6	0	High	4.5	113.6
	0	Low	33.3	212.8
	50		14.3	322.6
CS	0	High	6.4	19.0
	0	Low	35.7	66.7
	100		26.3	66.7

E8C10, Primary mixed (containing glia and neurons) nerve cell cultures from chick embryo cerebral hemispheres. E8CN6, Primary exclusively neuronal cell cultures (18). CS, Crude synaptosomal fractions (P2).
In the case of CS, the concentration of choline (100 μM) was arbitrarily chosen, since it is impossible to know the physiological concentration of choline in these organelles.

---

[1]With regards to the choline pool the physiological concentrations are easily controlled in cell cultures since they correspond to a concentration of choline in the incubation medium equivalent to those found in the growth medium 1 day after its change (around 30–50 μM choline).

corresponding to the low-affinity one. These results were confirmed using synaptosomal preparations from rat brain by ourselves (15) and others (12).

The uptake of choline is Na^+-dependent (5), but, as it was recently shown in synaptosomes (23), the transport of choline is less affected by the absence of Na^+ than the synthesis of acetylcholine. These results are explained by the strong reduction of choline acetyltransferase activity in the absence of Na^+ or, more generally, in low ionic strength media (4).

The uptake of choline has also been reported to be energy-dependent on the basis of the inhibitory action produced by some metabolic inhibitors (KCN, dinitrophenol, etc...) (5). The measurement of the energies of activation of the transport of choline and of the synthesis of its metabolites in nerve cells and in synaptosomes showed, however, an interesting result since, when the cells or the organelles were incubated with 0.5 μM choline (in the range of the high-affinity system), a low energy of activation was measured at "physiological" temperatures and, after a breaking point around 22°C, a second energy of activation with a much higher value could be observed. When nerve cells or synaptosomes were instead incubated with 100 μM choline only one energy of activation could be measured of a rather low value (24).

These data made possible the suggestion that choline is transported across the nerve cells membrane by a facilitated diffusion-like process dependent upon the energy offered by the Na^+ electrochemical gradient (15).

Most studies on the transport of metabolites are mainly centered on the influx of the metabolite inside the cell (inward flux). However, quite often in eukaryotic cells, inward movements are coupled to outward movements (efflux) and the latter may be important enough—even at short time of incubation—to be capable of altering the kinetics of the influx.

The efflux of choline was measured using mixed neuronal cultures preincubated 1 hr with 0.5, 50, and 200 μM [^{14}C]choline. After thorough washing of the label the cells were incubated with 0, 0.5, 50, and 200 μM of unlabeled choline (for each concentration of label). The results presented in Fig. 5 show that after increasing the concentration of unlabeled choline, an increase is observed in the efflux of labeled material (90–95% of the radioactivity found in the medium has been identified as choline). This suggests the possible presence of a homoexchange phenomenon, which becomes particularly relevant at high concentrations of choline and at times of incubations relatively long (after 5 min).

STUDIES ON THE METABOLISM OF NEUROTRANSMITTERS

Once defined the basic characteristics of the transport of tyrosine and of choline, studies were undertaken to measure the metabolism of these precursors in relation to the synthesis of catecholamines and of acetylcholine.

Catecholamines

The synthesis of biogenic amines has been analyzed by incubating neurons in the presence of 100 μM [^{14}C]tyrosine for various time periods. The results showed

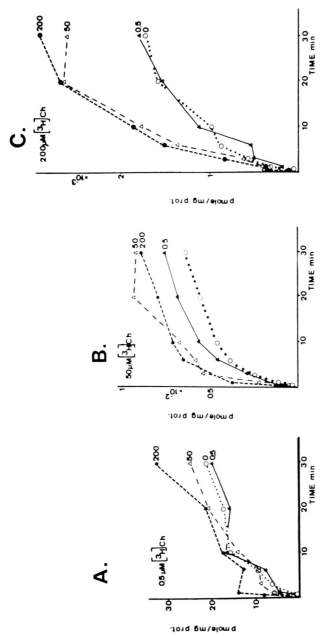

FIG. 5. Efflux of choline from mixed nerve cell cultures. Ten-day-old cultures from 8-day-old embryos, seeded on plastic Petri dishes precoated with polylysine, were preloaded with **(A)** 0.5, **(B)** 50, and **(C)** 200 μM [³H]choline for 2.5 hr in Krebs-Ringer-phosphate and the radioactivity was measured in the media containing 0 (○····○), 0.5 (▲——▲), 50 (△----△), or 200 (●----●) μM of unlabeled choline (n = 5). Cellular integrity was checked by Trypan blue exclusion.

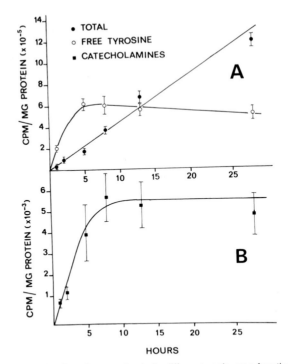

FIG. 6. Incorporation of radioactive tyrosine in its different pools, as a function of time. Seven-day-old neuronal cultures were incubated with 100 μM [U-¹⁴C]tyrosine (Amersham, specific activity, 10 mCi/mmol) in a MEM medium containing no unlabeled tyrosine (MEM—amino acid kit, Gibco) and 2% fetal calf serum (Gibco). In these conditions the concentration of unlabeled tyrosine—contributed by the fetal calf serum (tyrosine concentration ~ 60 μM)—was 1.2 μM. After various times of incubation the cultures were collected, homogenized, and the radioactivity determined in a fraction of the homogenate (**A** ●————●). The remaining homogenate was treated with ice-cold 0.4 N perchloric acid, and centrifuged (10,000 g for 10 min). Radioactivity of the free tyrosine pool was measured on the acid-soluble supernatant (**A** ○————○). Aliquots of this supernatant were brought to pH 8.6 with a 3 M Tris-buffer containing $Na_2S_2O_5$ (0.6%) and EDTA (0.6%), adsorbed onto alumina columns, and catecholamines were eluted with 3 ml of 0.2 N acetic acid. Eighty percent of the radioactivity found in this eluate was identified as dopamine by thin-layer chromatography on cellulose plates in n-butanol:water:glacial acetic acid (120:50:30) (**B** ■————■). Each point is the mean of three values ± SEM.

(Fig. 6A and B) a linear accumulation of [¹⁴C]tyrosine during the 27 hr of incubation, a saturation of the free tyrosine compartment as well as of the catecholamines compartments (in this experiment DOPA and dopamine were not separated; the latter, however, usually represents 80–85% of the total and, as we have previously mentioned, there is very little synthesis of noradrenaline in these cells). The slight decrease observed in the labeling of the varous tyrosine compartments after 20 hr of incubation (Fig. 6A and B) may be justified by the consumption of the exogenous tyrosine.

When neurons were incubated for 8 hr with various concentrations of [¹⁴C]tyrosine, an exponential incorporation was observed concerning the total uptake of [¹⁴C]tyrosine

(Fig. 7A). The macromolecular pool (perchloric acid-precipitated compounds) saturated with about 40 μM [^{14}C]tyrosine (Fig. 7A) similarly to the catecholamines pool (which, however, was saturated with higher concentrations of [^{14}C]tyrosine) (Fig. 7B).

These preliminary results offer the possibility of previewing the study of the turnover of dopamine with particular reference to its compartment.

Choline

It has been shown that the most important metabolite of choline in nerve cells is phosphorylcholine (15,16) and in synaptosomes acetylcholine (25). This finding might be correlated to a higher content of choline kinase in the cell body and of choline acetyltransferase in the nerve terminals, and was confirmed when primary neuronal cultures were incubated with different concentrations of choline (0.5, 10, 50, 150 μM) and the various choline-containing compartments analyzed as a function of time (15). The results indicated that neurons, when incubated with concentrations of choline far from the physiological ones, showed an abnormal metabolism of endocellular choline, suggesting non-steady-state conditions of the pool of choline. The synthesis of acetylcholine, however, was stimulated by increasing concentra-

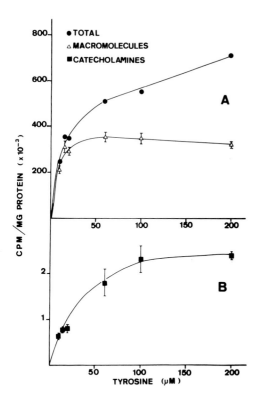

FIG. 7. Incorporation of radioactive tyrosine in the macromolecular and the catecholamine pools as a function of tyrosine concentrations.

tions of the substrate. When cells were incubated with 150 μM choline (a concentration three- to sixfold higher than the physiological one), acetylcholine synthesis was stimulated, reached a maximum of incorporation at 30 min, and afterwards the radioactive labeling decreased. This, while suggesting the possibility that synthesis of the neuromediator could be stimulated by addition of more choline in the incubation medium, also indicated a nonphysiological steady state of the choline pool (as it was judged from the bell-shaped curve of incorporation).

Upon its entry choline was immediately metabolized (mainly phosphorylated) and some compartments took a long time to reach saturation, while the free choline compartment was saturated within a few minutes. Total incorporation increased linearly. This finding should draw some attention to the use of uptake measurements as an index for the transport of choline, especially when the time of incubation is relatively long.[2] It should, moreover, be recalled that at a relatively long incubation time homoexchange phenomenon became more and more relevant.

CONCLUSIONS

Isolated neurons in culture appear to behave, from a biochemical point of view, with a remarkable similarity to what is known about their metabolism *in vivo*. The simplicity of the model suggests its use in the study of the complex biochemical events occurring in cell-to-cell recognition that are leading to the establishment of functional circuitries by the differentiation of cellular contacts into chemically active synapses. But before approaching these intricate phenomena some information may be obtained on relatively "simple" biochemical events. Hence the observation made on the transport studies that have been reviewed may suggest the following conclusions.

Great care should be taken in analyzing the transport of metabolizable substances. Thus roughtly two types of transport have been revealed in the course of these studies. In the first, dopamine was found to be transported by a highly specific mechanism without any apparent correlation to its metabolism. Its transport appears to be energy-dependent and future experiments may clarify the role of Na^+ that may be cotransported with dopamine or give the necessary energy simply by establishment of the electrochemical driving force.

The second type to which belong the transports of GABA, choline, and possibly tyrosine appeared to be dependent on the metabolism of these substances. Only one mechanism seems to mediate these transports of a facilitated diffusion type

---

[2]It might be useful at this point to define precisely the difference between uptake and transport used in this review. In the case of metabolizable substances the rate values obtained by uptake measurements, i.e., the measurement of the total amount of metabolite entered into the cell per unit of time —regardless of its metabolic fate—are highly affected by metabolism, by efflux movements and by the time factor which, for experimental reasons, usually exceeds 1 min. The rates of transport might instead be approached in a close approximation in measuring the transfer of the metabolite from the milieu to its free endocellular compartment and subtracting the possible efflux movement present.

and, especially in the case of choline, low energy-dependent, being driven by the electrochemical gradient of Na^+. A certain relationship has also been found between the inward and outward fluxes since a homoexchange of choline was observed. It is interesting to notice in this respect that recent experiments have suggested that the outward flux of choline might be driven by other electrochemical gradients, possibly K^+. It is then suggestive to imagine that the balance between Na^+ and K^+ fluxes may regulate the supply of choline for cellular needs.

In any case, the experiments that have been herein described do not support the hypothesis of the existence of a specific mechanism of transport that might be rate-limiting in the synthesis of acetylcholine in neurons. Similar results obtained with synaptosomal preparations in our laboratory (22) and in others (11) reach very much the same conclusion.

ACKNOWLEDGMENTS

This work has been supported by grants from the INSERM (ATP no. 79.81.113) and the DGRST (Aide no. 80 E.875).

REFERENCES

1. Augusti-Tocco, G., and Sato, G. (1969): Establishment of functional clonal lines of neurons from mouse neuroblastomas. *Proc. Natl. Acad. Sci. USA*, 64:311–315.
2. Booher, J., and Sensenbrenner, M. (1972): Growth and cultivation of dissociated neurons and glial cells from embryonic chick, rat and human brain in flast cultures. *Neurobiology*, 2:97–105.
3. Cleland, W. W. (1967): The statistical analysis of enzyme kinetic data. *Adv. Enzymol.*, 29:1–32.
4. Froissart, C., and Massarelli, R. (1981): Placental choline acetyltransferase purification and properties. In: *Cholinergic Mechanism*, edited by G. Pepeu and H. Ladinsky, pp. 91–95. Plenum Press, New York.
5. Jope, R. S. (1979): High affinity choline transport and acetylCoA production in brain and their roles in the regulation of acetylcholine synthesis. *Brain Res. Rev.*, 1:313–344.
6. Kuhar, M. J., and Murrin, L. C. (1978): Sodium-dependent high affinity choline uptake. *J. Neurochem.*, 30:15–21.
7. Levi, G., and Raiteri, M. (1976): Synaptosomal transport processes. *Int. Rev. Neurobiol.*, 19:51–74.
8. Louis, J. C., Pettmann, B., Courageot, J., Rumigny, J. F., Mandel, P., and Sensenbrenner, M. (1981): Developmental changes in cultured neurons. An ultrastructural and neurochemical study. *Exp. Brain Res.*, 42:63–72.
9. Louis, J. C., Vincendon, G., Massarelli, R., and Dreyfus, H. (1981): Development of dopaminergic properties in cultured neurons from chick embryo cerebral hemispheres. *Biochem. Soc. Trans.*, 9:104–105.
10. Lundberg, J., Bylock, A., Goldstein, M., Hansson, H. A., and Dählstrom, A. (1977): Ultrastructural localization of dopamine-β-hydroxylase in nerve terminals of the rat brain. *Brain Res.*, 120:549–552.
11. Marchbanks, R. M. (1981): Interaction of choline transport with acetylcholine release and synthesis. In: *Cholinergic Mechanisms*, edited by G. Pepeu and H. Ladinsky, pp. 489–496. Plenum Press, New York.
12. Marchbanks, R. M., and Wonnacott, S. (1979): Relationship of choline uptake to acetylcholine synthesis and release. In: *The Cholinergic Synapse*, edited by S. Tuček, pp. 77–88. Elsevier, Amsterdam.
13. Martin, D. L. (1976): Carrier-mediated transport and removal of GABA from synaptic regions. In: *GABA in Nervous System Function*, edited by E. Roberts, T. N. Chase, and D. B. Tower, pp. 347–386. Kroc Foundation Series, Raven Press, New York.

14. Massarelli, R. (1978): Uptake of choline in nerve cell cultures: Correlation with the endogenous pool of choline. In: *Cholinergic Mechanisms and Psychopharmacology*, edited by D. J. Jensen, pp. 539–550. Plenum Press, New York.
15. Massarelli, R., and Wong, T. Y. (1981): Choline uptake in nerve cell cultures and in synaptosomal preparations is regulated by the endogenous pool of choline. In: *Cholinergic Mechanisms*, edited by G. Pepeu and H. Ladinsky, pp. 511–520. Plenum Press, New York.
16. Massarelli, R., Wong, T. Y., Froissart, C., and Robert, J. (1979): Choline uptake and metabolism by nerve cell cultures. In: *The Cholinergic Synapse*, edited by S. Tuček, pp. 89–96. Elsevier, Amsterdam.
17. Nelson, P. G. (1975): Nerve and muscle cells in culture. *Physiol. Rev.*, 55:1–61.
18. Pettmann, B., Louis, J. C., and Sensenbrenner, M. (1979): Morphological and biochemical maturation of neurons cultured in the absence of glial cells. *Nature*, 281:378–380.
19. Porcellati, G., Gaiti, A., Woelk, H., De Medio, G. E., Brunetti, M., Francescangeli, E., and Trovarelli, G. (1978): Membrane-bound base exchange reactions in animal tissues. In: *Advances in Experimental Medicine and Biology, Vol. 101: Enzymes of Lipid Metabolism*, pp. 287–299. Plenum Press, New York.
20. Schubert, D., Humphreys, S. Baroni, C., and Colin, M. (1969): *In vitro* differentiation of a mouse neuroblastoma. *Proc. Natl. Acad. Sci. USA*, 64:316–323.
21. Varon, S. (1975): Neurons and glia in neural cultures. *Exp. Neurol.*, 48:93–134.
22. Wong, T. Y., Dreyfus, H., Harth, S., Louis, J. C., Mandel, P., and Massarelli, R. (1981): Role of sialocompounds in the uptake of choline in synaptosomes. *C. R. Acad. Sci. [D] (Paris)*, 293:31–34.
23. Wong, T. Y., Dreyfus, H., and Massarelli, R. (1981): Transport and metabolism of choline in synaptosomes: Ionic requirement. *Biochem. Soc. Trans.*, 9:84–85.
24. Wong, T. Y., Louis, J. C. Vincendon, G., and Massarelli, R. (1981): Transport and metabolism of choline in synaptosomes: Energy requirement. *Biochem. Soc. Trans.*, 9:83–84.
25. Yamamura, H. I., and Snyder, S. H. (1973): High affinity transport of choline into synaptosomes of rat brain. *J. Neurochem.*, 21:1355–1374.

Neural Transmission, Learning and Memory,
edited by R. Caputto and C. Ajmone Marsan.
Raven Press, New York © 1983.

Compartmentation of Monoaminergic Synaptic Vesicles. Physiological Implications

A. Pellegrino de Iraldi

*Instituto de Biología Celular, Facultad de Medicina, Universidad
Nacional de Buenos Aires, Buenos Aires, Argentina*

After the discovery by von Euler and Hillarp (13) that noradrenaline was present in a particulated fraction of bovine splenic nerves, the ultrastructure of monoaminergic neurons was intensively studied. These studies led to the description of two types of vesicles: a predominant population of clear and granular vesicles of 40 to 60 nm diameter and a minor population of 80 to 90 nm diameter in nerve endings and varicosities of the peripheral nervous system (PNS) (4,11) and in the central nervous system (CNS) (21,36). Both types of vesicles were also found in the perikaryon (12) and the large ones in the nerve trunks (17).

Histochemical, pharmacological, and biochemical similarities and differences have been reported between both kind of vesicles. Even though monoamines have been located in both of them, they seem to play different roles in neurotransmission. Many lines of evidence support the concept that small vesicles are directly involved in the synthesis of the neurotransmitter and its release upon the arrival of the nerve impulse. The role of large vesicles in the nerve terminals is not yet clearly understood; they have been interpreted as a storage site for a resistant pool of amines (15).

This chapter is concerned with the anatomical and functional organization of small vesicles, using as a model the pineal nerves of the rat, which are known to contain noradrenaline and serotonin (42) coexisting in their synaptic vesicles (23,38).

MORPHOLOGICAL ORGANIZATION OF GRANULAR VESICLES

On morphological grounds monoaminergic synaptic vesicles were characterized, from their first description (11), using osmium tetroxide fixations, by the presence of an electron-dense core separated from the vesicle membrane by an electronlucent space (Fig. 1A). It was soon demonstrated by histochemical and pharmacological methods that the dense granules contain biogenic amines (3,33,42). The clear space was disregarded or considered as an artifact of the fixation techniques. The analytical and systematic study of small vesicles in different experimental conditions, and with different histochemical techniques, led us to propose that the clear space is

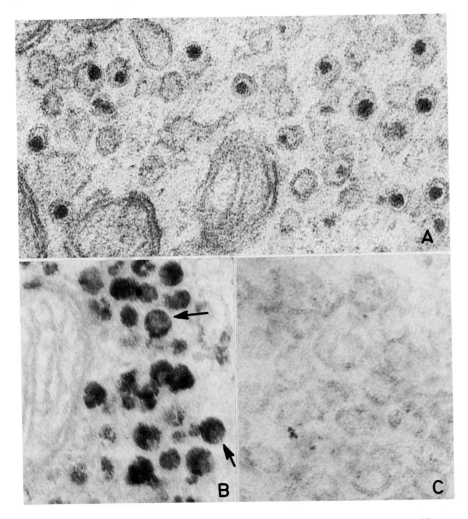

FIG. 1. A: Small synaptic vesicles of rat pineal nerves fixed in OsO₄. Dense cores of different sizes in contact with the vesicle membrane are apparent in half of the vesicles. In these granulated vesicles an electronlucent space (the matrix) separates the core from the vesicle membrane. In half of the vesicles the dense core is absent. **B:** The same vesicles fixed in zinc iodide-osmium tetroxide mixture (ZIO). The matrix is electron-opaque and the cores *(arrows)* appear faintly stained. **C:** ZIO reaction was carried out after treatment *in vitro* with *N*-ethylmaleimide. The inhibition of -SH groups abolished ZIO reaction. ×240,000.

an important and distinct component of the vesicle, which is formed by two compartments: the dense core and the clear space, which we called the matrix (39–41).

According to that proposal both compartments have a different functional significance, the matrix being involved in the synthesis and the release of the neurotransmitter and the core in its storage (30–32). In osmium tetroxide fixations (Fig. 1A) we observed that the size of both compartments is variable and inversely related: i.e., the smaller the core, the larger is the matrix and vice versa. The core may even disappear, giving place to a small clear vesicle exclusively formed by the matrix. It has been calculated that even when the core reaches its maximum size, the matrix is around three times larger. Thus the matrix is a constant component of the small granular vesicle and the core is a transient one (31,41). The core is always linked to the vesicle membrane, being directly in contact or connected to it by a pedicle (41), the width of which is about twice the thickness of the vesicle membrane.

This configuration suggests that the core is an invagination of the vesicle membrane and marks a special locus in the vesicle membrane the functional significance of which has not yet been elucidated. Further, it suggests that the size of the vesicle must change inversely with the size of the core. Measurements made after electrical stimulation (33) show a highly significant increase in the vesicle diameter that could be interpreted as an unfolding of the vesicle membrane. However, under other conditions of depletion of biogenic amines, such as repeated doses of tyramine (40) and high potassium concentration (35), only a tendency to increase in the size of the vesicles was observed. Further, the incubation in a solution containing Na^+ as the main cation, which does not depletes monoamines, also tends to increase the vesicle diameter (35). Thus the diameter of the synaptic vesicles could not be directly correlated with the release of the amines stored in the core.

Small and scarce cores are seen in the nerves of organs with a predominant "tonic" functioning (i.e., in small arteries) and abundant and large cores in organs with an important "phasic" function (i.e., in the vas deferens and the pineal gland) (31).

ZIO REACTION IN THE VESICLE MATRIX

When a mixture of zinc iodide and osmium tetroxide (ZIO) was used (Fig. 1B), a reverse image was obtained and the matrix appeared denser than the core in small vesicles (37). This change was not observed in large vesicles, which present the same appearance as in osmium tetroxide fixation. Although *in vitro* assays (39) have shown that ZIO reacts with different compounds, giving a black precipitate (which could explain the electron-density of different types of synaptic vesicles) the ZIO reaction was shown to be due to the presence of reactive -SH groups, possibly belonging to protein molecules within the vesicles (30,43). The ZIO reaction is temperature- and time-dependent and varies in different types of synaptic vesicles (30). In monoaminergic vesicles is affected by drugs interfering with the uptake, storage, and synthesis of monoamines (32,39). The fact that the inhibitors of the synthesis of monoamines located in the vesicle affect the ZIO reactive sites in the vesicle matrix can be taken to suggest that the enzymes involved in the monoamine synthesis are located in that compartment (32). This interpretation is in line with the speculations by Udenfriend (48) on the integration of norepinephrine-synthesizing enzymes in a subcellular structure (the granular vesicle) that also binds noradrenaline and has been considered elsewhere (31).

TWO POOLS OF AMINES IN MONOAMINERGIC VESICLES

On pharmacological, electrical stimulation, and biochemical evidences at least two pools of amines have been defined in nerve terminals: an "easily releasable," "recently synthesized," or "functional pool" (26) and a "tightly bound" or "reserve pool" (49). The functional pool has been hypothetically placed in the axoplasm, in synaptic vesicles closest to the plasma membrane of sympathetic nerve endings, or in the large granular vesicles which would be recently synthesized. The reserve pool has been located in the small granular vesicles, in a pool of vesicles far from the plasma membrane, or in a pool of "old" small vesicles derived from the large ones (7). A compartmentation of noradrenaline pools in adrenergic granules or vesicles has also been postulated (16). Studies made in our laboratory (31,33) have shown that endogenous amines are distributed—in the granular vesicles of the pineal nerves of the rat—in two pools, which can be characterized by histochemistry and electrical stimulation: a loosely bound pool located in the matrix and a tightly bound pool located in the core. The behaviour of both pools under electrical stimulation and in resting conditions is compatible with the idea that the amines stored in the core form a reserve pool and the amines stored in the matrix correspond to a functional pool which can be released "spontaneously" and by electrical stimulation, being replaced by the transmitter newly synthesized or by the amines stored in the core. Thus this pool is reduced by electrical stimulation but does not disappear, whereas the amines tightly bound, stored in the core, are suddenly released by electrical stimulation. Both amines stored in the vesicles of the pineal nerves (noradrenaline and serotonin) follow the same behaviour under electrical stimulation (31,33). A similar distribution is adopted by the false transmitter formed by the administration of 5-hydroxydopamine (5-OH-DA), which is 5-hydroxynoradrenaline (5-OH-NA) (31,33). The release of the false transmitter may easily be followed at the electron microscope because of the intense osmiophilia induced in the vesicles by the storage of 5-OH-NA (47). After a prolonged treatment with 5-OH-DA, noradrenaline is substituted by the false transmitter that specifically fills the vesicles of adrenergic nerve terminals (47), being loosely bound in the matrix and tightly bound in the core (31,38). In our laboratory we have studied the release of the false transmitter *in vivo*, at rest and under electrical stimulation (31,33), in rats treated according to Tranzer and Thoenen (47): several doses of 20 mg/kg of 5-OH-DA were injected i.p. over a period of 48 hr. As seen in Fig. 2A, 1 hr after the last injection most of the vesicles appeared filled with an osmiophilic material. At 5 hr after the last injection (Fig. 2B) the osmiophilia was restricted to the core; the matrix was electronlucent. Electrical stimulation applied to the afferent trunks of both superior cervical ganglia (sq pulses 1 msec, 25V, 25 Hz, for 30 min), 1 or 5 hr after the last injection, depletes the osmiophilic material from the matrix and the core (Fig. 2C). Thus the false transmitter stored in the matrix is preferentially depleted at rest while electrical stimulation acts on both compartments. Emptied vesicles remain in the terminal. Exocytotic images are not observed.

More recently (35) the release of the false transmitter by high potassium was studied. Pineal glands of rats treated with 5-OH-DA as previously described were

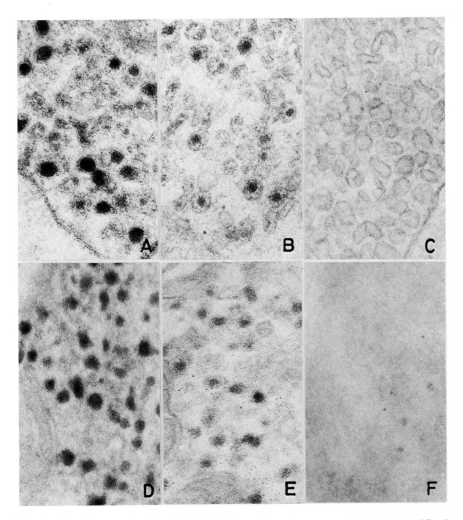

FIG. 2. Pineal nerves of rats treated with 5-hydroxydopamine over a period of 48 hr and fixed in glutaraldehyde-osmium tetroxide. **A:** One hour after the last injection, many vesicles are totally stained and a minor proportion shows dense cores. **B:** Five hours after the last injection. The matrix of the vesicles is electronlucent. In many vesicles the core is electron-dense. **C:** After electrical stimulation applied 30 min after the last injection the vesicles are electronlucent. **D, E, and F:** Nerve endings incubated in Tyrode solutions: **D:** in TyNa, **E** in TyK and **F** in TK + 2 mM CaCl$_2$. In **D** most of the vesicles are totally stained or show a dense core. In **E** most of the vesicles show a dense core; no totally stained vesicles are seen. In **F** the osmiophilia has almost disappeared. Only a few and faint cores remain. Compare **A** with **D**, **E** with **B**, and **F** with **C**. ×120,000.

incubated at room temperature for 30 min in (a) Tyrode solution with Na$^+$ as predominant cation, without Ca^{2+} (TyNa); (b) Tyrode solution with K$^+$ as predominant cation, without Ca^{2+} (TyK); and (c) TyK + 2 mM CaCl$_2$ (TyKCa). The composition of TyNa was: NaCl, 0.8g; KCl, 0.02 g; MgCl$_2$, 0.02 g; PO$_4$HNa$_2$,

0.005 g; NaHCO$_3$, 0.1 g; glucose, 0.1 g; deionized water, 100 ml. In TyK, NaCl was substituted by an equivalent amount of KCl. Fixation was done in glutaraldehyde (33). As shown in Fig. 2D, in the glands incubated in TyNa, the osmiophilia induced by the false transmitter is retained; many vesicles are totally stained showing the others a dense core. (Compare with Fig. 2A.) In the nerves of glands incubated in TyK without Ca^{2+} (Fig. 2E), the osmiophilia was restricted to the cores being the matrix electron lucent. (Compare with Fig. 2B.) In the glands incubated in TyKCa osmiophilic vesicles could be observed in some terminals; however in most of them only a few small faint cores were evident (Fig. 2F) (Compare with Fig. 2C.) These results seem to indicate that Na$^+$ protects the storage of the false transmitter in the vesicles; that high K$^+$ release the transmitter contained in the matrix in the absence of Ca^{2+} and that high K$^+$ plus Ca^{2+} acts on both compartments, depleting the matrix and the core in some way like electrical stimulation. These findings are in line with the knowledge that the presence of Na$^+$, in the extracellular fluid, is required for the retention of stored noradrenaline by nerve endings and that calcium ions are required for the release of neurotransmitter by the nerve impulse (2,9,25). Electrical stimulation and TyKCa activation considerably differed in the preservation of the vesicle membrane in glutaraldehyde-osmium tetroxide fixation (compare Figs. 2C and 2F). The significance of this difference has not yet been investigated.

The effect of high K$^+$ without Ca^{2+} was also compared with the effect of electrical stimulation in glands fixed directly in osmium tetroxide dissolved in a balanced solution (31) containing different ions and polyvinylpyrrolidone, which will be called O-P. We have previously shown (31,33) that electrical stimulation reduces the size and the frequency of dense cores revealed with O-P. Figure 3A shows a control fixed immediately after killing the animals and B after electrical stimulation of the afferent trunks of both superior cervical ganglia. In addition to the change in the cores, electrical stimulation produces a significant increase in the size of the vesicles and a dilution of the axoplasm. More recently (35) pineal glands incubated at room temperature in TyNa (Fig. 3C) and in TyK without Ca^{2+} were fixed in O-P. High K$^+$ reduces somewhat the size of the cores, but their frequency related with the number of vesicles (compare with Fig. 3B) is maintained. The axoplasm appeared as more diluted than with electrical stimulation, and the nerve endings or varicosities are considerably enlarged. Measurements made of the mean diameter of the vesicles seem to indicate that the vesicles are enlarged after TyNa and TyK incubations but the increment was not significant. The dilution of the axoplasm observed after electrical stimulation or high K$^+$ incubation was not apparent in glutaraldehyde-osmium tetroxide fixation (see Figs. 2C and 2F, respectively).

A CALCIUM BINDING SITE IN THE CORE COMPARTMENT MODIFIABLE BY ELECTRICAL STIMULATION AND POTASSIUM AND SODIUM IONS

Taking into account that Ca^{2+} is thought to be involved in the integration of the storage complexes of monoamines and that a Ca^{2+}-dependent mechanism is also

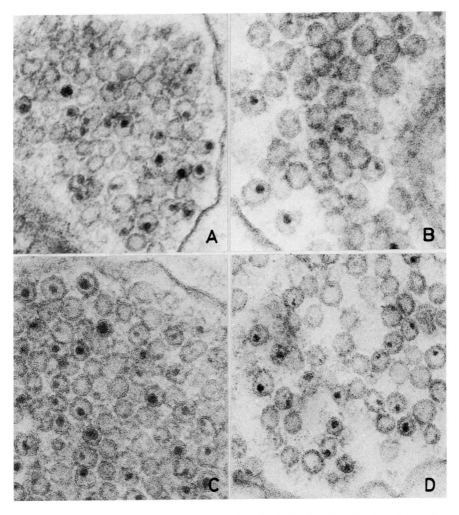

FIG. 3. Nerve endings from rat pineal nerves fixed in OsO_4. **A:** without treatment. **B:** After electrical stimulation of the afferent trunks of both superior cervical ganglia. **C:** Incubated in TyNa and **D:** in TyK. In **B** the vesicles are significantly enlarged, and the cores are decreased in size and frequency. Compare with **A**. Under high K^+ **(D)** the size of the cores is diminished (compare with **C**) but they are clearly evident. $\times 120,000$.

implicated in the release of neurotransmitters (9,25), we have investigated (34) the effect of Ca^{2+}-containing solutions on the morphology of synaptic vesicles from rat pineal nerves in control and electrical stimulated glands. We used the methodology applied by other authors to different types of cholinergic vesicles (5,29) based on the employment of Ca^{2+}-containing fixation solutions. Our studies showed (34) that a Ca^{2+} electron-dependent dense particle (C-EDP) is present within the small and large synaptic vesicles of rat pineal nerves. Apparently this particle occupies the same site as the osmiophilic cores characteristic of this type of vesicle.

Although the electron opacity produced by Ca^{2+} was enhanced by OsO_4, it could be established that osmium affinity could be independent of calcium deposits in the vesicle core.

Although different buffers may be used to dilute the fixatives, the better results were obtained with collidine buffer in the schedule proposed by Pappas and Rose (29): fixation in 3% glutaraldehyde in 80 mM collidine buffer, pH 7.2, overnight; washing in the same buffer for 4 hr and postfixation in 1% OsO_4 in collidine buffer for 2 hr, with the addition of $CaCl_2$ in all the solutions. The procedure was carried out at 4°C. The particle could be discerned in unosmicated tissues, indicating that the electron opacity was produced by the presence of Ca^{2+}. If Ca^{2+} was omitted, the electron-dense particles did not appear. The C-EDPs considerably decreased in size and number and even disappeared altogether following electrical stimulation, indicating that Ca^{2+} affinity is significantly altered by depolarisation and suggesting that this change has a role in the release of the neurotransmitter. More recently (35) the effect of high K^+ and Na^+ on this Ca^{2+} binding site was studied in our laboratory.

In a first experiment (Fig. 4) pineal glands were incubated for 30 min at room temperature, in TyNa (A), TyNa + 50 mM $CaCl_2$ (B) and TyK + 50 mM (D and E). Fixation was done in A without $CaCl_2$ and in C, D, and E with 50 mM $CaCl_2$. It was observed that the electron-dense particle was absent when Ca^{2+} was omitted in the incubation medium and the fixation solutions (Fig. 4A). They were more abundant, larger, and denser in TyK + 50; mM $CaCl_2$ than in TyNa + 50 mM $CaCl_2$ (Figs. 4C and 4B, respectively). Electron-dense deposits were also increased in the cytoplasmic mitochondria (Fig. 4D), while only small deposits or a diffuse density could be observed in nerve ending mitochondria.

In a second experiment the glands were incubated for 30 min at room temperature in TyK or TyNa, without $CaCl_2$, and fixed in solutions containing 50 mM $CaCl_2$. It was observed that the C-EDPs were almost absent or did not appear in TyK incubations (Fig. 5A) and were small but clearly evident in TyNa incubation (Fig. 5B). To determine if the change introduced in the Ca^{2+} binding site by the incubation in high potassium was reversible, we conducted a third experiment in which the glands were incubated first in TyK for 30 min and then in TyNa for an additional 30 min. It was observed that the C-EDPs reappeared (Fig. 5C). In other cases the glands were incubated for 1 hr in TyNa and fixed in calcium-containing solutions. It was observed that the Ca^{2+} binding site was considerably increased in size in the synaptic vesicles (Fig. 5D).

These results show that high K^+ without Ca^+ changes the Ca^{2+} site of the vesicle core, as the electrical stimulation does. However, if the incubation is made in TyK + 50 mM $CaCl_2$ calcium deposits were considerably increased in the synaptic vesicles and cytoplasmic mitochondria, as if the ion was entering through the plasma membrane. They also show that Na^+ has a great effect on the Ca^{2+} affinity of the vesicle, increasing considerably the Ca^{2+} deposits therein. This result can be correlated with the fact that 5-OH-NA is retained in the vesicles incubated in TyNa (Fig. 2D) and is consistent with the knowledge that Na^+ hinders the release of the neurotransmitter (2).

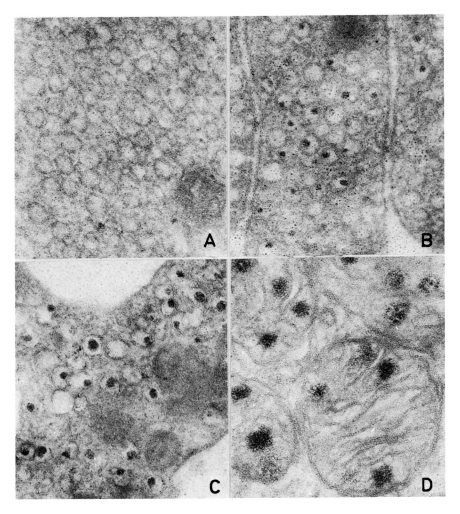

FIG. 4. A: Nerve ending incubated in TyNa without Ca^{2+}. **B:** Nerve ending incubated in TyNa + 50 mM $CaCl_2$; **C:** Nerve ending. **F:** Cytoplasmic mitochondria incubated in TyK + 50 mM $CaCl_2$. Fixation was done in glutaraldehyde-collidine-OsO_4, in **A** without $CaCl_2$ and in **B**, **C**, and **D** with 50 mM $CaCl_2$. The vesicles, electronlucent in **A**, show an electron-dense particle in **C** and **D**. Large calcium deposits are seen in cytoplasmic mitochondria. × 120,000.

The fact that Ca^{2+} binds to the core seems to emphasize its role in a storage site for the biogenic amines, taking into account that Ca^{2+} integrates the storage complex of biogenic amines.

MECHANISMS OF NEUROTRANSMITTER RELEASE AND COMPARTMENTATION

According to the calcium hypothesis (25,28), synaptic transmission is controlled fundamentally by the neurotransmitter secreted in response to a rapid depolarisation-

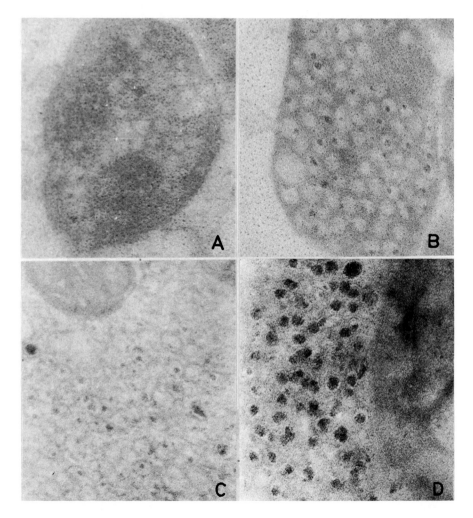

FIG. 5. Rat pineal nerves incubated in solutions without calcium and fixed in solutions containing 50 mM CaC1$_2$. The incubation was made in **A**, in TyK and in **B**, in TyNa, for 30 min.; in **C**, 30 min in TyK and 30 min in TyNa and in **D** 60 min in TyNa. In **A** no electron-dense particles are observed inside the vesicles; small spots are clearly evident in **B** and **C** and large dense cores in **D**. ×120,000.

triggered calcium influx (25,28). The release of neurotransmitter at rest is less Ca^{2+}-dependent (24). Elevated K$^+$ pulses, often used to mimic the depolarising effect of action potentials, may produce the efflux of neurotransmitter in the absence and in the presence of Ca^{2+} in the extracellular fluid, and a Ca^{2+}-dependent and a Ca^{2+}-independent release of the neurotransmitter are distinguished (19). Our experiments (35) seem to indicate that Ca^{2+}-independent release is primarily concerned with the neurotransmitter located in the matrix, and the calcium-dependent release with the neutotransmitter stored in the core. The efflux of neurotransmitter at rest may be equated with the effect of elevated K^+ in the absence of Ca^{2+} and the releasing effect of electrical stimulation with that of elevated K^+ in the presence of Ca^{2+}. That means that in each case a different pool of neurotransmitter is primarily involved. However, as can be expected, it seems that a simple relationship between each kind of stimulus and each vesicle compartment must be excluded. Thus electrical stimulation and high K^+ in the presence of Ca^{2+} also affect the matrix and the reduction of size cores produced by high K^+ in the absence of Ca^{2+} suggests that the amines stored in the core could be progressively released. Both compartments are integrated in a functional unit. In this context it is interesting that in cortical synaptosomes, Ca^{2+}-dependent and Ca^{2+}-independent efflux of GABA, in response to elevated K^+ pulses, arise not only via different flux mechanisms but also different GABA pools (19). Further, K^+ in the absence of Ca^{2+} changes the Ca^{2+} binding site, decreasing the Ca^{2+} affinity of the core compartment (Fig. 5A) and as a consequence the storage of amines in the core must be influenced by K^+ alone. On the contrary, Na^+ has an important role in the retention of the amines by adrenergic nerve endings (2). In our experiments (35) with high Na^+, 5-OH-NA is retained in the matrix and the core, suggesting that Na^+ is acting on both compartments. At the level of the core, calcium affinity is increased and this probably could favour the storage of the amines.

Thus, two different but interlocked mechanisms for releasing the neurotransmitter are the functional counterpart of the anatomical duality of small monoaminergic synaptic vesicles. This functional duality adds further support to the concept that in adrenergic nerves the quantal packet (6) corresponds to a fraction of the neurotransmitter contained in the vesicle (16,18,46), which is provided at rest by one compartment, possibly the matrix, and by both compartments during electrical stimulation (31).

The possible fates of the neurotransmitter released from each compartment has been considered elsewhere (31).

THE SYNAPTIC VESICLE, A SPECIFIC ORGANELLE FOR NEUROTRANSMISSION

The exact role of synaptic vesicles in neurotransmission has been a matter of controversy for the last years (22). This controversy is usually maintained in the conceptual frame of neurosecretion and the vesicles are conceived either explicitly or implicitly as secretory vesicles. Almost from the time of their discovery (10) the hypothesis was made that the transmitter quanta of acetylcholine, observed by Fatt and Katz (14) at the neuromuscular end plates, was preformed within the synaptic vesicle, from where would be released in an all-or-none fashion (24). This release would be accomplished by exocytosis, after fusion of the vesicle membrane with the plasma membrane. The vesicle membrane would be recycled through the plasma membrane (20). These concepts were also extended to adrenergic vesicles (1,45).

This conception implies that synaptic vesicles must disappear after being stimulated. This is a point of disagreement in the literature. It was observed very early

(10) that the vesicle population may be either increased or decreased by nerve stimulation; and different results have been reported in different preparations. The number of vesicles per unit area has been taken as a hint of the change in the total number of synaptic vesicles (1,10,22) in different experimental conditions. This criterion has the drawback that the axoplasm may be diluted or concentrated by different treatments, including the fixation technique, leading to erroneous appreciations. Further, every component of the cell is in a dynamic equilibrium and its development related with the functional requirements. In consequence, their quantitative variations do not give information about their nature but only about their participation, direct or indirect, in a regulatory process.

Our experiments (31,33–35) clearly show that stimulated vesicles may remain in the nerve endings or varicosities after electrical (31,33,34) or high K^+ (35) stimulation, supporting the concept that the neurotransmitter can be released without destruction of synaptic vesicles by exocytosis. The fate of the vesicles has been followed with different markers such as 5-OH-NA, Ca^{2+} deposits, and osmiophilic dense cores (31,33–35).

The persistence of stimulated synaptic vesicles is in line with the knowledge about the life span of vesicle constituents, leading to the conception that the vesicles are reused (8,27,44).

These facts and the morphological and functional organization of the monoaminergic vesicles led us to propose (31) that the small synaptic vesicle is a specific organelle for neurotransmission and not a merely secretory granule. The original findings here reported are in agreement with that proposal.

CONCLUSIONS

Morphological and histochemical observations in different experimental conditions seem to indicate that the small monoaminergic synaptic vesicles contain two compartments, each of which has a different pool of monoamines: (a) a loosely bound, easily releasable pool in the outer compartment or matrix, and (b) a tightly bound, more resistant pool in the central compartment or core. These two pools subserve, respectively, a tonic and a phasic release of the neurotransmitter, correlated with a tonic or phasic stimulation of the receptor. The monoamines synthesised in the matrix could be released or stored in the core. The storage compartments could also take part in the regulation of monoamine synthesis by feedback inhibition.

Two different but interlocked mechanisms for releasing the neurotransmitter are operative in both compartments. A Ca^{2+}-independent release is primarily concerned with the neurotransmitter located in the matrix and a Ca^{2+}-dependent efflux with the neutotransmitter stored in the core, but both mechanisms affect finally both compartments. The efflux of neurotransmitter at rest could be equated with Ca^{2+}-independent release and Ca^{2+}-dependent release with electrical stimulation. The release, slow in the first case, would be accelerated in the second one.

On the basis of the fate of synaptic vesicles after electrical and high K^+ stimulation, the proposal is made that the small synaptic vesicle is a specific organelle for neurotransmission.

SUMMARY

On morphological and histochemical evidence obtained in different experimental conditions, two compartments can be conceived in the small monoaminergic synaptic vesicles: the core and the matrix, corresponding respectively to the electron-dense core and the electronlucent space observed between the core and the vesicle membrane in osmium tetroxide fixations. The sizes of both compartments are inversely related: i.e., the smaller the core the larger the matrix and vice versa. The core may even disappear, giving place to a small electronlucent vesicle made exclusively by the matrix. Thus the matrix is a constant component of the vesicle and the core a transient one. The core is always linked to the vesicle membrane. The function of this linkage has not yet been elucidated. The amines synthesized in the matrix could be release or stored in the core.

Each compartment has a different pool of amines: a loosely bound, easily releasable pool in the matrix and a tightly bound, more resistant pool in the core. These two pools subserve, respectively, a tonic and a phasic release of the neurotransmitter, correlated with a tonic or a phasic stimulation of the receptor. The core is more developed in organs with a phasic functioning.

A Ca^{2+} binding site may be revealed in the core, modifiable by electrical stimulation, high K^+ and high Na^+. Ca^{2+} deposits in the matrix would be integrating the storage complexes of the amines and could have a role in regulating Ca^{2+} concentration in the axoplasm.

Two different but interlocked mechanisms for releasing the neurotransmitter would be operative in both compartments: a Ca^{2+}-independent release primarily concerned with the neurotransmitter contained in the matrix and a Ca^{2+} dependent efflux primarily related with the neurotransmitter stored in the core. Na^+ would be important for the retention of the amines in both compartments.

Based on this morphological and functional compartmentation, the persistence of stimulated vesicles in the nerves, demonstrated with different markers and in the life span of vesicle constituents, the proposal is made that the small synaptic vesicles are a specific organelle for neurotransmission.

ACKNOWLEDGMENTS

I am grateful to J. Pablo Corazza for his collaboration in the experimental work first reported in this chapter; Engineer Luis Zimmermann and Mrs. Margarita López de Cáceres for their skillful technical assistance, and Adriana Contreras for the electron micrographs. The original work contained in this chapter was supported by a grant from the Consejo Nacional de Investigaciones Científicas y Técnicas, CONICET, Argentina. Financial support for the Electron Microscope Service is greatly acknowledged to the Faculty of Medicine of Buenos Aires.

REFERENCES

1. Basbaum, C. B., and Heuser, J. E. (1979): Morphological studies of stimulated adrenergic axon varicosities in the mouse vas deferences. *J. Cell Biol.*, 80:310–325.

2. Blaszkowski, T. P., and Bogdanski, D. F. (1971): Possible role of sodium and calcium ions in retention and physiological release of norepinephrine by adrenergic nerve endings. *Biochem. Pharmacol.*, 20:3281–3294.
3. Bloom, F. (1972): Electron microscopy of the catecholamine containing structures. In: *Catecholamines*, edited by H. Blashko and E. Muscholl, pp. 46–78. Springer-Verlag, Berlin.
4. Bondareff, W. (1965): Submicroscopic morphology of granular vesicles in sympathetic nerves of rat pineal body. *Z. Zellforsch. Microsk. Anat.*, 6:211–218.
5. Boyne, A. F., Bohan, R. P., and Williams, T. H. (1974): Effects of calcium-containing fixation solutions on cholinergic synaptic vesicles. *J. Cell Biol.*, 63:773–779.
6. Burnstock, G., and Helma, M. E. (1962): Spontaneous potentials at synaptic nerve endings in smooth muscle. *J. Physiol. (Lond.)*, 160:446–460.
7. Dahlström, A. (1973): Adrenergic transmission. Introduction and review. *Brain Res.*, 62:441–460.
8. Dahlaström, A., and Häggendal, J. (1966): Some quantitative studies on the noradrenaline content in the cell bodies and terminals of a synaptic adrenergic system. *Acta Physiol. Scand.*, 67:278–288.
9. De Potter, W. P. (1976): *Peripheral Sympathetic Neurotransmission.* Arscia Utigaven, N.V., Brussels.
10. De Robertis, E. (1964): *Hystophysiology of Synapses and Neurosecretion*, lst ed. Pergamon Press, Oxford.
11. De Robertis, E., and Pellegrino de Iraldi, A. (1961): A plurivesicular component in adrenergic nerves. *Anat. Res.*, 139:299.
12. Eränkö, L. (1972): Ultrastructure of the developing sympathetic nerve cell and the storage of catecholamines. *Brain Res.*, 46:159–175.
13. Euler, U. S. von, and Hillarp, N. A. (1956): Evidence for the presence of noradrenaline in submicroscopic structures of adrenergic axons. *Nature*, 177:44–45.
14. Fatt, P., and Katz, B. (1952): Spontaneous subthreshold activity at motor nerve endings. *J. Physiol. (Lond.)*, 117:109–128.
15. Fillenz, M. (1977): The factors which provide short-term and long-term control of transmitter release. *Progr. Neurobiol.*, 8:251–278.
16. Folkow, B., and Häggendal, J. (1970): Some aspects of the quantal release of the adrenergic tramitter. In: *New Aspects of Storage and Release Mechanisms of Catecholamines*, edited by H. J. Schümann and G. Kroneberg, pp. 91–97. Bayer Symposium II. Springer-Verlag, Berlin.
17. Geffen, L. B., and Livett, B. G. (1971): Synaptic vesicles in sympathetic neurons. *Physiol. Rev.*, 51:98–157.
18. Geffen, L. B., Livett, B. G., and Rush, R. A. (1970): Immunohistochemical localization of chromogranins in sheep sympathetic neurons and their release by nerve impulses. In: *New Aspects of Storage and Release Mechanisms of Catecholamines*, edited by H. J. Shümann and G. Kroneberg, pp. 58–77. Bayer Symposium II. Springer Verlag, Berlin.
19. Haylock, J. W., Levy, W. B., Denner, L. A., and Cotman, C. W. (1978): Effects of elevated (K^+) on the release of neurotransmitter from cortical synaptosomes: Efflux or secretion? *J. Neurochem.*, 30:113–1125.
20. Heuser, J., and Reese, T. (1973): Evidence for recycling of synaptic vesicle membrane during transmitter release at the frog neuromuscular junction. *J. Cell Biol.*, 57:315–344.
21. Hökfelt, T. (1968): *In vitro* studies on central and pepipheral monoamine neurons at the ultrastructural level. *Z. Zellforsch. Mikrosk. Anat.*, 91:1–74.
22. Irael, M., Dunant, Y., and Manaranche, R. (1979): The present status of the vesicular hypothesis. *Prog. Neurobiol.*, 13:237–275.
23. Jaim Etcheverry, G., and Zieher, L. M. (1968): Cytochemistry of 5 hydroxytryptamine at the electron microscope level. II. Localization in the autonomic nerves of rat pineal gland. *Z. Zellforsch.*, 86:393–400.
24. Katz, B. (1966): *Nerve, Muscle and Synapse.* McGraw-Hill, New York.
25. Katz, B., and Miledi, R. (1967): Ionic requirements of synaptic transmitter release. *Nature (Lond.)*, 215:651.
26. Kopin, I. J., Breese, G. R., Krauss, K. R., and Weise, V. K. (1968): Selective release of newly synthesized norepinephrine from the cat spleen during sympathetic nerve stimulation. *J. Pharmacol. Exp. Ther.*, 161:271–278.
27. Lapetina, E. G., Lunt, G. G., and De Robertis, E. (1970): The turnover of phosphatidyl choline in rat cerebral cortex membranes *in vivo*. *J. Neurobiol.*, 1:295–302.

28. Llinás, R., Stenberg, I. Z., and Walton, K. (1976): Presynaptic calcium currents and their relation to synaptic transmission: Voltage clamp study in squid giant synapse and theoretical model for the calcium gate. *Proc. Natl. Acad. Sci. USA*, 73:2918–2922.
29. Pappas, G. D., and Rose, S. (1976): Localization of calcium deposits in the frog neuromuscular junction at rest and following stimulation. *Brain Res.*, 103:362–365.
30. Pellegrino de Iraldi, A. (1977): Significance of the Maillet method (ZIO) for cytochemical studies of subcellular structure. *Experientia*, 33:1–10.
31. Pellegrino de Iraldi, A. (1980): Compartmentation of synaptic vesicles in autonomic neurons: Morphological correlates of neurotransmitter pools in monoaminergic synapses; the vesicles as dual quantal elements in transmitter storage and release. In: *Histochemistry and Cell Biology of Autonomic Neurons, SIF Cells, and Paraneurons*, edited by O. Eränkö et al., pp. 255–268, Raven Press, New York.
32. Pellegrino de Iraldi, A., and Cardoni, R. (1979): ZIO staining in synaptic vesicles of the rat pineal nerves after inhibition of serotonin and noradrenaline synthesizing enzymes. *Cell Tissue Res.*, 200:91–100.
33. Pellegrino de Iraldi, A., and Corazza, J. P. (1981): Two pools of amines in synaptic vesicles of rat pineal nerves. *Rev. Can. Biol.*, 40:101–109.
34. Pellegrino de Iraldi, A., and Corazza, J. P. (1981): A calcium binding site modifiable by electrical stimulation in the monoaminergic vesicles of rat pineal nerves. *Cell Tissue Res.*, 16:625–635.
35. Pellegrino de Iraldi, A., and Corazza, J. P. (1982):Efecto del K^+, el Na^+ y el Ca^{2+} sobre el almacenamiento de 5-OH-noradrenalina (5-OH-NA) en las vesículas sinápticas de los nervios pineales de la rota. *Actos Physiol. Latin. Am.*, (in press).
36. Pellegrino de Iraldi, A., Farini Duggan, J., and De Robertis, E. (1963): Adrenergic synaptic vesicles in the anterior hypothalamus of the rat. *Anat. Res.*, 145:521–531.
37. Pellegrino de Iraldi, A., and Gueudet, R. (1968): Action of reserpine on the osmium tetroxide-zinc iodide reactive sites of synaptic vesicles in the pineal nerves of the rat. *Z. Zellforsch. Mikrosk. Anat.*, 91:178–185.
38. Pellegrino de Iraldi, A., Gueudet, R., and Suburo, A. M. (1971): Differentiation between 5-hydroxytryptamine and catecholamines in synaptic vesicles. *Prog. Brain Res.*, 34:161–170.
39. Pellegrino de Iraldi, A., and Suburo, A. M. (1971): Two compartments in the granulated vesicles of the pineal nerves. In: *The Pineal Gland*, edited by G. E. W. Wolstenholme and J. Knight, pp. 177–195. Ciba Foundation Symposium, Churchill Living-stone, Edinburgh.
40. Pellegrino de Iraldi, A., and Suburo, A. M. (1972): Effect of tyramine on the compartments of granulated vesicles of rat pineal nerve endings. *Eur. J. Pharmacol.*, 19:251–259.
41. Pellegrino de Iraldi, A., and Suburo, A. M. (1972): Morphological evidence of a connection between the core of granulated vesicles and their membrane. *Neurobiology*, 2:8–11.
42. Pellegrino de Iraldi, A., Zieher, L. M., and De Robertis, E. (1965): Ultrastructure and pharmacological studies of nerve endings in the pineal organ. In: *Structure and Function of the Epiphysis Cerebri*, edited by J. Ariëns Kappers and J. P. Schadé, *Progress in Brain Res. Vol. 10*, pp. 389–422, Elsevier, Amsterdam, London, New York.
43. Reinecke, M., and Walther, C. (1978): Aspects of turnover and biogenesis of synaptic vesicles at locust neuromuscular junctions as revealed by zinc iodide-osmium tetroxide (ZIO) reacting with intravesicular -SH groups. *J. Cell Biol.*, 78:839–855.
44. Rodriguez de Lores Arnaiz, G., Alberici de Canal, M., and De Robertis, E. (1971): Turnover of proteins in subcellular fractions of rat cerebral cortex. *Brain Res.*, 31:179–184.
45. Smith, A. D., and Winkler, H. (1972): Fundamental mechanisms in the release of catecholamines. In: *Catecholamines*, edited by H. Blaschko and E. Muscholl, pp. 538–617. Springer Verlag, Berlin.
46. Stjärne, L. (1970): Quantal or graded secretion of adrenal medullary hormone and sympathetic neurotransmitter. In: *New Aspects of Storage and Release Mechanisms of Catecholamines*, edited by H. J. Schümann and G. Kronenberg, pp. 112–127. Bayer Symposium II. Springer-Verlag, Berlin.
47. Tranzer, J. P., and Thoenen, H. (1967): Electron microscopic localization of 5-hydroxydopamine (3,4,5-trihydroxyphenylethylamine) a new "false" sympathetic transmitter. *Experientia*, 23:743–745.
48. Udenfriend, S. (1968): Physiological regulation of noradrenaline biosynthesis. In: *Adrenergic Neurotransmission*, edited by G. E. W. Wolstenholme and M. O. O'Connor, pp. 3–11. Ciba Foundation Study Group No. 33, Churchill, London.
49. Wurtman, R. J. (1966): *Catecholamines*. Little, Brown, Boston.

Neural Transmission, Learning and Memory,
edited by R. Caputto and C. Ajmone Marsan.
Raven Press, New York © 1983.

Immunocytochemistry of Serotoninergic Neurons in the Central Nervous System of Monkeys

J. Pecci Saavedra, T. Pasik, and P. Pasik

Department of Neurology, Mount Sinai School of Medicine of the City University of New York, New York; and Instituto de Biología Celular, Facultad de Medicina, University of Buenos Aires, Buenos Aires, Argentina

In 1964, Dählstrom and Fuxe discovered the presence of serotonin (5-HT)-containing neuronal bodies and ample ascending and descending projections in the rat brain stem by means of the Falck-Hillarp formadelhyde-induced fluorescence (FIF) technique. Their results stimulated a number of other laboratories to further the research on the 5-HT systems in other species, such as cat (28), squirrel monkey (14,20), and macaque (32). Radioautographic labeling of serotoninergic cell bodies and fibers by means of intraventricular or local application of [^{3}H]-5-HT was also used for studying this system (1,3,5,10,12,17). Finally, biochemical determinations of 5-HT in the nervous system were performed by several investigators since the early studies of Amin et al. (2) and Bogdansky et al. (6); the precision of the regional distribution was improved greatly with the application of microtechniques (24,30,31).

The availability of antibodies to various enzymes related to neurotransmitter synthesis (DBH, DOPA decarboxylase, tryptophan hydroxylase) allowed the immunocytochemical (16,18) identification of specific neurons and their axons including 5-HT neurons (21,27). The introduction of antibodies to serotonin by Steinbusch et al. (33) prompted a number of recent studies of the 5-HT system (7,19,23). Antiserotonin antibodies used in conjunction with the PAP technique of Sternberger (34) can reveal a more precise localization of 5-HT both at the light and electron microscopic levels. An advantage of the method is that no exogenous 5-HT (cold or radioactive) is needed for detection, a in the FIF technique to enhance definition, or in radioautography to be uptaken by specific cells. In fact, the immunocytochemical technique allows the identification of endogenous 5-HT even without pharmacological pretreatment. In the present chapter some recent findings on the serotoninergic neurons of the raphe and their projections are presented and discussed in relation to the participation of the serotoninergic system in various CNS functions.

MATERIALS AND METHODS

General

Adult monkeys *(Macaca fascicularis)* were used for this study. The animals were pretreated with a MAO inhibitor, Pargyline (75 mg/kg), and a dose of L-tryptophan (100 mg/kg) given 120 min and 30 min before sacrifice, respectively. The monkeys were perfused under deep barbiturate narcosis, after a brief rinse with saline solution, with a mixture of 4% pure formaldehyde and 0.25% glutaraldehyde in 0.12 M phosphate buffer, at a pH of 7.4 for 30 min. The excised brain and spinal cord, devoid of meninges, were kept in the same fixative for 2 hr, at 4°C, and then cut in an Oxford vibratome at 30 μm. A protocol for preembedding immunocytochemical staining with the peroxidase-antiperoxidase (PAP) complex was adapted from Sternberger (34) and Pickel (26). Sections were treated with 0.2% Triton X-100 during 15–30 min before incubation with the primary antibody for 12 to 14 hr in dilutions of 1:500, 1:800, 1:1,000, and 1:2,000. Development of the reaction was performed with diaminobenzidine tetrahydrochloride and hydrogen peroxide during 5 to 6 min under microscopic control. All procedures were carried out at 4°C. Following the PAP technique, the sections were postfixed in 1% osmium tetroxide for 1 hr, treated with uranyl acetate, embedded in Epon-araldite, and flat-mounted between two plastic coverslips. Thus, observation with the light microscope was possible before selecting the block to be cut with the ultramicrotome. Other sections were mounted for light microscopy without osmication. Serial thin sections were mounted on formvar coated slot grids and double stained with uranyl acetate and lead citrate.

Specificity of the Method

Controls for specificity included incubation with absorbed serotonin antisera obtained by addition of either 100 μg of 5-HT, or 0.5 ml of diluted antigen complex to 0.5 ml of diluted antiserum (1:1,000). In some cases removal of the specific antibody was assured by coprecipitating the antigen-antibody complexes with anti-BSA serum, centrifugation for 30 min, and using the supernatant. Additional proofs of specificity were provided by incubation with the higher dilutions of the antibody, which resulted in excellent staining of well-known groups of 5-HT neurons and their ascending and descending projections, lack of labeling of dopaminergic cells (e.g., in the substantia nigra pars compacta) or of noradrenergic neurons, e.g. (in the locus coeruleus) and heavy staining of carcinoid tumor cells.

Antibodies of 5-HT produced in rabbits using 5-HT creatinine sulfate combined with bovine serum albumin (BSA) by employing pure formaldehyde as coupling agent.[1] This complex was reproduced in our laboratories according to the protocol

---

[1] Initial amounts were kindly supplied by Dr. Robert Elde. For further experiments, the antiserum was purchased from Immunonuclear Corp. (Stillwater, Minnesota).

of Ranadive and Sehon (29), to be used in the absorptions of the 5-HT antiserum *(see above).* The absorption spectrum of the complex is illustrated in Fig. 1, which also shows spectra for BSA and 5-HT. Calculations based on the extinction coefficients and absorbances reveal that the final product is a soluble complex in which 38 molecules of the hapten (5-HT) are conjugated with each molecule of BSA.

RESULTS

Light Microscope Observations

Figures 2 through 4 illustrate in serial sections the extensive serotoninergic system of neurons in the brain stem of the monkey. The main nuclei in which 5-HT labeled neurons are found belong to the raphe group: n. raphe dorsalis, n. centralis superior, n. raphe pontis, n. raphe magnus, n. raphe pallidus, and n. raphe obscurus. There are also collections of cells in the pedunculopontine tegmentum that have been considered as lateral extensions of n. centralis superior (Fig. 2, top). The size of the 5-HT neurons ranges between 20 and 35 μm and in many cases they are multipolar or bipolar (Fig. 5, top). Stained cells of n. raphe pallidus and n. raphe obscurus are, as a rule, somewhat smaller than those of rostrally situated nuclei. With the present technique it is possible to follow their dendrites and axons with the light microscope for some distances as in a Golgi-impregnated preparation. It is not unusual to observe the axons emerging from a proximal dendrite.

In addition to the classic serotoninergic groups just described, some labeled neurons, 15 to 25 μm in diameter, are found in the supraoptic region of the hypothalamus, in the area of both the n. paraventricularis, next to a very rich

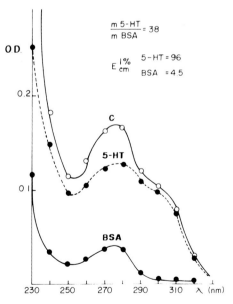

FIG. 1. Ultraviolet absorbtion spectra between 230 and 310 nm for bovine serum albumin (BSA), serotonin (5-HT), and 5-HT-BSA complex (c). Curves (c) and (BSA) were measured. Curve (5-HT) was calculated as the difference between (c) and (BSA). Values for the maximal optical densities in (c) and in (5-HT) are in accord with data in the literature. O.D., Optical density; λ (nm), wavelength. $E_{cm}^{1\%}$: calculated extinction coefficients. The data obtained permit the conclusion that each molecule of BSA binds 38 molecules of 5-HT, as shown in the upper right corner.

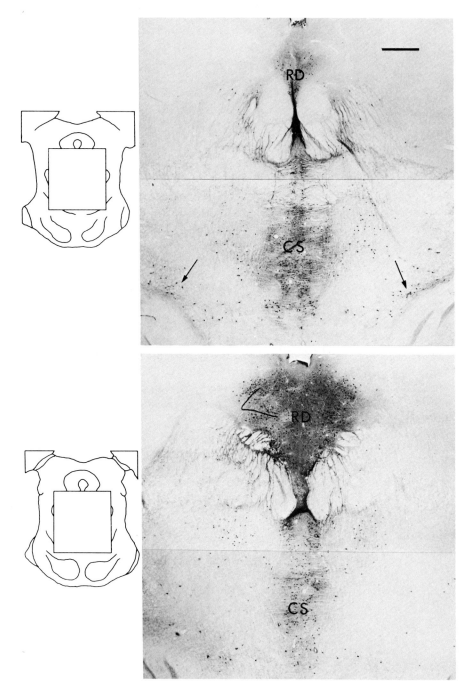

FIG. 2. Sections of monkey brainstem showing the distribution of labeled neurons in n.raphe dorsalis (RD) and n.centralis superior (CS) with its lateral extensions *(arrows)*. Scale **(top)** applies also to Figs. 3 and 4 and is equal to 1 mm. The sketches with framed areas on the **left** of each photograph indicate the level of the section as well as the region covered by the photograph.

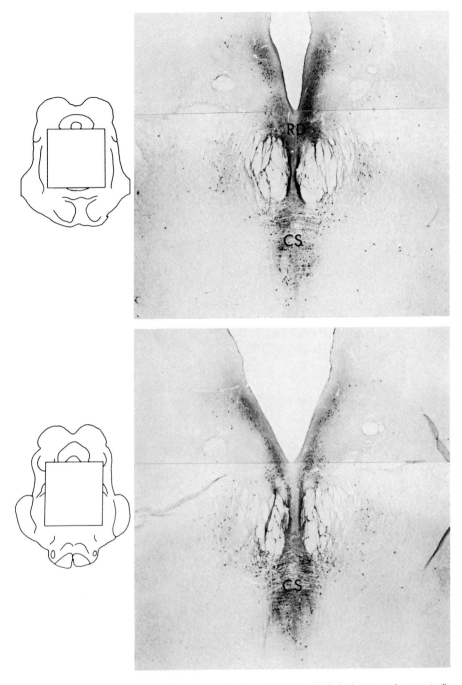

FIG. 3. Sections of monkey brainstem showing the distribution of labeled neurons in n.centralis superior (CS). See legend to Fig. 2 for further details.

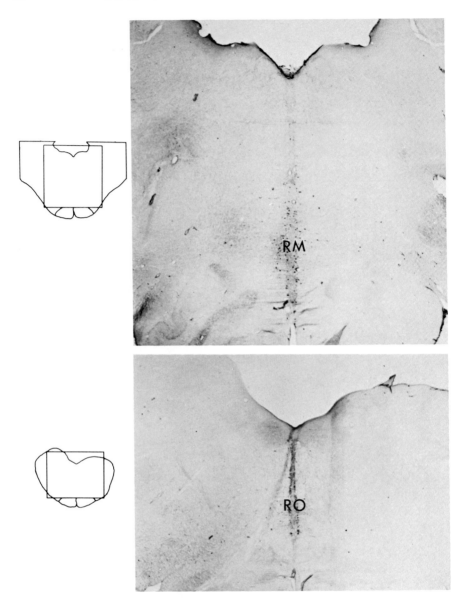

FIG. 4. Sections of monkey brainstem showing the distribution of labeled neurons in n.raphe magnus (RM) and n.raphe obscurus (RO). See legend to Fig. 2 for further details.

capillary plexus, and the n. supraopticus. The proportion of these labeled neurons is only a fraction of the well-known group of "neurosecretory" cells.

The neurons in the raphe complex are surrounded by a rich immunostained fiber plexus running longitudinally on both sides of the midline (Figs. 2 and 3). Although most of the elements are interpreted as labeled axons, it is very possible that many

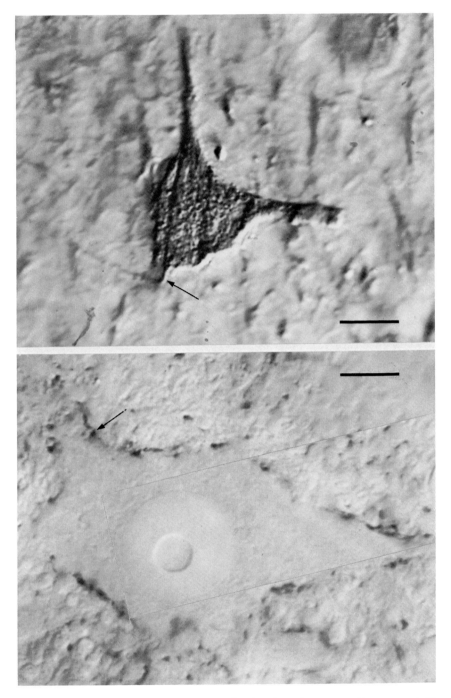

FIG. 5. Top: Labeled neuron of n.raphe dorsalis taken from the same section as seen in Fig. 2, bottom. Proximal regions of the dendrites and emerging axon *(arrow)* are labeled as well. Nomarski optics. Scale: 10 μm. **Bottom:** Numerous axosomatic contacts made by labeled boutons of the type marked by *arrow* on an α-motoneuron in Rexed lamina IX of the lumbar spinal cord. Nomarski optics. Scale: 10 μM.

of them represent sections of dendrites of the same longitudinal orientation.

Plexi of labeled axons are recognized in several forebrain structures namely hippocampus, amygdaloid complex, n. accumbens, septal nuclei (Fig. 6, bottom), caudate nucleus, putamen, globus pallidus and hypothalamus (Fig. 6, top). In the brainstem, some well-stained plexi are found in the substantia nigra, locus coeruleus, and n. interpeduncularis.

The sections of the spinal cord at the cervical, dorsal, and lumbar levels show a dense plexus of immunostained fibers and terminals in Rexed's laminae I, II, VII, VIII, IX, and X. Fibers in the dorsal horn, particularly in the convexity of the substantia gelatinosa Rolandi, are of somewhat thinner caliber than those found in the ventral horn and periependymal central gray. In the ventral horn, a very dense plexus of various caliber fibers, with average diameters of 1 μm, is observed surrounding the motoneurons (Fig. 5, bottom) and forming basket-like complexes around the perikarya and proximal dendrites. A similar configuration can be seen around cells of the lateral septal nuclei (Fig. 6, bottom). Preterminal fibers are fine and beaded and in transverse sections resemble synaptic boutons in contact with perikaryal surfaces (Fig. 5, bottom). In the white matter, positively stained fibers are detected as isolated brown dots in the anterolateral funiculus, or forming loosely packed small fascicles dispersed among unstained fibers. Longitudinally sectioned fibers are seen entering the gray matter. The cells immersed in the serotoninergic plexus are identified as α-motoneurons on the basis of their sizes and shapes. Other neurons of smaller size, possibly γ-motoneurons or Renshaw cells are also observed in close relationship with the stained fibers.

Electron Microscope Observations

Ultrastructural features of the reaction products are notably different in perikarya and dendrites as compared with axon terminals. The label found in somata and dendrites of the raphe region is less abundant and gives the cytoplasm a fine granular appearance. Some of the deposits are in close apposition to microtubules and to membranes of the endoplasmic reticulum (Fig. 7). The axonal profiles, present in the target structures, show densely packed, relatively large, and coarse deposits filling the thin branches and varicosities of preterminal and terminal fibers (Fig. 8). The label is found in synaptic vesicles, surrounding the microtubules, and occasionally on the external mitochondrial membrane. The higher intensity of the immunostain in axon terminals may be the result of a higher concentration of 5-HT in the axons or, less likely, to a lesser transmitter loss during the procedures. In all cases of stained somata, dendrites, axons, or synaptic terminals, the reaction product is strictly confined within the limits of the plasmalemma. No diffusion of the label to neighboring processes has ever been observed.

Specific electron microscopic findings include the presence of labeled and unlabeled dendrites in the neuropil of n. centralis superior (Fig. 7, bottom), which confirmed the existence of nonserotoninergic neurons in the raphe system. The plexi of labeled beaded axons in the n. accumbens, pallidum, caudate, and putamen

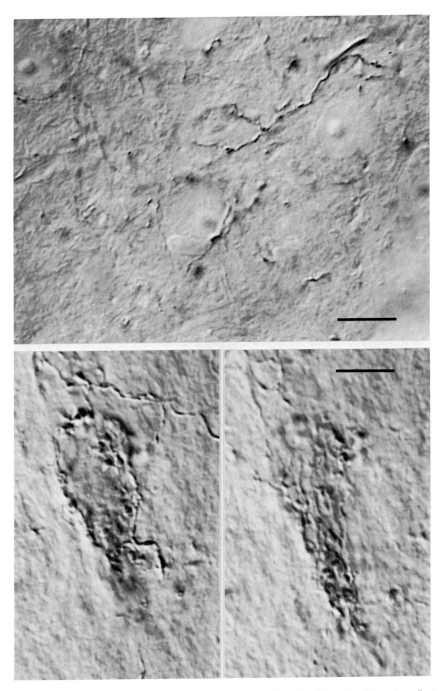

FIG. 6. Labeled terminal fibers in the hypothalamus **(top)** and the lateral septal nucleus **(bottom)**. The latter is shown in two views at different planes of focus revealing a basket-like formation enclosing a pear-shaped soma. Nomarski optics. Scale: 10 μm.

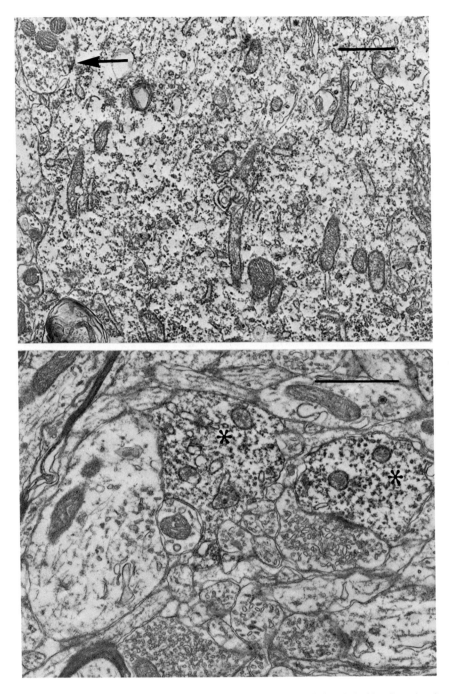

FIG. 7.   Top: Part of a perikaryon from n.centralis superior, heavily labeled with a fine granular material. An axosomatic synapse is formed by an unstained axonal profile at arrow. Scale: 1 μm **Bottom:** Neuropil of the same region showing the coexistence of labeled *(asterisks)* and unlabeled dendritic elements. No labeled axonal profiles were recognized. Scale: 1 μm.

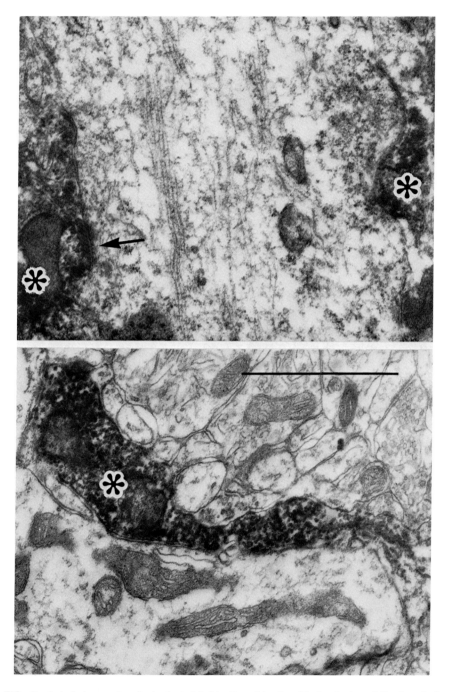

FIG. 8. Labeled axon terminals *(asterisks)* in Rexed lamina IX of spinal cord **(top)** and of caudate nucleus **(bottom)**. An asymmetric synaptic contact is made with the proximal portion of a dendrite at *arrow*. Scale: 1 μM.

correspond well with the light microscopic observations. (Fig. 8, bottom). Moreover, they conform to the axons with thin beaded branches identified in the neostriatum in Golgi material (13), i.e., thin axons of diameters below 1 μm with branches of less than 0.3 μm and varicosities of 0.5 to 1.2 μm in size. Other plexi of similar patterns are also recognized in the locus coeruleus, the substantia nigra, ventral hypothalamic areas, and in the spinal cord. In the latter structure, the ventral horn shows the presence of abundant labeled profiles, identified as of axonal nature on the basis of their ultrastructural features. Many of them are seen forming axosomatic and axodendritic synapses on motoneurons (Fig. 8, top). The contacts belong to the asymmetric type. It is usual to observe two or three such terminals on a transverse section of a primary dendrite. No synapses are seen between labeled profiles and other synaptic vesicle-containing elements.

DISCUSSION

This study demonstrates that an extensive serotoninergic system of neurons can be revealed by immunocytochemistry in the brain stem of macaques with rostral extensions into the hypothalamus. The distribution of these 5-HT neurons in the raphe nuclei is similar to that described in the rat (11), cat (28), and squirrel monkey (20). The different groups known in the literature with the nomenclature B1 to B9 were all found in the macaque, indicating that it is a phylogenetically very stable component of the CNS. The serotoninergic system of the raphe has been postulated to participate in mechanisms of sleep, thermoregulation, endocrine, motor, and sexual functions. It is conceivable that the anatomical basis for such functions, which are basic for species survival, should be very stable through phylogenesis.

The presence of serotoninergic neurons in the hypothalamus has been proposed from the results of fluorescence and radioautographic investigations (4,10,17,22) and found unquestionably in our study with immunocytochemical labeling. Several other lines of evidence support their existence. Thus, surgical isolation of the hypothalamus failed to show a complete disappearance of local 5-HT (9,37). The hypothalamic content of 5-HT in some areas was more reduced after local injections of 5-7 dihydroxytryptamine than when the neurotoxic agent was deposited in the raphe nuclei (35). Apparently, there are some differences as to the exact location of these neurons within the hypothalamus. In previous works in rats, the 5-HT somata were found in the n. dorsomedialis (4,10,17,22), and this was recently confirmed immunocytochemically (15). Our study shows that in macaque, 5-HT neurons appear in the area of the n. paraventricularis and supraopticus. We should like to propose that these neurons migrate from the brain stem and that their ultimate destination may not be the same in different species.

The results presented here show that in the macaque, the serotoninergic system projects numerous fibers caudally and rostrally to several target structures. Descending fibers from the raphe nuclei to the spinal cord were demonstrated by Brodal et al. (8) in the cat by retrograde degeneration studies. In the rat, Bowker et al. (7) identified the cells projecting to the spinal cord by double labeling with retrograde transport of horseradish peroxidase or wheat germ agglutinin and immunocytochemistry with serotonin antibodies. The origin of this pathway was restricted to the raphe neurons of the medulla, pons and periaqueductal gray of the midbrain. Our monkey brain stem sections indeed showed intense staining of these groups and corresponding projections to the spinal cord, with no stained neurons below the medulla or stained fibers in the spinal roots.

Concerning the functional significance of serotoninergic innervation of motoneurons, our observations of labeled axons containing round vesicles and forming asymmetric synapses suggest an excitatory action of 5-HT, which is contrary to earlier neurophysiological findings implying an inhibitory effect (25). More recently, however, a long-lasting facilitatory influence on motoneurons was reported after iontophoretic application of serotonin, and it was postulated that 5-HT acts as a modulator enhancing the effects of other excitatory inputs (38). It should be noted that the phenomenon of modulation, which is characterized by a relatively long-lasting effect, lack of direct drive on the affected neuron, and influence of relatively large territories, is generally explained as a result of local diffusion of the transmitter through the extracellular clefts and slow chemical inactivation, without the need for conventional synapses.

A similar configuration of asymmetric junctions was found in the synapses made by 5-HT labeled axons in the neostriatum. If the above-mentioned considerations applied also to this structure, it would corroborate the excitatory action of serotonin recently demonstrated in the caudate-putamen of the rat (36).

Some methodologic considerations are noteworthy. The specificity of the staining used in this study was firmly demonstrated by the absorptions performed for the controls and by the additional criteria mentioned in Materials and Methods. The immunocytochemical reactions were successful, probably because the formaldehyde fixation acted on the 5-HT giving conjugates with tissue proteins, thus preserving its antigenicity. A rapid fixation at high perfusion pressure was routine in this work to prevent the loss of 5-HT by diffusion, which never occurred when the speed was controlled and processing performed at 4°C. The specificity of the reaction was also clear at the electron microscope level where the label was confined within the limits of the plasmalemma in all cell somata and processes. Since no diffusion of the stain to neighboring elements or extracellular space was observed it was concluded that 5-HT remained trapped in the containing structures. The use of Triton X-100 previous to the incubation clearly contributed to the penetration of the primary antibody and reagents employed in the PAP procedure. If omitted, the stain was poor and limited to the superficial layers of the vibratome sections or blocks. Some degree of ultrastructural alterations was common in the Triton X-100 treated material. However, for the purpose of our study, such disruptions were of minor significance because the majority of cells and processes looked normal and could be easily recognized in the electron micrographs. The appearance and preservation of the light microscope sections were excellent.

SUMMARY

An antibody to 5-HT and Sternberger's PAP technique were applied for immunocytochemical localization of serotoninergic neurons in the central nervous system of Macaca Fascicularis monkeys. In the brain stem, labeled cell somata were found in n. raphe dorsalis, central gray, n. centralis superior, n. raphe pontis, n. raphe magnus, n. raphe pallidus, n. raphe obscurus, and in the tegmentum. Other stained neurons were found in hypothalamic areas. The axons and proximal dendrites were also labeled. Plexi of labeled axons were recognized in the n. accumbens, g. pallidum, n. caudate, putamen, septum, hippocampal complex, amygdala, and hypothalamus. Positively stained fibers were also found in laminae I, II, VII, VIII, IX, and X of the cervical, dorsal, and lumbar spinal cord. Electron microscopic observation of the labeled neurons revealed that the reaction product found in somata and dendrites of the raphe region is finely granular whereas in axons and terminals is coarse and larger. In the synaptic terminals the immunostain is found in synaptic vesicles, microtubules and attached to the outer mitochondrial membrane. In all cases the reaction product is confined within the limits of the plasmalemma with no diffusion to neighboring processes or extracellular space. Configuration of 5-HT synaptic terminals identified with this methodology corresponds to the asymmetric type, postulated as excitatory in different territories.

ACKNOWLEDGMENTS

This work was supported in part by the Clinical Center for Research in Parkinson's and Allied Disorders, N.I.H. Grants NS-11631, and the Consejo Nacional de Investigaciones Científicas y Técnicas.

The authors gratefully acknowledge the participation of Dr. Michael D. Gottlieb and Ms. Gay R. Holstein in the early stages of this work, and the skillful assistance of Minerva Feliciano, Marilyn Ilvento, and Victor Rodríguez.

The PAP complex was generously supplied by Dr. L. Sternberger.

REFERENCES

1. Aghajanian, G. K., and Bloom, F. E. (1966): Localization of tritiated serotonin in rat brain by electron microscopic autoradiography. *J. Pharmacol. Exp. Ther.*, 156:23–30.
2. Amin, A. H., Crawford, T. B. B., and Gaddum, J. H. J. (1954): The distribution of substance P and 5-hydroxytryptamine in central nervous system. *J. Physiol. (Lond.)*, 126:596–618.
3. Azmitia, E. C., and Segal, M. (1978): An autoradiographic analysis of the differential ascending projections of the dorsal and median raphe nuclei in the rat. *J. Comp. Neurol.*, 179:641–668.
4. Beaudet, A., and Descarries, L. (1979): Radioautographic characterization of a serotonin-accumulating nerve cell group in adult rat hypothalamus. *Brain Res.*, 160:231–243.
5. Bloom, F. E., Hoffer, B. J., Siggins, G. R., Barker, J. L., and Nicoli, R. A. (1972): Effects of serotonin on central neurons: microiontophoretic administration. *Fed. Proc.*, 31:97–106.
6. Bogdansky, D. F., Weissbach, H., and Udenfriend, S. (1956): The distribution of serotonin 5-hydroxytryptophan decarboxylase and monoamine oxidase in brain. *J. Neurochem.*, 1:272–278.
7. Bowker, R. M., Westlund, K. N., Steinbusch, H. W. M., and Coulter, J. D. (1980): Origins and terminations of serotonergic projections to the spinal cord. *Neurosci. Abstr.*, 6:101.
8. Brodal, A., Taber, E., and Walberg, P. (1960): The raphe nuclei of the brain stem in the cat. II. Efferent connections. *J. Comp. Neurol.*, 114:239–259.

9. Brownstein, M. J., Palkovits, M., Tappaz, M. L., Saavedra, J. M., and Kizer, J. S. (1976): Effect of surgical isolation of the hypothalamus on its transmitter content. *Brain Res.*, 117:287–295.

10. Chan-Palay, V. (1977): Indolamine neurons and their processes in the normal rat brain and in chronic diet-induced thiamine deficiency demonstrated by uptake of ^{3}H-serotonin. *J. Comp. Neurol.*, 176:467–494.

11. Dahlström, A., and Fuxe, K. (1964): Evidence for the existence of monoamine containing neurons in the central nervous system. I. Demonstration of monoamines in the cell bodies of brain stem neurons. *Acta Physiol. Scand. (Suppl. 237)*, 62:1–55.

12. Descarries, L., Beaudet, A., and Watkins, K. C. (1975): Serotonin nerve terminals in adult rat neocortex. *Brain Res.*, 100:563–588.

13. DiFiglia, M., Pasik, T., and Pasik, P. (1978): A Golgi study of afferent fibers in the neostriatum of monkeys. *Brain Res.*, 152:341–347.

14. Felten, D. L., Laties, A. M., and Carpenter, M. B. (1974): Monoamine-containing cell bodies in the squirrel monkey brain. *Am. J. Anat.*, 139:153–166.

15. Frankfurt, M., Lauder, J. M., and Azmitia, E. C. (1982): The immunocytochemical localization of a serotonin containing cell group in the rat hypothalamus. *Neurosci. Lett. (in press)*.

16. Fuxe, K., Goldstein, M., Hökfelt, T., and Joh, T. H. (1971): Cellular localization of dopamine-β-hydroxylase and phenylethanol-amine-*N*-methyl transferase as revealed by immunocytochemistry. In: *Histochemistry of Nervous Transmission. Progress in Brain Research, Vol. 34*, edited by O. Eränko, pp. 127–138. Elsevier, Amsterdam.

17. Fuxe, K., and Ungerstedt, U. (1968): Histochemical studies on the distribution of catecholamine and 5-hydroxytryptamine after intraventricular injection. *Histochemie*, 13:16–28.

18. Hökfelt, T., Fuxe, K., Goldstein, M., and Joh, T. H. (1973): Immunohistochemical localization of three catecholamine synthetizing enzymes: Aspects on methodology. *Histochemie*, 33:231–254.

19. Hökfelt, T., Ljungdahl, A., Steinbusch, H., Verhofstad, A., Nilsson, G., Brodin, E., Pernow, V., and Goldstein, M. (1978): Immunohistochemical evidence of substance P-like immunoreactivity in some 5-hydroxytryptamine-containing neurons in the rat central nervous system. *Neuroscience*, 3:517–538.

20. Hubbard, J. E., and Di Carlo, V. (1974): Fluorescence histochemistry of monoamine-containing cell bodies in the brain stem of the squirrel monkey *(Saimiri sciureus)*. II. Catecholamine-containing groups. *J. Comp. Neurol.*, 153:369–384.

21. Joh, T. H., Shikimi, T., Pickel, V. M., and Reis, D. J. (1975): Brain tryptophan hydroxylase purification of, production and antibodies to, and cellular and ultrastructural localization in serotoninergic neurons of the rat midbrain. *Proc. Natl. Acad. Sci. USA*, 72:3575–3579.

22. Kent, D. L., and Sladek, J. R. (1978): Histochemical, pharmacological and microspectrofluorometric analysis of new sites of serotonin localization in the rat hypothalamus. *J. Comp. Neurol.*, 180:221–236.

23. Lanerolle, N. C. de, and LaMotte, C. (1980): Light and EM localization of substance P, met-enkephalin and 5-HT in human and monkey spinal cord. *Neurosci. Abstr.*, 6:353.

24. Palkovits, M., Brownstein, M. J., and Saavedra, J. M. (1974): Serotonin content of the brain stem nuclei in the rat. *Brain Res.*, 80:237–249.

25. Phillis, J. W., Tebecis, A. K., and York, D. H. (1968): Depression of spinal motoneurons by noradrenaline, 5-hydroxytryptamine and histamine. *Eur. J. Pharmacol.*, 4:471–475.

26. Pickel, V. M. (1982): Immunocytochemical methods. In: *Neuroanatomical Tract-Tracing Methods*, edited by L. Heimer and M. J. Robards, pp. 483–509. Plenum Publishing, New York.

27. Pickel, V. M., Joh, T. H., and Reis, D. J. (1977): A serotoninergic innervation of noradrenergic neurons in nucleus locus coeruleus: Demonstration by immunocytochemical localization of the transmitter specific enzymes tyrosine and tryptophan hydroxylase. *Brain Res.*, 131:197–214.

28. Poitias, D., and Parent, A. (1978): Atlas of the distribution of monoamine-containing nerve cell bodies in the brain stem of the cat. *J. Comp. Neurol.*, 179:699–718.

29. Ranadive, N. S., and Sehon, A. H. (1967): Antibodies to serotonin. *Can. J. Biochem.*, 45:1701–1710.

30. Saavedra, J. M. (1977): Distribution of serotonin and synthetizing enzymes in discrete areas of the brain. *Fed. Proc.*, 36:2134–2141.

31. Saavedra, J. M., Palkovits, M., Brownstein, M. J., and Axelrod, J. (1974): Serotonin distribution in the nuclei of the rat hypothalamus and preoptic region. *Brain Res.*, 77:157–165.

32. Sladek, J., and Garver, D. L. (1976): Serotonin containing perikarya and pathways in the stump-tailed macaque *(Macaca arctoides)*. *Neurosci. Abstr.*, 2:475.

33. Steinbusch, H. W. N., Verhofstad, A. A. J., and Joosten, H. W. J. (1978): Localization of serotonin in the central nervous system by immunohystochemistry. Description of a specific and sensitive technique and some applications. *Neuroscience*, 3:811–819.
34. Sternberger, L. A. (1979): *Immunocytochemistry*, 2nd ed. Wiley, New York.
35. Van der Kar, L. D., Lorens, S. A., Vodraska, A., Allers, G., Green, M., Van Orden, D. E., and Van Orden, L. S. (1980): III. Effect of selective midbrain and diencephalic 5,7-dihydroxytryptamine lesions on serotonin content in individual preopticohypothalamic nuclei and on serum LH level. *Neuroendocrinology*, 31:309–315.
36. Van der Maelen, C. P., Bonduki, A. C., and Kitai, S. T. (1979): Excitation of caudate-putamen neurons following stimulation of the dorsal raphe nucleus in the rat. *Brain Res.*, 175:356–361.
37. Vermes, I., Molnas, D., and Telegdy, G. (1973): Hypothalamic serotonin content and pituitary-adrenal function following hypothalamic deafferentation. *Acta Physiol. Acad. Sci. Hungar.*, 43:239–245.
38. White, S. R., and Neuman, R. S. (1980): Facilitation of spinal motoneurone excitability by 5-hydroxytryptamine and noradrenalin. *Brain Res.*, 188:119–127.

Neural Transmission, Learning and Memory,
edited by R. Caputto and C. Ajmone Marsan.
Raven Press, New York © 1983.

GABA Receptor Function

G. Toffano

Department of Biochemistry, Fidia Research Laboratories, Abano Terme, Italy

The role of γ-aminobutyric acid (GABA) as a major inhibitory neurotransmitter in the mammalian central nervous system (CNS) is now well documented. Electrophysiological studies provided the most compelling evidence to support a role for GABA as a neurotransmitter. Stimulation of neuronal cells containing GABA results in the hyperpolarisation of postsynaptic cells similar to that produced by exogenous application of GABA. However, mainly in the spinal cord cells, GABA produces a depolarising response, probably because the intracellular chloride concentration in these presynaptic terminals exceeds that present in the extracellular space (for reviews, see 24, 39, 42).

Since GABA-containing neurons are abundant in virtually all regions of mammalian CNS, one might predict that they will influence and will be influenced by most of the other neurotransmitters involved in central neurotransmission. As a consequence, a disturbance of the GABAergic transmission in the CNS plays a role in several human neurological and neuropsychiatric diseases such as Huntington's disease (15), Parkinsonism (26), schizophrenia (41), epilepsy (29), dementia (2), and anxiety (11).

The possibility that a number of these disorders may be treated with agents stimulating the GABAergic neurotransmission prompted great attempts to discover and develop specific GABA-mimetic drugs (22,25,30).

However, drugs, by interfering with neurotransmitter metabolism or receptors, may have a limited therapeutic value or may induce side effects, mainly after chronic use, as a result of a synaptic plasticity. This plasticity is probably centered on the mechanisms that continuously change the responsiveness of postsynaptic receptors where neurotransmitters bind to initiate the biological response.

An important family of drugs that indirectly maximizes GABA receptor function are the benzodiazepines (BDZ), which are widely used for their anxiolitic, anticonvulsant, and muscle relaxant properties and because they produce little or no toxicity (10,11). BDZ facilitate GABAergic transmission at postsynaptic levels by interfering with the modulation mechanism of the system exerted by endogenous ligand(s), possibly mimicking a cotransmitter system (3,9,18,31,40,45). However, the attempt to design new drugs provided with this action requires a better knowledge of the composition and the regulation of the GABA receptor, which appears as a complex structure composed of a variety of independent, but interrelated, sites.

[³H]GABA BINDING AND ENDOGENOUS MODULATORS

An approach to understanding the regulation of those GABA recognition sites associated with GABA receptors and the mechanism of drugs altering the GABAergic system at the postsynaptic level is the measurement of [³H]GABA binding to specific recognition sites on synaptic plasma membranes (13,19,36).

To study the complete spectrum of the regulation of GABA recognition sites, the experiments must be carried out in a Na^+-free medium and with membranes repeatedly frozen, thawed, and washed with buffer after incubation with 0.05% Triton X-100 (14,46,47). This procedure allows the maximal binding capacity of the membrane preparation and unmasks a population of binding sites that, without such a treatment, fails to be expressed (Table 1).

Triton X-100, by extracting components embedded in the fluid mosaic structure of brain membranes, removes from GABA receptor complex also a protein with the capacity to inhibit the binding of [³H]GABA termed GABA-modulin (46,47). GABA-modulin, an uncompetitive inhibitor of high-affinity binding for [³H]GABA, has a molecular weight of about 15,000, is relatively thermostable, digested by trypsin and pronase, GABAese-resistant and ammonium sulfate-precipitable, and does not bind [³H]GABA or [³H]diazepam per se (27).

In addition to GABA-modulin other endogenous components, which can be removed by Triton X-100, interfere with the high-affinity [³H]GABA binding. In this respect, a certain contribution in the regulation of [³H]GABA binding has been attributed to GABA itself (35), a number of small-molecular-weight materials (28,50) and phospholipids, particularly phosphatidylethanolamine (17,21). However, we found (48) that it is unlikely phosphatidylethanolamine polar head that directly competes with endogenous GABA for binding to the protein receptor.

MULTIPLE GABA RECEPTORS

The appearance of two binding sites for [³H]GABA in appropriate experimental condition raises the question of whether they express separate receptors or represent a conformational change of the same receptor.

Using anatomical and biochemical criteria, it was suggested that the low- and high-affinity binding sites for GABA are separate entities (19). An uneven distri-

TABLE 1. *[³H]GABA binding to crude synaptic plasma membrane preparation from rat cerebellum*

Tissue	B_{max1} (pmoles/mg protein)	K_{D1} (nM)	B_{max2} (pmoles/mg protein)	K_{D2} (nM)
Fresh	4.4	300	Not detectable	Not detectable
Frozen + Triton X-100	5.28	130	1.8	20

Membrane preparation and [³H]GABA binding assay were performed as previously described (26).

bution of high- and low-affinity binding sites for GABA was found in different brain areas. The total GABA receptor density is higher in the cerebellum, cerebral cortex, and hypothalamus and relatively lower in the striatum and substantia nigra. However, the density of high affinity GABA binding sites in substantia nigra (SN) is, at least, as great as that measured in other brain areas. As a result, the ratio of density of the high-affinity to the low-affinity binding sites is the highest in SN, where it is approximately 8–10 times higher than in cerebellum or in cerebral cortex.

In addition, GABA binding increases in the SN following denervation of GABA receptor produced by surgical lesion of the striato-nigral descending connections. Scatchard plot analysis revealed that the increase involved exclusively the high affinity component of GABA binding. The B_{max} of high-affinity [^{3}H]GABA binding increased from 1.1 pmole/mg protein (intact side) to 1.75 pmole/mg protein (lesioned side). No significant change in the K_D values was observed. The induced supersensitivity of a population of SN pars reticulata neurons was recently confirmed with an electrophysiological approach in rats after striatal lesions (49). To determine whether the lack of agonist-receptor interaction was responsible for the increase in the number of GABA binding after deafferentation of SN, rats with brain hemi-transection were injected twice daily with 400 ng of muscimol, a GABA agonist, into the lateral ventricle by means of chronically implanted cannules. The intra-ventricular administration of muscimol for 7 days prevented the lesion-induced increase in GABA binding in the deafferented SN and failed to alter the binding in the intact part (Table 2).

From these data one may infer that the two sites represent two independent classes of GABA receptors and that the high affinity component is the most related with GABAergic transmission. This possibility was recently confirmed by Olsen et al. (37) by studying the different sensitivity rate of heat denaturation of the two binding affinity subpopulations.

GABA/BDZ COMPLEX

Further complication in the definition of GABA receptor is provided by the evidence that part of the recognition sites for BDZ are located in the same post-synaptic membranes containing those for GABA. The coexistence of recognition

TABLE 2. [^{3}H]GABA binding in rat substantia nigra 20 days after hemitransection

	Specifically bound [^{3}H]GABA (fmoles/mg protein)	
Treatment	Intact side	Lesioned side
Control	480 ± 75	930 ± 95
Muscimol (400 ng twice daily intraventricularly)	450 ± 85	520 ± 75

Lesions and binding assay were performed as previously described (22).

sites for GABA and BDZ was demonstrated biochemically in membranes either prepared from rat brain (16) or cultured cells (1), and morphologically in GABAergic synapses (33). A functional interaction exists between BDZ and GABA receptors (17,44), although they might reside on separate macromolecules with different physiochemical properties (27).

Specific classes of binding sites for BDZ are present in the brain tissues (for reviews see 5,10,34). Their neuronal localization was shown in biochemical experiments using lesioning techniques, but a presynaptic localization or the presence in nonGABAergic synapses cannot be completely excluded. A good correlation was established between the affinity of several BDZ for the binding sites *in vitro* and their pharmacological potency *in vivo* in tests that predict clinical effects in man, namely inhibition of pentazol convulsions, cat muscle relaxant effect, Geller-anticonflict activity, and others. BDZ binding sites present in liver, kidney membranes, and serum albumin are clearly different from those detected in brain. No pharmacological effects have yet been attributed to peripheral BDZ binding sites (4).

Because of the presence of specific binding sites for BDZ, the presence of endogenous ligand is suspected by analogy with morphine, enkephalins, and opiate receptors. Extracts of brain tissues were fractioned in various ways and tested for their capacity to displace [^{3}H]diazepam from its binding sites. Some of these compounds were isolated and characterized. Among them hypoxanthine, inosine, and nicotinamide have a rather poor affinity to the BDZ receptor (32,43), and it is still unknown whether, in the brain, they reach an appropriate concentration at the receptor sites. β-Carboline-3-carboxylic acid ethyl ester has a high affinity for BDZ receptors and assumes a pharmacological interest although is not a brain constituent, but rather a product formed during tissue extraction (6). The biosynthetic pathways leading to β-carbolines involve tryptophan and tryptamine. It cannot be excluded that low amount of norharman, harman, tetrahydroharman, and 6-hydroxytetrahydronorharman, evidentiated in blood platelets and brain tissue may have a physiological role. Various brain fractions contain inhibitory activity of [^{3}H]diazepam binding susceptible to proteolysis (8,12,18). These peptides and proteins have a molecular weight ranging from 1,500 to 40–70,000. Other less characterized inhibitors seem to be present in the brain (12,23,38). Recently, Massotti et al. (27) have isolated and characterized from rat brain an endogenous competitive inhibitor of [^{3}H]diazepam binding termed DBI that differs from all the previously described ones. This compound has a molecular weight of 1,800–10,000, is thermostable and sensitive to tryptine and pronase digestion, indicating a proteic nature.

Therefore, GABA receptor unit appears constituted by several membrane components coupled into a functional entity that includes the GABA binding sites, the Cl^- ionophore, GABA-modulin, BDZ binding sites, and DBI. All of them are located at postsynaptic level with the exception of DBI, which may residue also presynaptically. On this supramolecular structure it is difficult to predict how a drug can alter GABAergic transmission at postsynaptic level.

MOLECULAR INTERACTION BETWEEN
GABA AND BDZ RECEPTORS

The physiological role played by the different GABA-receptor unit constituents is still unknown. A useful approach for understanding its functioning seems to be the dissection and the reconstitution of the unit, step by step, to study the molecular interaction between the single components (27).

Still unsolved is the question of how BDZ, by stimulating BDZ binding sites, can maximize GABA receptor function. It is possible that BDZ, by regulating membrane fluidity by a mechanism similar to that proposed by Hirata and Axelrod (20), might influence GABA receptor responsiveness. The finding that BDZ increase membrane fluidification and phospholipid methylation in astrocytoma cells (44) prompted us to investigate whether phospholipid methylation is a molecular event involved in the action of BDZ. We found that phospholipid methylation increases both [³H]diazepam and [³H]GABA binding (7). Preincubation of crude synaptic plasma membranes with SAM (*s*-adenosylmethionine) results in a dose-dependent increase of [³H]diazepam binding (Table 3), due to an increase of the apparent $B_{max.}$ In contrast, the increase of [³H]GABA binding is due to the unmasking of a population of binding sites with the characteristics of the high affinity, the effect is antagonised by *s*-adenosylhomocistein. These results, which are awaiting further confirmation, suggest a sort of relationship between membrane fluidity, phospholipid methylation, [³H]diazepam, and [³H]GABA binding. An increased membrane fluidity may enhance the mobility of proteins located in the GABA-BDZ receptor domain and, as a consequence, maximize GABA receptor response.

CONCLUSIONS

GABA receptor unit appears as a supramolecular structure that includes Cl^- channel, GABA recognition sites, GABA-modulin, BDZ receptor sites, and a pu-

TABLE 3. *Effect of phospholipid methylation on*
[³H]diazepam binding

Addition		Specifically bound [³H]diazepam (fmoles/mg protein)
None		381
SAM	1 μM	568 (+49%)
	10 μM	600 (+57%)
	50 μM	725 (+90%)
	100 μM	775 (+103%)

Fresh crude S.P.M. from rat cerebellum were preincubated with or without different amount of SAM for 30 min at 37°C. The reaction was stopped by cooling. After centrifugation, the pellet was resuspended in Tris buffer and [³H]diazepam binding assayed with 4.5 nM[³H]diazepam (19).

tative ligand for the BDZ receptor. These various subunits appear to be necessary for the function of GABA postsynaptic receptor, and reside postsynaptically with the only exception of the putative ligand for BDZ receptors which may be located presynaptically. The physiological role of these constituents and their molecular interaction are still under investigation. It is difficult on this unit to predict how a drug alters GABAergic transmission at a postsynaptic level, since an effect on each of these constituents may result in an altered GABA receptor response. The possibility that BDZ maximize GABA receptor responses by affecting membrane properties has to be evaluated.

However, in this model, worthy of attention is the possibility of devising new psychotropic drugs acting on the modulatory system without affecting directly the binding sites. These drugs may not obstruct synaptic function and, as a consequence, fail to trigger those compensatory mechanisms that lead to side effects.

REFERENCES

1. Baraldi, M., Guidotti, A., Schwartz, J. P., and Costa, E. (1979): GABA receptors in clonal cell lines: A model for study of benzodiazepine action at molecular level. *Science*, 205:821–823.
2. Bird, E. D. (1977): In: *Neurotransmission and Disturbed Behavior*, edited by H. M. Van Praag and J. Bruinvels, pp. 140–149. Bohn, Scheltema and Holkema, Utrecht.
3. Braestrup, C., and Nielsen, M. (1980): Searching for endogenous benzodiazepine receptor ligands. *TIPS*, 1:424–427.
4. Braestrup, C., Nielsen, M., and Olsen, C. E. (1980): Urinary and brain β-carboline-3-carboxylates as potent inhibitors of brain benzodiazepine receptors. *Proc. Natl. Acad. Sci. USA*, 77:2288–2292.
5. Braestrup, C., and Squires, R. F. (1977): Specific benzodiazepine receptors in rat brain characterized by high affinity [^{3}H]diazepam binding. *Proc. Natl. Acad. Sci. USA*, 74:3805–3808.
6. Braestrup, C., and Squires, R. F. (1978): Brain specific benzodiazepine receptors. *Br. J. Psychiatry*, 133:249–260.
7. Calderini, G., Battistella, A., Di Perri, B., Balzano, M., Aldinio, C., and Toffano, G. (1981): Modification of ^{3}H-GABA and ^{3}H-diazepam binding sites in different rat brain areas at different ages. In: *Second Capo Boi Conference on Neuroscience*, June 7–10, Capo Boi (Cagliari), Abstr. 10.
8. Colello, G. D., Hockenbery, D. M., Basmann, H. M., Fuchs, S., and Folkers, K. (1978): Competitive inhibition of benzodiazepine binding by fractions from porcine brain. *Proc. Natl. Acad. Sci. USA*, 75:6319–6323.
9. Costa, E. (1979): The role of gamma-aminobutyric acid in the action of 1,4-benzodiazepines. *TIPS*, 1:41–44.
10. Costa, E., and Guidotti, A. (1979): Molecular mechanisms in the receptor actions of benzodiazepines. *Annu. Rev. Pharmacol. Toxicol.*, 19:531–545.
11. Costa, E., Guidotti, A., and Toffano, G. (1978): Molecular mechanisms mediating the action of diazepam on GABA receptors. *Br. J. Psychiatry*, 133:239–248.
12. Davis, L. G., and Cohen, R. K. (1980): Identification of an endogenous peptide-ligand for the benzodiazepine receptor. *Biochem. Biophys. Res. Commun.*, 92:141–148.
13. Enna, S. J., and Snyder, S. H. (1975): Properties of gamma-aminobutyric acid (GABA) receptor binding in rat brain synaptic membrane fractions. *Brain Res.*, 100:81–86.
14. Enna, S. J., and Snyder, S. H. (1977): Influence of ions, enzymes and detergents on gamma-aminobutyric acid receptor binding in synaptic membranes of rat brain. *Mol. Pharmacol.*, 13:442–453.
15. Enna, S. J., Stern, L. Z., Wastek, G. J., and Yamamura, H. I. (1977): Neurobiology and pharmacology of Huntington's disease. *Life Sci.*, 20:205–211.
16. Gavish, M., and Snyder, S. H. (1980): Benzodiazepine recognition sites on GABA receptors. *Nature*, 287:651–652.

17. Giambalvo, G. T., and Rosenberg, P. (1976): The effects of phospholipases and proteases on the binding of gamma-aminobutyric acid to junctional complexes of rat cerebellum. *Biochim. Biophys. Acta*, 436:741–756.

18. Guidotti, A., Gale, K., Suria, A., and Toffano, G. (1979): Biochemical evidence for two classes of GABA receptors in rat brain. *Brain Res.*, 172:566–577.

19. Guidotti, A., Toffano, G., and Costa, E. (1978): An endogenous protein modulates the affinity of GABA and benzodiazepine receptors in rat brain. *Nature*, 257:553–555.

20. Hirata, F., and Axelrod, J. (1980): Phospholipid methylation and biological signal transmission. *Science*, 209:1082–1090.

21. Johnston, G. A. R., Allen, R. D., Kennedy, S. M. E., and Twitchin, B. (1979): Systematic study of GABA analogues of restricted conformation. In: *GABA-Neurotransmitter*, edited by P. Kroskgaard-Larsen, J. Schell-Kruger and H. Kofod, pp. 149–164. Academic Press, New York.

22. Johnston, G. A. R., and Kennedy, S. M. E. (1978): GABA receptors and phospholipids. In: *Amino Acids as Chemical Transmitters*, edited by F. Fonnum, pp. 507–516. Plenum Press, New York.

23. Karobath, M., Speck, G., and Schönbeck, G. (1978): Evidence for an endogenous factor interfering with ³H-diazepam binding to rat brain membranes. *Eur. J. Pharmacol.*, 49:323–326.

24. Kroskgaard-Larsen, P., Honore, T., and Thyssen, K. (1979): GABA receptor agonists: Design and structure-activity studies. In: *GABA-Neurotransmitter*, edited by P. Kroskgaard-Larsen, J. Schell-Kruger and H. Hofod, pp. 201–216. Academic Press, New York.

25. Kroskgaard-Larsen, P., Schell-Kruger, J., and Kodof, H. (eds.) (1979): *GABA-Neurotransmitter*. Academic Press, New York.

26. Lloyd, K. G., Möhler, H., Heitz, P., and Bartholini, G. (1975): Distribution of choline acetyltransferase and glutamate decarboxylase within the substantia nigra and in other brain regions from control and parkinsonian patients. *J. Neurochem.*, 25:789–795.

27. Massotti, M., Guidotti, A., and Costa, E. (1981): Characterization of benzodiazepine and gammaaminobutyric recognition sites and their endogenous modulators. *J. Neurosci.*, 1:409–418.

28. Mazzari, S., Leon, A., Massotti, M., Guidotti, A., and Costa, E. (1980): Assaying GABAmodulin activity in brain extracts: Resolution of inherent difficulties. In: *Psychopharmacology and Biochemistry of Neurotransmitter Receptors*, edited by R. W. Olsen and H. I. Yamamura, pp. 607–615. Elsevier-North Holland, Amsterdam.

29. Meldrum, B. S. (1975): Epilepsy and gamma-aminobutyric acid mediated inhibition. *Int. Rev. Neurobiol.*, 17:1–36.

30. Metcalf, B. W., Jung, M. J., Lippett, B., Casara, P., Bohlen, P., and Schechter, P. (1979): Gamma-acetylenic GABA and gamma-vinyl GABA—two enzyme-activated irreversible inhibitors of GABA aminotransferase. In: *GABA-Neurotransmitter*, edited by P. Kroskgaard-Larsen, J. Schell-Kruger, and H. Kofod, pp. 236–246. Academic Press, New York.

31. Möhler, H. (1981): Benzodiazepine receptors: Are there endogenous ligands in the brain? *TIPS*, 2:116–119.

32. Möhler, H., and Okada, T. (1978): Biochemical identification of the site of action of benzodiazepines in human brain by ³H-diazepam binding. *Life Sci.*, 22:985–996.

33. Möhler, H., Polc, P., Cumin, R., Pieri, L., and Kettler, R. (1979): Nicotinamide is a brain constituent with benzodiazepine-like actions. *Nature*, 278:563–565.

34. Möhler, H., Wu, J. Y., and Richards, J. G. (1981): Benzodiazepine receptors: Autoradiographical and immunocytochemical evidence for their localization in regions of GABAergic synaptic contacts. In: *Advances in Biochemical Psychopharmacology. Vol. 26: GABA and Benzodiazepine Receptors*, edited by E. Costa, G. Di Chiara, and G. L. Gessa, pp. 139–146. Raven Press, New York.

35. Napias, C., Bergman, M. O., Van Ness, P. C., Greenlee, D. V., and Olsen, R. W. (1980): GABA binding in mammalian brain: Inhibition by endogenous GABA. *Life Sci.*, 27:1001–1011.

36. Olsen, R. W., Bergman, M. O., Van Ness, P. C., Lummis, S. C., Watkins, A. E., Napias, C., and Greenlee, D. V. (1981): Gamma-aminobutyric acid receptor binding in mammalian brain. Heterogeneity of binding sites. *Mol. Pharmacol.*, 19:217–227.

37. Olsen, R. W., Ticku, M. K., Van Ness, P. C., and Greenlee, D. (1978): Effects of drugs on gamma aminobutyric acids receptors, uptake, release, and synthesis *in vitro. Brain Res.*, 139:277–294.

38. Paul, S., Marangos, P., Brownstein, M., and Skolnick, P. (1980): Demonstration and characterization of an endogenous inhibitor of GABA-enhanced [³H]diazepam binding from bovine cerebral cortex. In: *Advances in Biochemical Psychopharmacology. Vol. 26: GABA and Benzodiazepine*

Receptors, edited by E. Costa, G. Di Chiara, and G. Gessa, pp. 103–110. Raven Press, New York.

39. Pepeu, G., Kuhar, M. S., and Enna, S. J. (eds) (1980): *Receptors for Neurotransmitters and Peptide Hormones.* Raven Press, New York.
40. Poddar, M. K., Urquhart, D., and Sinha, A. K. (1980): Diazepam binding in brain after sleep and wakefulness. *Brain Res.*, 193:519–528.
41. Roberts, E. (1972): A hypothesis suggesting that there is a defect in the GABA system in schizophrenia. *Neurosci. Res. Progr. Bull.*, 10:468–480.
42. Roberts, E., Chase, T. N., and Tower, D. B. (eds) (1976): *GABA in the Nervous System Function*, Raven Press, New York.
43. Skolnick, P., Syapin, P. J., Paugh, B. A., Moncada, V., Marangos, P. J., and Paul, S. M. (1979): Inosine, an endogenous ligand of the brain benzodiazepine receptor, antagonizes pentylenetetrazole-evoked seizures. *Proc. Natl. Acad. Sci. USA*, 76:1515–1518.
44. Strittmatter, W. J., Hirata, F., Axelrod, J., Mallorga, P., Tallman, J. F., and Henneberry, R. C. (1979): Benzodiazepines and β-adrenergic receptor ligands independently stimulate phospholipid methylation. *Nature*, 282:857–859.
45. Tallman, J. F., Thomas, J. W., and Gallager, D. W. (1978): GABAergic modulation of benzodiazepine binding site sensitivity. *Nature*, 274:383–386.
46. Toffano, G., Aldinio, C., Balzano, M., Leon, A., and Savoini, G. (1981): Regulation of GABA receptor binding to synaptic plasma membrane of rat cerebral cortex: The role of endogenous phospholipids. *Brain Res.*, 222:95–102.
47. Toffano, G., Guidotti, A., and Costa, E. (1978): Purification of an endogenous protein inhibitor of the high affinity binding of gamma-aminobutyric acid to synaptic membranes of rat brain. *Proc. Natl. Acad. Sci. USA*, 75:4024–4028.
48. Toffano, G., Leon, A., Massotti, M., Guidotti, A., and Costa, E. (1980): GABA-modulin: A regulatory protein for GABA receptors. In: *Receptors for Neurotransmitters and Peptide Hormones*, edited by G. Pepeu, M. J. Kuhar, and S. J. Enna, pp. 133–142. Raven Press, New York.
49. Waszczak, B. L., Hume, C., and Walters, J. R. (1981): Supersensitivity of substantia nigra pars reticulata neurons to GABAergic drugs after striatal lesions. *Life Sci.*, 28:2411–2420.
50. Yoneda, Y., and Kuriyama, K. (1980): Presence of a low molecular weight endogenous inhibitor of ^{3}H-muscimol binding in synaptic membranes. *Nature*, 285:670–673.

Neural Transmission, Learning and Memory,
edited by R. Caputto and C. Ajmone Marsan.
Raven Press, New York © 1983.

Studies of the Isolated γ-Aminobutyric Acid Receptor-Like Constituent of Brain: Interaction with Benzodiazepines

A. Arce, S. C. Kivatinitz, D. M. Beltramo, and R. Caputto

Departmento de Química Biológica, Facultad de Ciencias Químicas, Universidad Nacional de Córdoba, Córdoba, República Argentina

There is evidence that γ-aminobutyric acid (GABA) is a major inhibitory neurotransmitter in both the invertebrate and vertebrate central nervous system (CNS); early studies on the GABA-receptor interaction were done with electrophysiological methods (16). The increase in Cl^- conductance as a function of GABA concentration was studied in several invertebrate preparations with the conclusion that two GABA molecules would be required for receptor activation at the neuromuscular junction of the crayfish (25), and three or four GABA molecules seemed to be required at the receptor site on locust muscle (5).

GABA receptors are probably situated at the outer surface of neuronal plasma membrane since neither in cortical neurons nor in Mauthner cells intracellular injection of GABA has any significant inhibitory action (16). To confirm this, sodium-independent postsynaptic binding has been demonstrated (31,34).

Washing, freezing, or detergent treatment of membrane preparations has been employed to remove endogenous GABA (12) or an endogenous proteic inhibitor of GABA binding (28). Using these methods a rather complex kinetic of GABA binding to membrane sites was demonstrated; Scatchard plots and Hill's coefficients analysis of the GABA saturation curves indicated the existence of one high-affinity component ($GABA_2$ type) and another with low-affinity ($GABA_1$ type) for GABA binding (8,13). However, a more complex situation was described by Winkler et al. (30) who showed at least four inflection points in his saturation curves, indicating the existence of several GABA interacting sites in brain membranes.

With pharmacological criterium, two GABA receptors $GABA_a$ and $GABA_b$ receptors have been described (15), baclofen was bound to $GABA_b$ receptor but not to $GABA_a$ receptor; in addition, bicuculline was bound to $GABA_a$ receptor but not to $GABA_b$ receptor. The existence of two different types of GABA receptors also emerged from the existence of different $GABA_1/GABA_2$ receptor ratios in different brain regions and because only the high-affinity site is regulated by an endogenous inhibitor (13). There are also presynaptic GABA receptors pharmacologically iden-

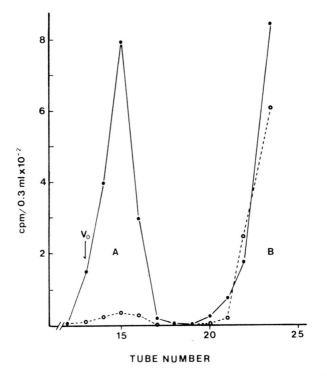

FIG. 1. Typical elution profiles of [³H]flunitrazepam-receptor complex (peak A) and free [³H]flunitrazepam (peak B) in a Sephadex G-25-150 column in the absence (●———●) or in the presence (○–––○) of 5 mM diazepam.

tical to postsynaptic GABA receptors (4); these presynaptic receptors, when activated by GABA agonist, inhibited GABA release.

Another interesting point is that drugs conformationally unrelated to GABA, as benzodiazepines (7,26) and barbiturates (17), showed GABA-enhancing actions. Electrophysiological studies showed that benzodiazepine effects could occur at least in part through an interaction with GABA enhancing the GABAergic transmission through an increase Cl⁻ influx at the postsynaptic junction (24); however, there was not a clear understanding of the mechanism at the molecular level.

Benzodiazepine binding to brain membrane sites can be modified by GABA and GABA agonists *in vivo* and *in vitro* (3,21); thus GABA and muscimol enhance the affinity of benzodiazepine receptors for their ligand (14,27,29) whereas bicuculline antagonizes this effect.

Binding sites for [³H]diazepam in peripheral tissues such as lung, liver and kidney have been described (3). They were different from the central ones because they have 5–30 times lower affinity and they exhibit a different specificity profile. In addition, two subpopulations of benzodiazepine receptors were found, one with high-affinity and another with low-affinity binding in brain membranes (32). Another study suggesting the existence of GABA-independent benzodiazepine receptors was done using quinoline derivatives that dissociated anticonflict from anticonvulsive properties of drugs acting on benzodiazepine receptors (18).

High affinity photolabelling with [³H]flunitrazepam of a specific protein of brain membranes was obtained, and this irreversible labelling had pharmacological properties similar to the reversible benzodiazepine receptor binding (20). Using similar methods a molecular heterogeneity was found in benzodiazepine receptor proteins (23). Several attempts of purification of GABA and benzodiazepine receptors were carried out but no reasonable grade of homogeneity was obtained (2,6,9,10,11,22,33).

Several compounds as inosine, hypoxanthine, nicotinamide, tromboxane A_2 and β-carbolines are proposed as putative endogenous ligands of the brain benzodiazepine receptor; however, there is no strong evidence supporting the existence of a native ligand of benzodiazepines. (For review see ref. 19).

THE ISOLATED GABA RECEPTOR-LIKE PEPTIDE

We have solubilized and purified a lipophilic peptide, a constituent of bovine brain, that was chromatographically and electrophoretically homogeneous, with molecular weight of 11,000 (1). The peptide nature is indicated by staining with ninhydrin of the chromatographic band or with Coomassie Blue of the SDS-polyacrylamide electrophoresis band, and because the binding activity was lost by the treatment with proteases. The protein was determined by the biuret method.

The kinetics of the specific GABA binding are complex and show four interacting sites. The values for the dissociation constants were: K_{D1} = 15 nM, K_{D2} = 92 nM, K_{D3} = 112 nM and K_{D4} = 0.66 mM. Those for maximal bindings were: 1×10^{-4}, 5×10^{-4}, 1×10^{-3} and 3 moles of bound GABA per mole of peptide, respectively.

Several compounds pharmacologically related to GABA show the capacity to displace [³H]GABA at the K_{D1} site; the IC_{50} values were, for GABA 99 nM, for muscimol 3 nM, for imidaloze acetate 720 nM, and for bicuculline more than 500,000 nM. In addition, muscimol displaced approximately 80% the bound GABA at the four sites when added at the same GABA concentrations assayed.

INTERACTION WITH BENZODIAZEPINES

We have evidence that the GABA receptor-like peptide also binds [³H]flunitrazepam reversibly and, if exposed to ultraviolet light, irreversibly. Further, the irreversible binding is enhanced in the presence of GABAergic agonist.

Binding and Photolabelling Assays

The incubation system contained, in a final volume of 0.25 ml, [³H]flunitrazepam (specific radioactivity, 84.8 Ci/mmole) at concentrations ranging from 0.4 to 200 nM, 50 μg for receptor peptide, and 50 nM Tris-citrate buffer, pH 7.1. (a) For the binding assay, the mixture was incubated at 0°C for 20 min; (b) For the photolabelling assay, the mixture was incubated at 0°C for various periods of time, ac-

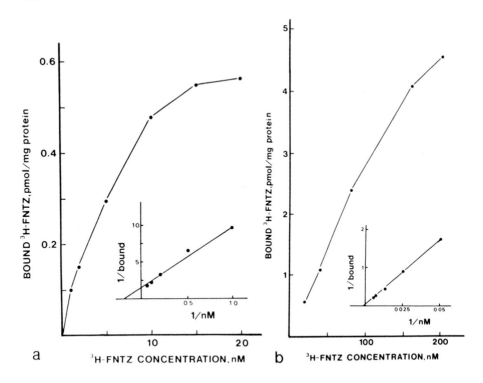

FIG. 2. Saturation curves of the specific [³H]flunitrazepam binding to the receptor peptide. **a:** The high-affinity site; **b:** The low-affinity site; [³H]flunitrazepam binding up to 20 nM [³H]flunitrazepam concentration is shown in the high-affinity site. The experiment was repeated once with almost identical results. The conditions were as indicated in text. In the Lineweaver-Burk plot the regression line at each site drawn through the experimental points was computer-fitted. The correlation coefficient for both sites was about 0.95.

cording to Möhler et al. (20). To separate the [³H]flunitrazepam-receptor complex from free [³H]flunitrazepam, after incubation for binding or photolabelling, the mixture was passed through a Sephadex G-25-150 column (0.8 × 24 cm) at a flux of 1.5 ml/min (Fig. 1). All operations were carried out between 0° and 4°C. The eluate was collected in 0.3-ml fractions and the radioactivities determined. Controls for zero incubation time and incubations in the presence of 5 mM diazepam were run to discount the nondisplaced [³H]flunitrazepam. Determinations were done in triplicate, the average deviations being less than 10%.

The kinetics studied of the [³H]flunitrazepam reversible binding (Fig. 2) showed two interacting sites, $K_{D1} = 5.1$ nM, which is in the same range of the $K_D = 1$ nM determined in brain membranes (19,33), and $K_{D2} = 3.3$ μM. The maximal bindings indicated in moles of bound [³H]flunitrazepam per mole of peptide were: $B_{max\ 1} = 6.6 \times 10^{-6}$, and $B_{max2} = 9.8 \times 10^{-4}$. We cannot discard the existence

TABLE 1. *Effect of GABA and related drugs on the [³H]flunitrazepam photolabelling of the GABA receptor-like peptide*

Additions	cpm of specifically incorporated [³H]FNTZ
None	5,208
GABA (4 μM)	9,010
Muscimol (15 nM)	7,405
Bicuculline (6 μM)	5,580

The peptide (50 μg) was incubated with [³H]flunitrazepam (3 nM) and irradiated with ultraviolet light during 1 hr, in the absence or presence of GABA, muscimol, or bicuculline.

of low-affinity and consequently very dissociable sites because the Sephadex column could not be an appropriate method for the measurement of these sites. However, when the photolabelling is used, the maximal incorporation of [³H]flunitrazepam was of 2 moles per mole of peptide. This value can be compared with the 3 moles of GABA bound per mole of peptide, at the K_{D4} site. It could be possible that the several interacting sites for GABA and flunitrazepam are expressions of different aggregations of a single primary structure.

The experimental observation of increase in [³H]flunitrazepam photolabelling induced by GABA and GABAergic compounds (Table 1) is compatible with the identity of flunitrazepam receptor with GABA receptor. This increase of [³H]flunitrazepam incorporation has pharmacological properties similar to reversible benzodiazepine binding and so it may be explained by GABAergic enhancement of [³H]flunitrazepam binding. Bicuculline did not affect the [³H]flunitrazepam labelling. This result is in agreement with the IC_{50} value of this GABA antagonist to displace GABA from the isolated peptide (1). Enhancement of [³H]flunitrazepam binding by GABA was observed in detergent-solubilized preparations from brain membranes, which contain benzodiazepines and GABA receptor sites; it was found that GABA and GABAergic compounds enhanced the benzodiazepine binding and that bicuculline did not affect it. Similar observations were reported with a preparation purified by affinity chromatography which contain GABA and benzodiazepine sites (10). However, there was no evidence that the preparation was homogeneous.

ACKNOWLEDGMENTS

This work was supported by grants from the Consejo Nacional de Investigaciones Científicas y Técnicas and the Secretaría de Estado de Ciencia y Tecnología, Argentina.

REFERENCES

1. Arce, A., Beltramo, D. M., Kivatinitz, S. C., and Caputto, R. (1981): Purification of a gamma-aminobutyric acid receptor-like constituent of bovine brain. *FEBS Lett.*, 127:149–153.
2. Asano, T., and Ogasawara, N. (1980): Solubilization of gamma-aminobutyric acid receptor from rat brain. *Life Sci.*, 26:1131–1137.

3. Braestrup, C., and Squires, R. F. (1977): Specific benzodiazepine receptors in brain characterized by high affinity ³H-diazepam binding. *Proc. Natl. Acad. Sci. USA*, 74:3805–3809.
4. Brennan, M. J. W., Cantrill, R. C., Oldfield, M., and Kroskgaard-Larsen, P. (1981): Inhibition of gamma-aminobutyric acid release by gamma-aminobutyric agonist drugs. *Mol. Pharmacol.*, 19:27–30.
5. Brookes, N., and Werman, R. (1980): Discrete states of responsiveness of a locust muscle gamma-aminobutyric acid receptor: The influence of extracellular ion concentrations. *Neuroscience*, 5:1669–1680.
6. Chude, O. (1979): Solubilization and partial purification of the GABA receptor from mouse brain and a binding assay for the solubilized receptor. *J. Neurochem.*, 33:621–629.
7. Costa, E., Guidotti, A., Mao, C., and Suria, A. (1975): New concepts on the mechanism of action of benzodiazepines. *Life Sci.*, 17:167–186.
8. Enna, S. J., and Snyder, S. H. (1977): Influence of ions, enzymes and detergents on gamma-aminobutyric acid receptor binding in synaptic membranes of rat. *Mol. Pharmacol.*, 13:442–453.
9. Fiszer de Plazas, S., and De Robertis, E. (1975): Isolation of hidrophobic proteins binding amino acids: Gamma-aminobutyric acid binding in the rat cerebral cortex. *J. Neurochem.*, 25:547–553.
10. Gavish, M., and Snyder, S. H. (1981): Gamma-aminobutyric acid and benzodiazepine receptors; Copurification and characterization. *Proc. Natl. Acad. Sci. USA*, 78:1939–1942.
11. Greenlee, D. V., and Olsen, R. M. (1979): Solubilization of gamma-aminobutyric acid receptor protein from mammalian brain. *Biochem. Biophys. Res. Commun.*, 88:380–387.
12. Greenlee, D. V., Van Ness, R. C., and Olsen, R. W. (1978): Endogenous inhibitor of GABA binding in mammalian brain. *Life Sci.*, 22:1653–1662.
13. Guidotti, A., Gale, K., Suria, A., and Toffano, G. (1979): Biochemical evidence for two classes of GABA receptors in rat brain. *Brain Res.*, 172:566–571.
14. Guidotti, A., Toffano, G., and Costa, E. (1978): An endogenous protein modulates the affinity of GABA and benzodiazepine receptors in rat brain. *Nature*, 275:553–555.
15. Hill, D. R., and Bowery, N. G. (1981): ³H-baclofen and ³H-GABA bind to bicuculline-insensitive GABAᵦ sites in rat brain. *Nature*, 290:149–152.
16. Krnjevic, K. (1976): Inhibitory action of GABA and GABA-mimetics on vertebrate neurons. In: *GABA in nervous system function*, edited by E. Roberts, T. N. Chase, and D. B. Tower, pp. 269–281. Raven Press, New York.
17. Leeb-Lundberg, F., Snowman, A., and Olsen, R. (1980): Barbiturate receptor sites are coupled to benzodiazepine receptors. *Proc. Natl. Acad. Sci. USA*, 77:7468–7472.
18. Le Fur, G., Mizoule, J., Bugevin, M. C., Ferris, O., Heaulme, M., Gauthier, A., Guérémy, C., and Uzan, A. (1981): Multiple benzodiazepine receptors: evidence of a dissociation between anticonflict and anticonvulsant properties by PK 8165 and PK 9084 (two quinoline derivatives). *Life Sci.*, 28:1439–1448.
19. Möhler, H. (1981): Benzodiazepine receptors: Are there endogenous ligands in the brain? *Trends Pharmacol. Sci.*, 2:116–118.
20. Möhler, H., Battersby, M. K., and Richards, J. G. (1980): Benzodiazepine receptor protein identified and visualized in brain tissue by photoaffinity label. *Proc. Natl. Acad. Sci. USA*, 77:1666–1670.
21. Möhler, H., and Okada, T. (1977): Benzodiazepine receptor: Demonstration in the central nervous system. *Science*, 198:849–851.
22. Peck, E. J., Schaeffer, J. M., and Clark, H. J. (1976): In presuit of the GABA receptor. In: *GABA in Nervous System Function*, edited by E. Roberts, T. N. Chase, and D. B. Tower, pp. 319–336. Raven Press, New York.
23. Sieghart, W., and Karobath, M. (1980): Molecular heterogeneity of benzodiazepine receptors. *Nature*, 286:285–287.
24. Speth, R. C., Johnson, R. M., Regan, J., Reisine, T., Yashi, K., Bresolin, N., Roeske, R., and Yamamura, H. I. (1980): The benzodiazepine receptor of mammalian brain. *Fed. Proc.*, 39:3032–3038.
25. Takeuchi, A. (1976): Studies of inhibitory effects of GABA in vertebrate nervous systems. In: *GABA in Nervous System Function*, edited by E. Roberts, T. N. Chase, and D. B. Tower, pp. 255–267. Raven Press, New York.
26. Tallman, J. F., Steven, M. P., Skolnick, P., and Gallager, D. W. (1980): Receptors for the age of anxiety: Pharmacology of the benzodiazepine. *Science*, 207:274–281.
27. Tallman, J. F., Thomas, J. W., and Gallager, D. W. (1978): GABAergic modulation of benzodiazepine binding site sensitivity. *Nature*, 274:383–385.

28. Toffano, G., Guidotti, A., and Costa, E. (1978): Purification of an endogenous protein inhibitor of the high affinity binding of gamma-aminobutyric acid to synaptic membranes of rat brain. *Proc. Natl. Acad. Sci. USA*, 75:4024–4028.

29. Wastek, G. J., Speth, R. C., Reisine, T. D., and Yamamura, H. I. (1978): The effect of gamma-aminobutyric acid on ^{3}H-flunitrazepam binding in rat brain. *Eur. J. Pharmacol.*, 50:445–447.

30. Winkler, M. H., Nicklas, W. J., and Berl, S. (1980): The complex binding of gamma-aminobutyric acid to a rat brain synaptic membrane preparation. *J. Neurochem.*, 32:79–84.

31. Wong, D. T., and Horng, J. S. (1976): Na$^+$-independent binding of GABA to the Triton X-100-treated synaptic membranes from cerebellum of rat brain. *Life Sci.*, 20:445–451.

32. Yokoi, I. (1981): Benzodiazepine receptor: Heterogeneity in rabbit brain. *Life Sci.*, 28:1591–1595.

33. Yosufe, M. A. K., Thomas, J. W., and Tallman, J. F. (1979): Solubilization of benzodiazepine binding site from rat cortex. *Life Sci.*, 25:463–470.

34. Zukin, S. R., Young, A. B., and Snyder, S. H. (1974): Gamma-aminobutyric acid binding to receptor sites in the rat central nervous system. *Proc. Natl. Acad. Sci. USA*, 71:4802–4807.

Neural Transmission, Learning and Memory,
edited by R. Caputto and C. Ajmone Marsan.
Raven Press, New York © 1983.

Formation and Differentiation of Synaptic Contacts in the Peripheral Nervous System

E. Giacobini

*Laboratory of Neuropsychopharmacology, Department of Biobehavioral Sciences,
University of Connecticut, Storrs, Connecticut 06268*

DEVELOPMENT OF PERIPHERAL SYNAPSES: PRE- AND POSTRECOGNITION EVENTS

The synapse is the site of a complex interaction between two or more nerve cells requiring a high degree of specialization in its structures. In contrast to *in vitro* conditions, synaptogenesis *in situ* represents a long-term process consisting of slow and complex structural and biochemical modifications (1).

On a chronological scale, these modifications occur not only during embryonic or fetal life, but also continue during the period following birth or hatching (2,3). It has been demonstrated that in some cases, such as in avian autonomic synapses, the process of synaptic growth and differentiation may proceed far beyond hatching with elaborate structural and biochemical changes (2,3). In light of these recent findings on peripheral cholinergic synapses, it seems questionable whether the adult synapse can be considered as a final and stable structure or rather one that might still undergo modifications throughout the entire life of the organism (2–4).

It is becoming increasingly evident that differentiation of synaptic structures represents a process controlled by multiple and complicated interactions mediated by signals moving in both directions across the synaptic gap. These interactions involve not only the growing fibers but also the target organ and the immediate environment as well. The present picture of synapse formation is still fragmentary and discontinuous. Synaptogenesis is like a story of which we know only a few and scattered episodes that often cannot be related to each other in time or cause.

For operational purposes, it seems convenient to consider the process of synapse formation within the frame of the period of general growth and differentiation of the neuron. We can arbitrarily separate those events preceding recognition and innervation of the target organ (ganglion cell, muscle, gland, or vessel) from those following it. On the other hand, a "synapse centered" vision of neuronal growth may be useful in dissecting out and analyzing each step of synaptogenesis to design experiments and test various hypotheses.

The events preceding recognition of the target organ take place mainly in the early embryonic or perinatal stages of development and consist of the migration of neuroblasts to specific sites as well as of neurotransmitter expression and differentiation (Fig. 1). The process of attraction and guidance of nerve fibers to their targets is poorly understood (Fig. 1). Phenomena such as cell death, selective survival and rescue, as well as normal development, all occur during this period (Fig. 1). The influence of target sites, as well as general phenomena of transynaptic regulation have been described in specialized reviews (5–9).

Following the process of recognition, which takes place in the late embryonic of perinatal period, the structural and chemical differentiation of the primitive terminals, as well as of the postsynaptic membrane, can be considered complete (Fig. 1). This particular phase of synaptogenesis includes important changes in receptor sensitivity, characteristics and number, and the establishment of functional neurotransmission (Fig. 1). The temporal relationship between the appearance of chemical and structural changes on one side, and the functional activity on the other, has been discussed in detail (10). Maintenance and regulation of neurotransmitter synthesis and inactivation, as well as the establishment of postjunctional membrane structure and activity, represents the main characteristic of the adult synapse. Several studies (2,3,5,7,8) suggest the presence of regulatory influences exerted by target organs and neurons as part of "trophic interactions" with the innervating fibers. Such interactions seem to be both modulatory and instructive for specific mechanisms of synapse formation (5,6,9–11).

	Migration
	Differentiation
Prerecognition	Attraction
	Survival—cell death
	Development
	Recognition
	Structural differentiation
Postrecognition	Function—regulation
	Maintenance—modulation
	Regeneration—degeneration
Maturation and aging	Cell death—aging

FIG. 1. Development of peripheral autonomic junctions—pre- and postrecognition events.

Biochemical signals provided by circulating or locally secreted hormones or peptides, neurotransmitters, and neuromodulators are involved in this process. In the case of functional emergency or in pathological conditions, mechanisms of regeneration, proliferation, or enzyme induction provide additional plasticity to the adult synapse. Such mechanisms can be mobilized at any stage of the postnatal life, including the aging period (4).

In the course of the present review, we shall discuss and emphasize some particular aspects related to early differentiation and growth of synaptic contacts and developmental signals occurring during synaptogenesis.

THE AVIAN CILIARY GANGLION-IRIS PREPARATION. A MODEL OF PERIPHERAL SYNAPTOGENESIS

The ciliary ganglion of the chick and its target organ, the iris (Fig. 2), provide a useful model for investigating the process of synapse formation and growth, starting from the earliest embryonic stages up to 7 years of age or later (2,3). For a comparison, in parallel investigations, the development of synapses and neurons was also examined in sympathetic and lumbar ganglia. The possibility of examining simultaneously cell bodies and nerve terminals in the same group of cells, belonging to a small (approximately 3,000) and homogeneous population of cholinergic neurons, represents a unique feature of this preparation (12,13). In this model, changes in biochemical parameters related to the metabolism of acetylcholine (ACh), the neurotransmitter of both ganglia and iris, can be correlated step by step to changes in neurotransmission and ultrastructure (10,14).

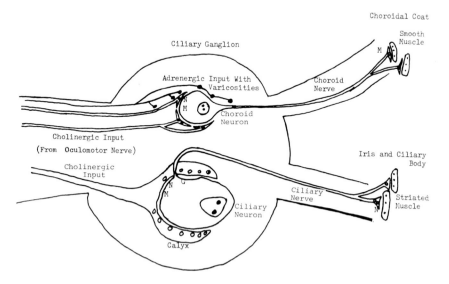

FIG. 2. Diagram of the chick ciliary ganglion and iris. N, Nicotinic receptors; M, muscarinic receptors; G, gap junctions.

A diagram of the ciliary ganglion-iris preparation of the chick is shown in Fig. 2. A scheme of the general development of chick sympathetic and parasympathetic ganglia is reported in Fig. 3. The data reported in the figure are to provide a temporal framework relating days of incubation (d.i.) to ganglionic development. A particularly interesting aspect of the development of the avian iris is the transformation from a neuroepithelial structure into a smooth muscle first, and then into a striated muscle. According to this diagram, based on data reported from the literature (2,3,10,12,14), the early stages of ganglionic development can be divided into three periods: (I) period of somal migration and differentiation, including the selection of the adult neurotransmitter system; (II) period of ganglionic and target organ innervation, involving axonal growth and penetration of fibers in the target organ; and a later period (III), which involves mainly the formation of synapses. This period has been subdivided by us (10) into four subsequent phases: innervation, neurotransmission, receptogenesis, and synaptic maturation (Fig. 4). The first phase of innervation can be considered to initiate in period II whereas the last phase of maturation extends itself to a longer period continuing after hatching. Period II includes phenomena such as cell death and the subsequent growth in volume of the ganglion cells. In the ciliary ganglion, cell death and the first phase of synaptogenesis coincide in time (14). It is particularly interesting to note that the cell death period starts toward the end of the period of innervation of the target organ (14). The

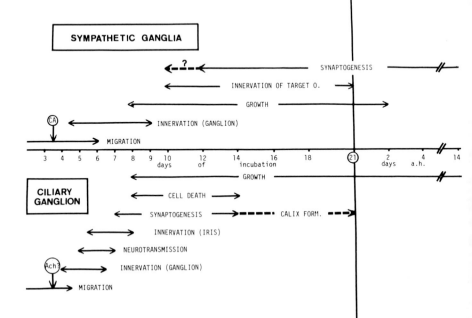

FIG. 3. General features of development of autonomic ganglia in the chick embryo.

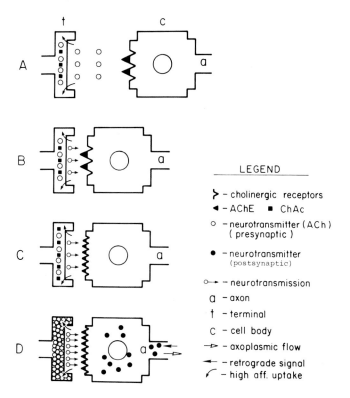

FIG. 4. Developmental sequence of the basic components of a peripheral cholinergic synapse. A, Phase of innervation; B, phase of neurotransmission; C, phase of receptogenesis, D, phase of biochemical and structural maturation.

diagram in Fig. 3 shows schematically that the following events are taking place sequentially: cellular migration, innervation of the ganglion, appearance of neurotransmission in the ganglion, innervation of the target organ formation of synapses (first in the ganglion and then in the iris), appearance of neurotransmission in the iris, and lastly, cell death. The number of ganglion cells, following the period of cell death remains constant during the entire life of the individual. In the present review, we shall concentrate upon the period of early differentiation of synaptic contacts and coupling to the target organ.

EARLY DIFFERENTIATION OF SYNAPTIC CONTACTS AND SYNAPTIC COUPLING TO THE TARGET ORGAN

The ontogeny of ACh receptors (AChRs) in the ciliary ganglion and iris has been examined in our laboratory by studying the appearance of α-bungarotoxin (α-BTX) binding sites in both organs *in vivo* (15) and *in vitro* (16). Variations in binding characteristics have been followed throughout the life of the animal (17). The α-BTX binding appears first in ganglia and then in the iris and is associated with nicotinic cholinergic receptors in both tissues (15). However, in the iris, previously to stage 30 (7 d.i.), a specific muscarinic-type of binding for (3-quinuclidinyl benzylate) ([^{3}H]QNB) can be demonstrated (15,17, and Giacobini et al., to be published). This is not surprising, as it has been previously shown that at this early stage of development the iris anlage of the chick eye is constituted by a smooth muscle (19). At the beginning of stage 31 (7 d.i.), growth cones are widely spread in the mesenchymal stroma overlying the pupil border (18,19). At the beginning of stage 34 (8 d.i.), ciliary nerve terminals appear to be in direct contact with the budding neuroepithelial cells which represent the first iris muscle anlage. Such a primitive contact is shown to be determinant for the nerve-dependent differentiation of the chick iris from smooth to striated muscle (19). It is interesting to note that a high affinity choline (Ch) uptake mechanism can be identified in the chick iris as early as 5 d.i. in conjunction with characteristic ultrastructural modifications of the iris bud (18). The evolution of the new characteristics of Ch uptake will continue at later stages.

Choline uptake has been shown to constitute an early and reliable biochemical marker for the presence of cholinergic innervation in the target organ (18). The development of the neuromuscular junction of the skeletal muscle which has been discussed by Dennis (11) shows remarkable similarities with the iris junction; therefore, analysis and comparison of both models allows a certain generalization of developmental events (Table 1).

In both organs, AChRs are present prior to innervation but are unevenly distributed. However, some localized areas of high receptor density (hot spots) are present (11). The presence of acetylcholinesterase (AChE) and choline acetyltransferase (ChAc) activities and high-affinity Ch uptake in presynaptic nerve terminals has been demonstrated (3) (Table 2). The growing terminals, which are endowed with a complete cholinergic machinery, are not guided or attracted to preexisting cholinergic receptor clusters (11).

TABLE 1. *Early differentiation of synaptic contacts*

PRIOR TO INNERVATION:
1. Receptors are present but are unevenly distributed.
2. Localized areas of high receptor density (hot spots) are present.
3. Growing terminals are *not* guided or attracted to preexisting receptor clusters.
4. Presence of AChE in presynaptic nerve terminals.

FOLLOWING INNERVATION:
1. Increased insertion and redistribution of receptors.
2. Modification of ion channels.
3. Appearance of high affinity transport mechanisms for precursors to neurotransmitter.
4. Appearance of junctional forms of AChE (dependent on target organ activity).
5. Reduction in duration of the synaptic potentials.

TABLE 2. *Developmental characteristics of cholinergic neurotransmission in the chick iris*

	Per iris			Percent of 3 d.a.h.		
Age	5 d.i.	10 d.i.	3 d.a.h.	5 d.i.	10 d.i.	3 d.a.h.
V_{max}[a]	9.9	25.9	29.0	34	90	—
Acetylcholine[b]	13.3	43.5	51.8	26	84	—
Choline[b]	247.0	131.9	291.0	85	45	—
ChAc[c]	0.8	12.5	833.0	0.1	2	100
AChE[e]	2.0	6.0	200.0	1	3	—
α-BTX Binding[d]	0	2.5	35.0	0	7	—
Neurotransmission[e]	0	50	100	0	50	—

[a]pmoles/5 min/iris (2).
[b]pmoles/iris (2).
[c]pmoles ACh synthesized or hydrolyzed/5 min/iris (2).
[d]fmoles/iris (15).
[e]Percent of 3 d.a.h. (14).

Following innervation, an increased insertion and neosynthesis of AChRs take place in the target organ simultaneous with a redistribution process (3,11,15). This phenomenon is associated to modifications of specific ion channels and to the reduction in duration of the synaptic potentials (11).

Two successive main synaptic events follow innervation. First, the consolidation of high-affinity carrier systems for precursors of neurotransmitter molecules with modifications of their kinetic and thermodynamic properties, as well as of sensitivity to specific inhibitors to ouabain and to Na^+ dependence (20).

Secondly, simultaneous to these postsynaptic phenomena is the appearance of junctional molecular forms of AChE that are dependent on target organ activity (21). The sequence of these early developmental events has been summarized in Table 1. Table 2 shows some of the developmental characteristics of cholinergic neurotransmission in the chick iris. For comparison, the data are reported on both a per iris and a percent of 3 days after hatching values.

THREE RULES OF SYNAPTOGENESIS

The available information on development of the neuromuscular junctions has been reviewed by Dennis (11). Together with the findings obtained by studies on ciliary ganglion-iris preparations (3,10), some preliminary hypotheses of synaptogenesis can be suggested (Table 3). The first hypothesis is that nerve fibers precede target organ differentiation, i.e., nerve terminals are present in the future synaptic region earlier than skeletal muscle fibers or iris muscle fibers (3,18). The primitive environment of these nerve fibers is represented by undifferentiated mesenchyma or stroma which will give rise to myoblasts. In the iris, the development of muscle cells is represented by a three-step metamorphosis involving complex structural and functional changes which are nerve-dependent (18,19). The time period and the nature of these inductive changes are unknown. Experiments could be designed to

TABLE 3. *Three rules of synaptogenesis*

I. NERVE PRECEDES TARGET ORGAN DIFFERENTIATION
Nerve terminals precede muscle fibers in the synaptic region.
Differentiation of myoblasts occurs in the presence of nerve terminals (inductive influence?).
II. NEUROTRANSMISSION PRECEDES SYNAPSE FORMATION
Appearance of EEPs upon stimulation → contraction.
Release of neurotransmitter in response to stimulation.
Spontaneous neurotransmitter release (MEEPs).
III. SYNAPSE FUNCTION PRECEDES SYNAPTIC SPECIALIZATION
Early contacts are structurally unspecialized.
Gap between pre- and postsynaptic cell can be wide.
Terminals lack clustered vesicles.
Synaptic cleft is irregular, synaptic folds are absent.
Postsynaptic receptors are scattered.

test this first hypothesis by delaying or abolishing the neural input *in situ* or by promoting myoblastic differentiation *in vitro* by means of neural factors. Such experiments would also help us to understand the difference between embryonic innervation and mature reinnervation following section or trauma in the nerve. In this respect, the avian iris could be of value in understanding not only the process of differentiation of myoblasts but also in evaluating presynaptic events such as appearance of specific carriers, or postsynaptic events such as changes in receptor characteristics and distribution.

As discussed in detail in a previous paper (10), neurotransmission seems to precede synapse formation (Table 3). This simply suggests that morphologically primitive synapses could be already functional during early phases of development. This concept is supported by direct morphological, biochemical, and functional evidence in the ciliary ganglion-iris preparation (Table 2). Evidence for spontaneous and stimulated release of neurotransmitter is supported by the presence of MEPPS and by the appearance of EPP upon stimulation followed by contraction of the embryonic skeletal muscle (11). It seems, therefore, plausible to think that synaptic function in the early stages of embryonic development may be primitive and incomplete, but still precede synaptic specialization (10) (Table 3). In reaching this third general conclusion, several characteristics of the primordial synapse should be kept in mind: the lack of ultrastructural presynaptic specialization, i.e., lack of segregated sites for storage and release of neurotransmitter, the lack of clustered vesicles, the wide and irregular synaptic cleft, the absence of postsynaptic folds, and the relatively low number and scattering of postsynaptic receptors.

Although much remains to be learned with regard to the physiological activity of primitive synapse, it is surprising how little structural specialization and how rudimentary is the neurotransmitter machinery required for functional activity. Table 2 compares developmental characteristics of cholinergic properties in neurotransmission junctions of the chick iris and emphasizes fundamental differences at three basically different stages of development.

DEVELOPMENTAL SIGNALS FOR SYNAPTIC DIFFERENTIATION

The major developmental changes briefly outlined in the previous sections strongly suggest the presence of inductive interactions between pre- and postsynaptic components of the developing synapse. The literature indicates that such interactions are numerous, or diverse nature, and occur at several critical periods of development. In Table 4, we have tentatively listed the possible effects of such mechanisms, as well as their possible site of origin and target. This scheme suffers from at least two oversimplifications: first, it subdivides the events into an early group and a late group, using as a point of separation the time at which recognition of the target occurs and innervation is shut off. Secondly, the communication system is described as being bidirectional with anterograde and retrograde signals carried through neural channels only. We are aware of the fact that developmental modulatory influences can be exerted by other neural and non-neural systems as well, such as the neuroglia, the vascular system, and the primitive endocrine system. In the particular case of the neuromuscular junction, the target itself can influence the presynaptic neuron by means of the electrical activity of the muscle fibers, and reciprocally, the presynaptic neuron can influence its target by means of the postsynaptic electrical activity (3). The role played by both pre- and postsynaptic receptors is still under examination; however, we known that modulatory influences originating from cho-

TABLE 4. *Developmental signals*

	Effect	Site of effect	Origin of signal	Direction
E A R L Y	Promotion of growth or survival of neuron	Cell body	Target organ	Retrograde
	Expression or modulation of neurotransmitter phenotype	Cell body	Target organ or environment	Retrograde
	Promotion of synaptic contacts	Synapse (muscle)	Noninnervated organ	Retrograde
	Shut off of innervation	Synapse (muscle)	Innervated organ	Retrograde
L A T E	Differentiation of target organ	Target organ (muscle)	Neurotransmission at target organ	Anterograde
	Differentiation of presynaptic contacts	Presynaptic sites (nerve)	Target organ	Retrograde
	Synthesis and regulation of membrane components	Postsynaptic sites (muscle)	Physiological activity of target organ	Local
	Synthesis and regulation of neurotransmitter enzymes	Cell body	Neurotransmission at target organ	Retrograde

linergic receptor interactions are important for the regulation of enzyme activities related to neurotransmitter metabolism (22). In addition, muscle activity modulates extrajunctional AChRs and deposition of AChE in developing end plates (11,16,21).

As we have previously discussed, neurotransmission constitutes an early phenomenon in synapse formation. It is therefore to be expected that it may serve as a signal for early differentiation and growth of the synapse.

Information on spontaneous activity of ganglionic and motor neurons during the embryonic period is scanty; however, subliminal excitatory activity could be effective enough to convey instructive signals to the developing synapse.

With regard to the chemical nature of the humoral signals, we are aware of at least three different groups of candidates: first, neurotransmitter molecules; secondly, polypeptides of various nature, including growth factors; and thirdly, hormones, such as corticosteroids. Each of these signals act at a defined period of development and probably on well-defined targets within the neuron. The passage of some signals as diffusible factors in a retrograde manner across the synaptic gap from the target to the nerve terminals represents an additional efficient mechanism of interneuronal communication.

In some cases, to exert their action, such factors would not need to penetrate intraneuronally or intraaxonally, but could interact with other macromolecules (e.g., receptors) on the external surface of the terminals. Through this mechanism, retrograde signals would not need to be carried through the axon to the cell body. With a similar mechanism, anterograde signals may be expected to act on various types of macromolecules located on the external surface of the muscle membrane. Presently, such mechanisms are still theoretical; however, recent studies using tissue culture seem to point in this direction.

The presence of local synaptic circuits and of terminal-terminal interactions should not be neglected, particularly in relation to mechanisms of competitive selection of fibers for innervation.

It is interesting to point out that in the diagram reported in Table 4, the great majority of signal systems seem to act through a retrograde pathway. This stresses the importance of the periphery on the differentiation and expression of neuronal attributes, a fact well known from the beginning of classical neuroembryology. It is difficult to say whether this concept is influenced by our present lack of knowledge with regard to anterograde factors and local synaptic phenomena.

The present picture of a developing peripheral synapse is far from clear. The information available, obtained mainly through biochemical and electrophysiological studies of the last decade, which have been condensed and schematized in the present review, provide, we believe, useful directions for future research in synaptogenesis.

ACKNOWLEDGMENTS

The investigations carried out in the author's laboratory were supported by PHS grants NS-11496, NS-11430, NS-15086, and NSF grant GB-41475 to E. G. and by grants from the University of Connecticut Research Foundation.

REFERENCES

1. Aloisi, M., and Mussini, I. (1979): Nerve dependent differentiation. The case of the avian iris muscle. In: *International Meeting Brain Development*, Selva di Fasano, Italy. Abstr.
2. Black, I. B., Coughlin, M. D., and Cochard, P. (1979): Factors regulating neuronal differentiation. *Soc. Neurosci. Symp.*, 4:184–207.
3. Black, I. B., and Patterson, P. H. (1980): Developmental regulation of neurotransmitter phenotype. *Current Top. Dev. Biol.*, 15:27–39.
4. Chiappinelli, V., and Giacobini, E. (1978): Time course of appearance of α-bungarotoxin binding sites during development of chick ciliary ganglion and iris. *Neurochem. Res.*, 3:465–478.
6. Chiappinelli, V., Giacobini, E., Pilar, G., and Uchimura, H. (1976): Induction of cholinergic enzymes in chick ciliary ganglion and iris muscle cells during synapse formation. *J. Physiol. (Lond.)*, 257:749–766.
7. Chiappinelli, V., Fairman, K., and Giacobini, E. (1978): Effects of nicotinic antagonists on the development of the chick lumbar sympathetic ganglia, ciliary ganglion and iris. *Dev. Neurosci.*, 1:191–202.
7. Dennis, M. J. (1981): Development of the neuromuscular junction: Inductive interactions between cells. *Annu. Rev. Neurosci.*, 4:43–68.
8. Giacobini, E. (1975): Neuronal control of neurotransmitters biosynthesis during development. *J. Neurosci. Res.*, 1:315–331.
9. Giacobini, E. (1978): Regulation of neurotransmitter biosynthesis during development in the peripheral nervous system. In: *Maturation of Neurotransmission*, edited by A. Vernadakis, E. Giacobini, and G. Filogamo, pp. 41–64. S. Karger AG, Basel.
10. Giacobini, E. (1979): Synaptogenesis: Chemistry, structure or function? Which comes first? In: *Neural Growth and Differentiation*, edited by E. Meisami and M. A. B. Brazier, pp. 153–167. Raven Press, New York.
11. Giacobini, E. (1980): Biochemical control of synapse formation *in vivo*. In: *Nerve Cells, Transmitters and Behaviour*, Pont. Acad. Scient. Scripta Varia 45:451–482.
12. Giacobini, E. (1980): Discrepancies and differences between nerve cells growing *in vitro* and *in situ*: A discussion. In: *Tissue Culture in Neurobiology*, edited by E. Giacobini et al., pp. 187–204. Raven Press, New York.
13. Giacobini, E. (1982): Aging of autonomic synapses. In: *Advances in Cellular Neurobiology, Vol. 3*, edited by S. Fedoroff and L. Hertz. Academic Press, New York, pp. 174–214.
14. Giacobini, E., and Chiappinelli, V. (1977): The ciliary ganglion: A model of cholinergic synaptogenesis. In: *Synaptogenesis*, edited by L. Tauc, pp. 89–116. Naturalia et Biologia, Paris.
15. Giacobini, E., and Marchi, M. (1981): Acetylcholine biosynthesis in developing cholinergic synapses. In: *Cholinergic Mechanisms*, edited by G. Pepeu. Plenum Press, New York, pp. 1–24.
16. Giacobini, E., Pilar, G., Suszkiw, J., and Uchimura, H. (1979): Normal distribution and denervation changes of neurotransmitter related enzymes in cholinergic neurones. *J. Physiol. (Lond.)*, 286:233–253.
17. Marchi, M., and Giacobini, E. (1981): Aging of cholinergic synapses in the peripheral autonomic nervous system. In: *Cholinergic Mechanisms*, edited by G. Pepeu. Plenum Press, New York, pp. 25–46.
18. Marchi, M., Hoffman, D. W., Giacobini, E., and Fredrickson, T. (1980): Age dependent changes in choline uptake of the chick iris. *Brain Res.*, 195:423–431.
19. Marchi, M., Hoffman, D. W., Mussini, I., and Giacobini, E. (1980): Development and aging of cholinergic synapses III. Choline uptake in the developing iris of the chick. *Dev. Neurosci.*, 3:185–198.
20. Marchi, M., Yurkewicz, L., Giacobini, E., and Fredrickson, T. (1981): Development and aging of cholinergic synapses. V. Changes in nicotinic cholinergic receptor binding in ciliary ganglia and irises of the chicken. *Dev. Neurosci.*, 4:258–266.
21. Scarsella, G., Toschi, G., Chiappinelli, V. A., and Giacobini, E. (1978): Molecular forms of acetylcholinesterase in the ciliary ganglion and iris of the chick. *Dev. Neurosci.*, 1:133–141.
22. Shainberg, A., Shahar, A., Burstein, M., and Giacobini, E. (1980): Effect of innervation on acetylcholine receptors in muscle cultures. In: *Tissue Culture in Neurobiology*, edited by E. Giacobini et al., pp. 25–33. Raven Press, New York.

Neural Transmission, Learning and Memory,
edited by R. Caputto and C. Ajmone Marsan.
Raven Press, New York © 1983.

Features of the Calcium Ion and Calmodulin-Dependent Protein Kinase Activity in Fragments of Synaptosomal Membranes from the Rat

*R. Rodnight, *H. Gower, **L. Martinez-Millan
and †D. De Souza

*Department of Biochemistry, Institute of Psychiatry, De Crespigny Park, London, U.K.;
**CSIC, Patronato "Alfonso el Sabio" Departamento de Anatomia, Zaragoza, Spain;
†Departamento de Bioquimica, Instituto de Biociencias—UFRGS Rue Sarmento Leite,
90000 Porto Alegre, RS, Brazil

Calcium ions are intimately involved in the two main facets of synaptic transmission: release of neurotransmitter from the presynaptic terminal and in modulation of the postsynaptic response (45,46,70). In both situations the actions of calcium ions are complex and probably involve cascades of molecular events, the nature of which is little understood at present. In this regard, two recent advances provide leads that may eventually contribute to the formulation of testable hypotheses: first, the realisation that many of the biological actions of calcium ions depend upon a calcium-binding protein, now generally known as calmodulin (10,37,68), and second the discovery of protein kinase enzymes activated by calcium ions. Two general types of Ca^{2+}-dependent protein kinase are known: (a) several protein kinases dependent upon calmodulin as well as Ca^{2+}; these include phosphorylase kinase (11), myosin light chain kinase (19,56), and a multifunctional protein kinase (89); (b) Ca^{2+}-dependent protein kinase that requires for full activity the presence of phosphatidylserine and diacylglycerols (41,83). Takai et al. (83) have designated this enzyme "protein kinase C."

Calmodulin is a ubiquitous low-molecular-weight (17,000) protein of highly conserved structure that binds four calcium ions per molecule. In addition to the protein kinases mentioned above, it mediates the activating effects of Ca^{2+} on the following enzymes: high K_m cyclic nucleotide phosphodiesterase, adenylate cyclase, guanylate cyclase, tryptophan hydroxylase (39,99), and the transport of Ca^{2+}-ATPase in erythrocyte membranes (17,57,88), sarcoplasmic reticulum (43), adipocytes (62), and the synaptic plasma membrane (40,78). Some of these activations may be secondary to protein kinase activation.

Tissue from brain is an especially rich source of calmodulin; the highest concentration occurs in the caudate nucleus and cerebral cortex. At the subcellular level both cell fractionation (23) and immunocytochemical studies (44,98) have shown that a considerable proportion (perhaps as much as 30%) of neuronal calmodulin is located in the postsynaptic densities. Some calmodulin is also found bound to neuronal plasma membranes, where it is presumably associated with calmodulin-dependent enzymes. Further, brain contains a Ca^{2+}-dependent calmodulin-binding protein, calcineurin, of molecular weight 80,000, which inhibits the activity of calmodulin-requiring enzymes (90). Some of the physiological functions of Ca^{2+}-calmodulin system are now becoming evident: it appears to be involved in the regulation of the balance between the synthesis and degradation of cyclic nucleotides and other metabolic processes; in the transport of calcium ions across cell membranes; and, through its action on specific protein kinases, in the regulation of the contractile process (19), cell motility (37,71), and microtubule assembly–diassembly (58). Other biochemical effects of calmodulin cannot at present be explained in terms of known physiological processes; in particular functional roles for a range of proteins, located in the plasma membrane, that are phosphorylated by Ca^{2+}-calmodulin-dependent protein kinase activity remain a mystery. These Ca^{2+}-calmodulin-dependent protein phosphorylating systems (comprising protein kinase-acceptor molecule-protein phosphatase) are ubiquitous (e.g., see ref. 42) but are enriched in synaptic structures and need now to be considered in more detail.

Protein phosphorylation and dephosphorylation involving hydroxy groups of amino acids are now recognised as ubiquitous biochemical reactions regulating numerous cellular processes (11,95); various aspects of the phenomenon have been extensively studied in the nervous system (for recent reviews see 18,25,65–68,96).

Of particular interest to the present theme is the occurrence in fragments of synaptosomal membranes of endogenous Ca^{2+}-calmodulin-dependent protein kinase activity toward membrane-bound proteins, first reported by Schulman and Greengard (73). Later work, both from Greengard's laboratory and others, has confirmed and extended this observation (15,24,31,32,36). The major advance concerns a pair of phosphorylated polypeptides now generally known as proteins Ia and Ib, possessing molecular weights (as determined by gel electrophoresis) between 76,000 and 86,000. These polypeptides are subunits of a single synapse-specific (12) polymeric protein that is located mainly, if not exclusively, in the limiting membrane of synaptic vesicles (3,86). Proteins Ia and Ib were first recognised in preparations of synaptic membranes as the major substrates for endogenous cyclic AMP-dependent protein phosphorylation (see ref. 25 for early literature). These substrates, and their associated kinases, have been extracted, purified, and characterised in detail (85–87). They are basic in nature with a high content of proline and glycine and both consist of a globular head and a collagen-like tail (84). The membrane-bound cyclic AMP-dependent protein kinase that catalyses their phosphorylation resembles the Type II enzyme (49,93). Later work (31,32,36) showed that proteins Ia and Ib are also phosphorylated by a membrane-bound Ca^{2+}-calmodulin-dependent protein kinases at multiple sites that are distinct from the sites accepting phosphate through cyclic AMP-dependent kinase action. Moreover, it was found that Ca^{2+} influx into ³²P-labeled respiring cerebral cortex slices (22) or synaptosomes (38) induced by exposure to high K$^+$ or veratradine led to an increased level of phosphorylation in intraterminal proteins Ia and Ib.

The other major acceptors for Ca^{2+}-calmodulin-dependent protein kinase activity in synaptic membranes have received as yet little attention. They consist of several high-molecular-weight (>90,000) components, and polypeptides of approximately 60,000, 57,000, and 50,000 M.W. In addition, brain membranes contain an acceptor of about 45,000 M.W., extensively studied by Gispen and co-workers (33,100,101), that is maximally phosphorylated in the presence of Ca^{2+} only, apparently via the protein kinase C of Takai et al. (83). In the present chapter we present data on the characteristics of these Ca^{2+}-activated phosphorylating systems and discuss their possible significance.

METHODS

Preparation of Synaptosomal Membrane Fragments

A modification of the procedure of Jones and Matus (34) was used to prepare membrane fragments from rat forebrain, but excluding the thalamus, septum, and midbrain. The nature of this preparation and the extent to which it is contaminated are considered later under Discussion. Animals were killed by decapitation; the brain tissue was dissected within 1 min and homogenized within 5 min of death. Ca^{2+} was omitted from the sucrose solutions and the fragments received an extra centrifugal wash with 4 mM imidazole HCl (pH 7.0) to decrease contamination with endogenous cytosolic Ca^{2+}. Preparations were stored at $-20°C$ in 50% (vol/vol) glycerol in 2 mM imidazole HCl (pH 7.0) at a protein concentration of 5 μg/ml. Under these conditions no loss in phosphorylating activity, including sensitivity to activating factors, was observed for periods of at least 12 months.

Labeling with [³²P]ATP

The basic medium, to which CaCl$_2$ and calmodulin were added, contained in a final volume of 80 μl: 30 mM Tris HCl (pH 7.4 at 37°C), 1 mM MgSO$_4$, 0.25 mM EGTA, 100 μM [γ-³²P]ATP (100–200 c.p.m./pmole) and 100 μg of membrane protein. The reaction was initiated by injecting protein into the preincubated medium at 37°C and stopped after 10 sec by injecting 20 μl of the usual SDS-mercaptoethanol solubilizing solution (30). Samples were not boiled.

Polyacrylamide Gel Electrophoresis

Previous methodology was followed (30). After electrophoresis gels were stained with Coomassie Blue, destained, dried under vacuum, and exposed for periods up to 24 hr to Kodak NS-2T X-ray film. After development the films were scanned in a densitometer to give a semiquantitative profile of the labeled proteins (see Fig. 1). Peak heights were measured from an arbitrary baseline.

Apparent molecular weights were derived from the means of mobilities determined in gels of six different acrylamide concentrations, using for standards the

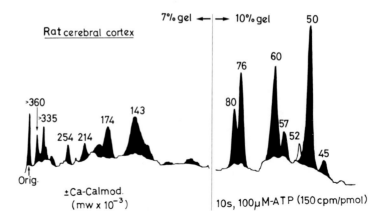

FIG. 1. Densitometric scans (expanded ×3) of radioautographs prepared from labeled synaptosomal membrane fragments incubated with 100 μM [³²P]ATP (150 c.p.m./pmole). The figures represent molecular weights × 10⁻³. Two gel systems were used: 7% for polypeptides above 100 daltons and 10% for acceptors of lower molecular weight. The black areas indicate stimulation by Ca²⁺ and calmodulin, or Ca²⁺ only in the case of the peak labeled 45 × 10⁻³, and were derived by superimposing scans of radioautographs from membranes labeled under basal conditions. Note the pronounced peak on the origin, which is only seen in material labeled in the presence of Ca²⁺ and calmodulin.

following proteins (approximate molecular weight): apoferritin (450,000), myosin (200,000), phosphorylase b (197,000), bovine serum albumin (68,000), and ovalbumin (45,000). The values are given in Table 1 and differ in some respects from those quoted by our group in previous publications (30,65–68), mainly because we were unaware in the earlier work of anomalies in the mobilities of certain standards and phosphopeptides (22a). Like all molecular weights determined by electrophoresis the present values are approximate; this applies especially to certain high-molecular-weight polypeptides, for which only minimal values could be deduced: to O_{3b}, for which a mean value for two component polypeptides is given and for α_5, which was found to possess a grossly abnormal free mobility.

Calmodulin was prepared from ox brain by the method of Walsh and Stevens (91), omitting the final DEAE column. The product yielded a single band on electrophoresis.

Calculation of "Available" Ca²⁺

This is defined as the sum of the free [Ca²⁺] and the [Ca²⁺] bound to calmodulin. To calculate it a computer program (61) was used incorporating 10 stability constants: $K_{Ca\text{-}EGTA}$; $K_{Mg\text{-}EGTA}$; $K_{H\text{-}EGTA}$; $K_{H_2\text{-}EGTA}$; $K_{Ca\text{-}ATP}$; $K_{Mg\text{-}ATP}$; $K_{H\text{-}ATP}$; $K_{H_2\text{-}ATP}$; $K_{Ca\text{-}calmodulin\,(av)}$; $K_{Mg\text{-}calmodulin\,(av)}$. Average stability constants for the binding of Ca²⁺ and Mg²⁺ to calmodulin were taken from Wolff et al. (97).

TABLE 1. *Major phosphorylating systems in synaptosomal membranes*

Designation	M.W. ($\times 10^{-3}$)[a]	Activating factor	Comments
O$_1$	> 360 (209)	cAMP, Ca-CM	—
O$_2$	> 335 (204)	Ca-CM	—
O$_{3a}$	> 300 (198)	cAMP	Microtubular associated protein-MAP$_2$ (49)
O$_{3b}$	254 (195)	cAMP, Ca-CM	Contains at least two components
α$_1$	214	cAMP, Ca-CM	Minor
α$_2$	189	cAMP	Minor
α$_3$	174 (162)	Ca-CM	Absent from cerebellum
α$_5$	143 (138)	cAMP, Ca-CM	Broad diffuse band; absent in cerebellum
α$_6$	139	cAMP	Poorly separated from α$_5$
β$_3$	80 (86)	cAMP, Ca-CM	Protein Ia (25,85)
β$_4$	76 (79)	cAMP, Ca-CM	Protein Ib (25,85)
β$_6$	60 (68)	Ca-CM	? DPH-L (14)
β$_7$	57 (62)	Ca-CM	Minor in cerebral cortex; major in cerebellum and colliculus
γ$_2$	54 (59)	cAMP	Regulatory subunit of cyclic AMP-dependent protein kinase (92)
γ$_3$	52 (54)	None	—
γ$_4$	50 (50)	Ca-CM	Absent in cerebellum; may be major postsynaptic density protein (8,24). ? DPH-M (14)
γ$_5$	45 (47)	Ca	B-50 (33,100). Anomalous free mobility; M.W. unreliable

[a]Values in parentheses are those previously suggested by our group (30,65–68).

RESULTS

General Characteristics of Endogenous Ca^{2+}-Activated Phosphorylation

Figure 1 illustrates densitometric scans of typical separations of synaptosomal membrane polypeptides phosphorylated by endogenous Ca^{2+}-activated protein kinases. Under the conditions used in this experiment (100 μM ATP of relatively low specific radioactivity) it is evident that the basal phosphorylation is minimal and mainly confined to the acceptor of 52,000 M.W. In contrast, if a low concentration of ATP of high specific radioactivity (e.g., <20 μM, >1,000 c.p.m./pmole) is used, some of the acceptors are appreciably phosphorylated under basal conditions, the stimulation given by Ca^{2+} and calmodulin is less dramatic and the phosphorylation of the 52,000 M.W. acceptor relative to the others is greater. Two factors are involved in this difference in pattern: first the contribution of endogenous contaminating Ca^{2+} and calmodulin is greater at low ATP concentrations, and second the affinity of the Ca^{2+}-activated protein kinases for ATP is some five times less than for the basal kinase that phosphorylates the 52,000 M.W. acceptor as well as for the cyclic AMP-dependent protein kinases.

Table 1 compares the main Ca^{2+}-dependent phosphorylating systems with the systems activated by cyclic AMP. The designations (O, α, β, and γ, etc.) follow previous practice (30,65–67); established equivalents from other laboratories are given in the last column. The polypeptides designated as O_1, O_2, α_5, β_3, and β_4 are phosphorylated by both Ca^{2+}-dependent and cyclic AMP-dependent kinase activities, but as mentioned above only in the case of β_3 and β_4 (or proteins Ia and Ib) has it been firmly established that the two kinases transfer phosphate to different sites on the same polypeptide chain (31,32,36). The other acceptors in this category may be mixtures, the complexity of which must await two-dimensional analysis. However, in the case of O_{3b} it is already clear that the two activities phosphorylate distinct polypeptides that are separable under certain conditions (R. Rodnight and H. Gower, *unpublished observations*).

The acceptor designated γ_5, which is equivalent to the B-50 polypeptide of the Utrecht group (33,100), is maximally phosphorylated in media containing >0.1 μM Ca^{2+} (free) and no further incorporation is given by calmodulin. However, preliminary experiments (H. Gower, *unpublished observations*) show that in the range 0.02 μM–0.1 μM Ca^{2+} (free) calmodulin does stimulate phosphorylation of this acceptor. As the two phosphorylations are not additive it appears probable that the same sites on the γ_5 acceptor may be phosphorylated by two kinases with different requirements.

In the remainder of this chapter we will refer to β_3 and β_4 collectively as protein I and to γ_5 as B-50, in view of the extensive work published on these acceptors by other laboratories who use these alternative designations. The other acceptors will be given the designations indicated in Table 1 followed by present estimates of molecular weight, using the symbol K to indicate 10^3.

Dependence on Mg²⁺ Concentration

The Ca^{2+}-dependent phosphorylating systems responded differently to a wide range of Mg^{2+} concentrations in the incubation media. Typical results are shown in Fig. 2 for the two components of protein I and for β_6(60K) and γ_4(50K); Mg^{2+} concentrations above 10 mM were progressively less effective in the case of protein I, but continued to stimulate in the case of the other two. It is interesting to note here that while protein I is predominantly presynaptic in location evidence presented below suggests that γ_4(50K) is mainly located in the postsynaptic densities. Of the remaining major systems, O_1(>360K), O_2(>335K), O_{3b}(254K), α_3(174K), and α_5(143K) gave an activation pattern similar to that observed with β_6(60K) and γ_4(50K), whereas B-50 was activated and inhibited similarly to protein I. Phosphorylation of all the acceptors in the cyclic AMP-dependent systems was uniformly inhibited by Mg^{2+} concentrations greater than 5 mM.

Although the 1 mM Mg^{2+} concentration used routinely in our incubation media is suboptimal for all systems it may be more physiological than the higher concentrations used by many workers: the free Mg^{2+} concentration in brain cytosol is considered to be approximately 1 mM (97).

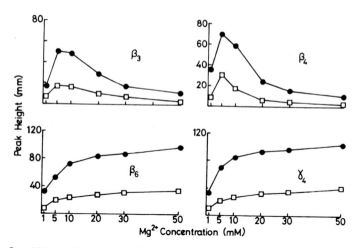

FIG. 2. Sensitivity of Ca²⁺-calmodulin-dependent labeling to Mg²⁺ concentration. Standard incubations of 10 sec were used, with an "available" Ca²⁺ concentration of 250 μM. β₃ and β₄ are the two subunits of protein I which is located in presynaptic areas; γ₄ is probably a major postsynaptic density protein. Peak heights were measured on densitometric scans within a linear range.

Sensitivity to Ca²⁺ and Calmodulin

In the presence of a free Ca²⁺ concentration greater than 1 μM calmodulin stimulated the phosphorylation of all acceptors except, as already noted, B-50. The optimum concentration of calmodulin was 4 μM, which is rather high compared with that used by other workers (73, but see 24). Inclusion of saponin in the medium did not increase sensitivity to calmodulin, suggesting that access to endogenous kinase is not a limiting factor in our experiments.

The sensitivity of the Ca²⁺-calmodulin-dependent kinases to "available" Ca²⁺ (free Ca²⁺ plus calmodulin-bound Ca²⁺) was similar for all acceptors and was remarkably steep in the range of pCa 7 to pCa 6, half-maximal stimulation being given by about 0.2 μM "available" Ca²⁺. Figure 3 illustrates this for protein Ib, β₆(60K) and γ₄(50K). Concentrations of "available" Ca²⁺ above 1 mM were progressively inhibitory.

Extrasynaptic and Subsynaptic Location of Ca²⁺-Dependent Phosphorylating Systems

The precise cellular location of protein phosphorylating systems may provide important clues as to their physiological function. However, preparations of synaptosomal membranes, as discussed below, are inevitably a mixture of pre- and postsynaptic membrane fragments and are contaminated to some extent with non-synaptic structures. In addition the possibility of artifactual change occurring during preparation has to be considered. Careful assessment employing a variety of stratagems is therefore required in investigating these aspects. Several approaches have been used, both by ourselves and others. These include: *in vivo* studies using

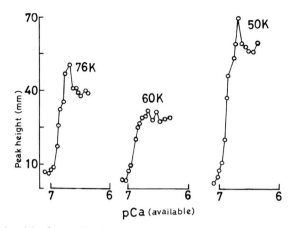

FIG. 3. Sensitivity of the Ca^{2+}-calmodulin-dependent labeling to Ca^{2+} concentration. Standard incubations of 10 sec were used, with a Mg^{2+} concentration of 1 mM. Peak heights were determined as described in the legend to Fig. 2.

neurotoxic agents, ontogenetic studies, and *in vitro* studies of intact synaptosomes and subfractionated synaptic membrane preparations.

The induction of brain lesions by the injection of neurotoxic agents has pointed to a predominantly neuronal location for both cyclic AMP-dependent and Ca^{2+}-calmodulin-dependent systems. The most striking results have been obtained with the neurotoxic agent kainic acid, which destroys neuronal perikarya but spares presynaptic terminals possessing soma remote from the lesion site and glial cells (26,74). Thus lesions made in the rat striatum by injection of 10 nmoles of kainic acid resulted in the loss of all the cyclic AMP-dependent (75) and Ca^{2+}-calmodulin-dependent (76) endogenous protein phosphorylation. We have confirmed these observations by using the same dose of kainic acid and observed that in contrast to the major loss of cyclic AMP- and Ca^{2+}-dependent systems obtained with this dose, phosphorylation of γ_3 (52 K) by basal protein kinase activity and B-50 by a Ca^{2+}-dependent kinase, are much less affected. Lower doses (5 nmoles per striatum) still resulted in complete loss of Ca^{2+}-calmodulin-dependent systems, but only a partial (about 60%) loss in cyclic AMP-dependent systems and no significant loss in γ_3 (52 K) and B-50. The possible significance of this result is discussed later in relation to information on the ontogeny of the B-50 system.

Ontogenetic studies have shown that many protein phosphorylating systems do not appear in the brain until after the onset of synaptogenesis. In the rat this stage of development is delayed until around the 12th day after birth (1). Lohmann et al. (47) found that the appearance of protein I was similarly delayed until after day 10, although the appropriate cyclic AMP-dependent protein kinase activity was present from birth (48). By contrast, neonatal guinea pig brain, in which synaptogenesis occurs *in utero*, contained near-adult levels of protein I (47). Later work from our laboratory (30) has extended these observations in the rat to other cyclic AMP-dependent systems and to the Ca^{2+}-dependent systems. With respect to the former, low levels of phosphorylation of the acceptors referred to by us as O_{3a} (>300K), O_{3b}(254K), α_2(189K), and α_5(143K) were observed in neonatal brain, after which a fairly steady increase was observed; however, O_{3b} and α_5 increased more rapidly than the others after day 10. The appearance of α_6(139K, a pronounced shoulder on the broad α_5 band) occurred coincidentally with protein I.

The ontogeny of the Ca^{2+}-calmodulin-dependent kinase activities also showed a variable pattern (Fig. 4): phosphorylation of α_3(174K) and γ_4(50K) was undetectable until day 15, but thereafter developed very rapidly; also, as expected, the Ca^{2+}-calmodulin-activated phosphorylation of protein I was similarly delayed. Activity toward β_6(60K) developed gradually from birth onward. The surprising result concerned the Ca^{2+}-only-dependent phosphorylation of B-50: this activity was more than three times higher in neonatal brain than in adult brain; between 1 and 10 days the level of phosphorylation of this acceptor increased further, after which it started to decline.

The available evidence indicates that the enhanced level of phosphorylation of B-50 reflects a high content of the acceptor protein in the immature brain, rather than an increased activity of its associated protein kinase. For example, electrophoretograms from immature brain stained by Coomassie Blue exhibit a major polypeptide that exactly corresponds in mobility to the phosphorylated band of B-50 and that declines to virtually undetectable levels in adulthood. It may be added that Ca^{2+} sensitivity for the phosphorylation of B-50 is the same in membranes made from infant brain as from adult brain. However, in one striking respect, the B-50 phosphorylation system in immature brain is different from that in adult. Up until 10 days of age the major part of the phosphorylating activity is recovered in a light fraction of membrane fragments that equilibrates in the gradient over 0.95 M sucrose, whereas in adult animals the activity is entirely confined to the synaptosomal membrane fraction that equilibrates over 1.1 M sucrose. In mature brain the equivalent "light" fraction consists almost entirely of myelin fragments that contain no

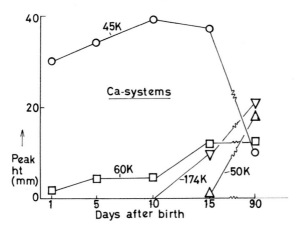

FIG. 4. Ontogenesis of some of the Ca^+-dependent phosphorylation systems. Data derived from Holmes and Rodnight (30).

trace of the B-50 system. It is of interest to note that high-affinity transport systems for γ-aminobutyric acid and glutamate are progressively associated with heavier particles during development (28).

With regard to the presynaptic as opposed to postsynaptic location of acceptors, a variety of approaches has been used, some of which are discussed below. Here we report a follow-up of an earlier study of the late Malcolm Weller (94) in which intact and lysed synaptosomes were labeled with [^{32}P]ATP under identical conditions in parallel. Our work confirms Weller's conclusion that virtually all cyclic AMP-dependent phosphorylation is occluded and requires lysis of the synaptosomal fraction for its manifestation; presumably, therefore, it is located within the synaptic terminal or (less likely) in vesicular structures derived from other membranes. By contrast, the activity of several of the Ca^{2+}-calmodulin-dependent systems, namely α_3 (174 K), α_5 (143 K), β_6 (60 K), and γ_4 (50 K), was hardly increased by lysis (Fig. 5), although this did not apply to the Ca^{2+}-calmodulin-dependent phosphorylation of protein I. With regard to the B-50 system present evidence indicates that this is only slightly phosphorylated in intact as compared with lysed synaptosomes.

DISCUSSION

Three aspects of the subject will be further considered: (a) the validity of using the subcellular approach for the study of Ca^{2+}-dependent protein phosphorylation; (b) the extrasynaptosomal location of phosphorylated polypeptides; (c) their subsynaptic locations; and (d) the extent to which functional implications can be drawn from present data.

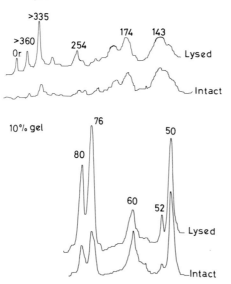

FIG. 5. Ca^{2+}-calmodulin-dependent labeling of acceptors in intact and lysed synaptosomes. Synaptosomes were isolated from a gradient and divided into two parts; one part was diluted with 0.32 M sucrose, centrifuged, and resuspended in 0.32 M sucrose to 5 mg of protein/ml; the other part was lysed by dilution with water, adjusted to 0.32 M sucrose by addition of 2 M sucrose, centrifuged, and resuspended in 0.32 M sucrose to 5 mg of protein/ml. Incubation conditions were as described in the legend to Fig. 1. Labeled samples were run on 5% and 10% gels in parallel.

Validity of the Subcellular Approach

There are several reasons for questioning the physiological relevance of protein phosphorylation reactions in membrane fragments: (a) Disruption of the cell may lead to association of kinases and phosphatases with unphysiological substrates; (b) protein dephosphorylation and/or proteolysis may occur during preparation; (c) redistribution of regulatory factors may occur; and (d) the fact that ATP may have access to both sides of the membrane may reasonably be considered unphysiological. Points (b) and (c) have been little explored, although De Lorenzo's group claim that significant proteolysis of components of certain Ca^{2+}-calmodulin-activated phosphorylation systems may occur postmortem (R. De Lorenzo, *personal communication*). Unfortunately, satisfactory inhibitors of protein dephosphorylation that do not interfere with subcellular fractionation procedures are not yet available. With regard to (d) the fact that ATP is probably released at synapses (63), either as a purinergic transmitter, or along with other transmitters, makes this double access situation less unphysiological than was once considered the case.

The problem posed by (a), however, is serious and has been considered in other tissues (7). Matus (52) has drawn attention to it with evidence that certain cytoplasmic proteins tend to stick to the postsynaptic densities after cell disruption. We have approached the problem by arguing that components of phosphorylating systems that become artificially associated with membrane fragments during subcellular fractionation may prove amenable to dissociation by centrifugally washing the fragments with high concentrations of neutral salts. Loss of phosphorylating capacity toward an acceptor by washing before labeling with ATP could then be interpreted as indicating extraction of the relevant protein kinase activity or of the acceptor or of both these components. To distinguish between the first two of these possibilities we also treated labeled membranes with salt solutions. Preliminary results indicate that the acceptor O_{3a} (>300 K) is loosely associated with the membrane fragments, since it is almost entirely removed, in both labeled and unlabeled material, by a single wash with 250 mM NaCl. A phosphorylated polypeptide with similar mobility and properties was observed in synaptosomal membranes made from bovine brain by Lohmann et al. (49) and was identified by these workers as a microtubule-associated protein (MAP_2). It is reasonable to conclude, therefore, that O_{3a} is not an integral membrane polypeptide, but represents MAP_2 derived from the cytoplasm that becomes attached to the surface of the plasma membrane during or after cell disruption. By contrast, the following acceptors were not significantly extracted by salt solutions either before or after labeling: O_{3b} (254 K), α_3 (174 K), α_5 (143 K), β_6 (60 K), and γ_4 (50 K); these are therefore polypeptides that are either tightly bound peripheral proteins, integral to the membrane structure, or components of associated structures such as the postsynaptic densities. Further, on present evidence it would seem that their associated protein kinases have similar tight or integral associations. The remaining acceptors gave intermediate results. Of particular interest is the finding that a single NaCl wash removed more than 50% of protein I both before and after labeling, and the loss was greater using membranes phosphorylated in the presence of Ca^{2+} plus calmodulin.

Extrasynaptosomal Location of Phosphorylated Polypeptides

The degree of contamination of synaptosomal membrane fractions has proved difficult to determine accurately, mainly because of a lack of satisfactory markers to distinguish synaptic plasma membrane fragments from axolemmal fragments. For this reason, following Dunkley (18), we have referred to our preparation as one of fragments of "synaptosomal membranes" rather than of the usual "synaptic plasma membranes." Electron microscopy of our preparation (68) shows it to consist of smooth membrane fragments, many of which have formed vesicles, frequent junctional elements, and occasional mitochondria, myelin fragments, and synaptic vesicles.

One way to assess the specificity of the Ca^{2+}-dependent protein phosphorylation pattern for synaptic membranes is to compare it with the phosphorylation pattern in other cellular components. Thus if a phosphorylated polypeptide proves characteristic or is enriched in a particular component, then only a very minor contamination of the synaptosomal membrane fraction with this particle will give a misleading impression. Together with others (20) we have examined phosphorylation patterns in the following extrasynaptic cell particles: mitochondria, myelin, ribosomes, nuclei, and nonsynaptic neuronal membrane fragments prepared from dorsal root ganglia.

Pure mitochondria (obtained by several low-speed centrifugal washings of the crude mitochondrial fraction from the gradient) exhibited on phosphorylation with $[^{32}P]$ATP only two phosphorylated polypeptides of molecular weights ~40,000 and ~32,000. The former has been identified by several workers (5,50,55) as the α-subunit of the enzyme pyruvate dehydrogenase (PDH) and the latter as a component of succinyl CoA-synthetase (81). Both polypeptides sometimes occur in trace amounts in preparations of synaptosomal membranes. This applies particularly to the PDH subunit, although the possibility of confusion with phosphorylated actin, which possesses an almost identical mobility, has to be considered (27,29). Although more work is needed to distinguish these two polypeptides, it is probable that the ~40,000 M.W. acceptor seen by most workers in relatively crude preparations is the α-subunit of PDH. Recent evidence (4,6), discussed below, suggests that this polypeptide, although of mitochondrial origin, may play an indirect role in modulating synaptic transmission in some situations.

As noted previously by several laboratories (e.g., 20,82), myelin fragments usually contain only endogenously phosphorylated acceptors of <30,000 M.W., including two components of myelin basic protein (82). However, some preparations do contain traces of a polypeptide of molecular weight about 48,000 phosphorylated by a cyclic AMP protein kinase; mixed with synaptosomal membranes this acceptor migrates to a position between γ_4 (50 K) and γ_5 (45 K), which makes it unlikely that it is identical with the regulatory subunit of cyclic AMP-dependent protein kinase, as suggested by Sulakhe et al. (82).

Ribosomes and nuclei prepared from brain and washed free of contaminating particles yield a distinctive pattern of endogenous phosphorylation, the overall level of which is much lower than in synaptosomal membranes and that cannot account for any of the typical acceptors observed in the latter. Membrane fragments prepared from rat dorsal root ganglia, a neural structure lacking synapses, contain polypeptides in the molecular weight range 20,000–35,000 that are phosphorylated mainly by basal protein kinase activity (68). No direct information is available on the level and pattern of phosphorylation in glial cell membranes, but indirect evidence suggests any contribution from this source to be negligible. In particular, the effectiveness of adequate doses of the neurotoxin, kainic acid, in abolishing the typical phosphorylation pattern (75,76) supports this conclusion, because membrane preparations made from kainate-treated tissue are presumably grossly contaminated with glial membrane fragments. Also, membrane preparations made from C-6 glioma cell cultures and astrocytoma tissue contain only a very low level of endogenous protein phosphorylating systems (R. Rodnight, *unpublished observations*). With the exception of the special case of O_{3a}, which we accept is MAP_2, there seems no reason to suspect that any of the phosphorylated polypeptides listed in Table 1 is derived to any significant degree from extrasynaptosomal sources.

Subsynaptic Location of Phosphorylated Polypeptides

For present purposes there are four locations we need to consider: synaptic vesicles, presynaptic membranes, postsynaptic membranes, and postsynaptic densities. The first two structures are presumably involved in transmitter release and the second two with postsynaptic functions, although the existence of presynaptic receptors complicates the situation. Of the polypeptides in Table 1 phosphorylated by Ca^{2+}-activated protein kinase activity evidence is available for the location of protein I, β_6 (60 K), γ_4 (50 K), and more controversially, for B-50.

The most definitive evidence relates to protein I, which, as mentioned in the introduction, appears to be mainly, if not exclusively, located in the limiting membrane of synaptic vesicles (3,86). Earlier reports (3) that protein I also occurs in postsynaptic densities now have to be treated with caution in view of the work of Matus (52), but should not be entirely discounted. It is also uncertain whether the presence of protein I is a universal feature of CNS synapses or restricted to certain types only (16). Our own work supports the conclusion that the protein I system has a presynaptic location and is absent in postsynaptic densities because in unlysed synaptosomes these structures may be presumed to be accessible to ATP (Fig. 5). The relatively high content of protein I in synaptosomal membrane fragments is more difficult to explain, however. It is true that the concentration of protein I in purified synaptic vesicle preparations is at least 20 times that in the membrane preparation (86), but this level would still require a considerable degree of contamination of the latter with vesicles to account for the apparent protein I content of membranes. One possibility would be that membrane-located protein I is derived from vesicles that have fused with the presynaptic membrane during excytosis, but no clear consensus exists as to whether vesicular proteins are so incorporated (2,80).

The presence of other polypeptide substrates for Ca^{2+}-calmodulin-dependent protein kinase activity in synaptic vesicles is somewhat controversial. We have not been able to detect in vesicles prepared by conventional methods any other acceptors apart from protein I and the basally phosphorylated $\gamma_3(52K)$. DeLorenzo and co-workers (13–15), on the other hand, present evidence for vesicles containing two substrates for Ca^{2+}-calmodulin-dependent kinase, designated DPH-L and DPH-M and with molecular weights of ~62,000 and ~52,000, respectively. The method used by these workers for preparing vesicles involves a long series of differential centrifugation in salt solutions and is therefore radically different from the usual gradient procedures in sucrose solutions. The DeLorenzo procedure does yield a vesicle preparation that apparently contains a relatively high content of neurotransmitters, but in our view is more likely by its nature to give a contaminated product. Whether the methodological difference accounts for the discrepancy in results is unclear at present, but it appears very likely that DPH-L and DPH-M are identical with the acceptors $\beta_6(60K)$ and $\gamma_4(50K)$ present in standard synaptosomal membrane preparations and that, from evidence summarised below, seem to be located primarily in the postsynaptic densities (24), and, at rather low concentrations, in the soluble fraction (59). Replication of the works of this group is urgently required as it forms the basis of an imaginative speculation (13) on molecular roles for Ca^{2+} and calmodulin in neurotransmitter release mechanisms.

The evidence for the main location of the major substrates for Ca^{2+}-calmodulin-dependent kinase activity (α_3-174K, β_6-60K, β_7-57K, and γ_4-50K) being in postsynaptic structures is of several kinds. Thus they are all absent in membrane preparations made from striatal tissue lesioned with kainic acid and they are all phosphorylated by exposure of intact synaptosomes to ATP (Fig. 5). Moreover, from the work of Siekevitz's group it appears that $\beta_6(60K)$, $\beta_7(57K)$, and $\gamma_4(50K)$ occur together with their associated kinases in high concentrations in pure preparations of postsynaptic densities made from cerebral cortex tissue, where they are assigned molecular weights of 62,000, 58,000, and 51,000, respectively (24). According to these authors the 51,000 M.W. acceptor may in fact be unique to postsynaptic densities and identical to the major, highly insoluble protein of these structures. This accords well with our observation (Fig. 4) that in the rat the development of this phosphorylating system is delayed until the onset of synaptogenesis and the appearance of synaptic densities. With regard to the 62,000 M.W. acceptor (β_6-60K, in our work) Grab et al. (24) have reported tentative evidence that this polypeptide may represent the catalytic subunit of the Ca^{2+}-calmodulin-dependent cyclic nucleotide phosphodiesterase: both polypeptides migrate to the same position on polyacrylamide gels and both bind calmodulin. Further evidence supporting a location for $\gamma_4(50K)$ in postsynaptic densities comes from regional studies: synaptosomal membranes prepared from rat cerebellum are deficient in this acceptor and/or its kinase (R. Rodnight and L. Martinez-Millan, *unpublished ob-*

servations), as are purified postsynaptic densities from this brain region (24). Cerebellar postsynaptic densities are also deficient in calmodulin and are structurally dissimilar from cerebral cortical densities (8). Synaptosomal membrane fragments from cerebral cortex and cerebellar cortex do, however, contain similar contents of phosphorylating activity toward β_6(60K), but in the cerebellar preparation we find that the β_7(57K) system is equal in activity to β_6(60K) *(unpublished observations; see Fig. 1 for the relative activities in cerebral cortical fragments). If β_6(60K) is indeed the catalytic subunit of a cyclic nucleotide phosphodiesterase, as Grab et al. (24) suggest, its wider distribution as well as its more gradual ontogeny (Fig. 4), would be understandable. One final word about the α_3 (174K) system, which may also turn out to be a component of postsynaptic densities. This is suggested because it is conspicuously absent in cerebellar membranes (67, see Fig. 2 of this paper, where the α_3 peak is labeled 162 $\times$ 10^{-3} M.W.) and because it also develops in parallel with the γ_4(50K) system (30).

The question of the cellular location of the B-50 system is a conundrum. Immunocytochemical evidence from the Utrecht group (60) using rat cerebellum indicates a high concentration in the synapse-rich molecular layer, relatively little in the granular layer and none in white matter. Mahler's group consider it has a presynaptic location (79) and our own studies are in some respects consistent with this conclusion: thus it is not labeled by ATP incubated with intact synaptosomes and it is consistently associated with light rather than heavy membrane fragments (R. Rodnight, *unpublished observations*). Also, the fact that the B-50 system survives kainate-induced lesions of the striatum could be interpreted as indicating a presynaptic location, although we originally thought that this experiment pointed to a location in oligodendroglia. However, a specific location in dopaminergic terminals is excluded by an observation that its activity is not decreased by lesions made with 6-hydroxydopamine. The main difficulty in ascribing a purely synaptic location to this phosphorylating system, however, lies in its presence, apparently in high concentration, in immature rat brain many days before the onset of synaptogenesis.

Speculations on Functional Implications

Sensitivity to Ca^{2+} is a striking feature of the Ca^{2+}-calmodulin-dependent protein kinase activity in synaptosomal membranes (Fig. 3). The very narrow range over which activation occurs, and its correspondence with intraneuronal free Ca^{2+} concentration, suggests that small fluctuations in the latter will result in major changes in the phosphorylation state of synaptic proteins. This appears to apply equally to protein I, which has a presynaptic location, and to γ_4(50K), which is located in some postsynaptic densities. However, the protein kinase activities responsible for phosphorylation in the two situations are distinguished by their sensitivities to Mg^{2+}, in that the presynaptically located protein I system is progressively inhibited by increasing concentrations of this cation. Preliminary evidence indicates that this effect of Mg^{2+} is competitive, since lower concentrations of free Ca^{2+} shift the optimum Mg^{2+} concentration to the left. This is of particular interest in view of the well-known fact that the process of transmitter release is inhibited, competitively with Ca^{2+}, by increasing extracellular Mg^{2+} concentration (64).

Two features of protein I—its location in vesicles and the sensitivity of its associated kinase to high Mg^{2+}—strongly suggest it is involved in some aspect of transmitter release. This conclusion is supported by the observations of Greengard's group (22,38) on the Ca^{2+}-dependent depolarisation-induced phosphorylation of protein I in brain slices and synaptosomes. We have replicated this work using field electrical stimulation of synaptosomes instead of high K^+ or veratradine as the depolarising agent (D. De Souza and R. Rodnight, *unpublished observations*). However, although some direct evidence for an involvement of Ca^{2+}-dependent protein phosphorylation in secretory process has been obtained from nonneuronal systems (72,77), it would be premature to assume that the Ca^{2+}-dependent phosphorylation of protein I is directly involved in a general mechanism of transmitter release in the CNS. Even if the exocytotic hypothesis is accepted there are obvious difficulties, for it seems possible that protein I is not a universal feature of all CNS synapses (16). Further, a hypothetical phosphorylation step has to take into account the speed of transmitter release for acetylcholine which, in the neuromuscular junction, is of the order of microseconds (45). It seems more likely therefore that protein I is concerned in some modulatory aspect of the release of certain transmitters, as suggested from experiments in *Aplysia* by Castellucci et al. (9), rather than in a universal mechanism of exocytotic release.

The possibility of membrane-located, rather than vesicle-located protein phosphorylation being an accessory factor in a release mechanism is worth a brief comment. Michaelson and Avissar (54) found that depolarisation-induced release of acetylcholine from *Torpedo* synaptosomes was associated under a variety of circumstances with the phosphorylation of a 100,000 M.W. protein, which they tentatively suggest may be a subunit of a Ca^{2+}-ATPase. Inhibition of the membrane Na^+, K^+-ATPase by Ca^{2+} has been proposed (53) as the first step in a mechanism for acetylcholine release, which would appear to be more relevant to a nonexocytotic hypothesis of transmitter release (51). The possibility that the Na^+, K^+-ATPase is regulated by the esteric phosphorylation of an hydroxyamino acid has been considered from time to time, but no satisfactory evidence has been forthcoming. It would be of interest to know whether the inhibition of Na^+, K^+-ATPase activity by Ca^{2+} is enhanced by calmodulin.

Turning to the postsynaptic site, even less is known in this situation about the molecular consequences of Ca^{2+} fluxes. As already noted, Ca^{2+} and calmodulin are concerned in the regulation of the metabolism of cyclic nucleotides through activation of the two cyclases and high-K_m cyclic nucleotide phosphoesterase, but it remains uncertain whether such regulation occurs as a direct consequence of Ca^{2+} entry associated with synaptic potentials or secondarily, e.g., following intracellular events that perturb the balance of Ca^{2+} stores. Nor is it known whether the effects of Ca^{2+} and calmodulin on these enzymes of cyclic nucleotide metabolism involve a phosphorylation step. It is of interest to note, however, that evidence for an effect of protein phosphorylation on the activity of Ca^{2+} channels is available: thus the intracellular injection of the catalytic subunit of a cyclic AMP-dependent protein kinase into bag cell neurones of *Aplysia* in cell culture enhanced Ca^{2+}-dependent action potentials (35).

The virtual absence in cerebellum of γ_4(50K), according to Grab et al. (24) a major postsynaptic density protein, is of particular interest, as it suggests that this polypeptide is specifically associated with certain types of synapse. Detailed regional studies of the location of this acceptor in relation to neurotransmitter content are needed. Is the absence of cholinergic synapses in the cerebellum of significance here?

Long-term potentiation and heterosynaptic facilitation are two aspects of synaptic transmission that conceivably may be regulated by the phosphorylation state of membrane protein. However, when the possibility was investigated in brain slices (6), changes in the phosphorylation state of a mitochondrial protein were observed. Thus electrical stimulation of hippocampal slices with pulses that resulted in long-term potentiation of synaptic transmission led to an increased phosphorylation of the α-subunit of PDH. This change in phosphorylation was assessed by a "post hoc" endogenous phosphorylation assay that showed that the appropriate stimulus conditions led, in a particulate fraction from the incubated tissues, to a decreased incorporation of ^{32}P from [^{32}P]ATP into PDH, presumably as a result of enhanced incorporation of cold phosphate having occurred in the intact tissue slice. The authors propose that long-term potentiation may be related to modulation of intracellular Ca^{2+} by neuronal mitochondria and that the enhanced phosphorylation of the PDH subunit following potentiation may be mediated by Ca^{2+} uptake. In support of this conclusion the drug trifluoperazine, which inhibits Ca^{2+}-calmodulin-dependent protein kinase activity, was found to block the effect of stimulation on both potentiation and the phosphorylation of the PDH subunit (21). However, the precise Ca^{2+}-calmodulin dependence of PDH kinase has not been firmly established.

The B-50 phosphorylation system possesses a number of features that set it apart from the other Ca^{2+}-dependent systems: maximum phosphorylation of the acceptor does not require calmodulin, and, as originally noted by Gispen's laboratory, the associated kinase activity is inhibited in a dose- and structure-dependent manner by fragments of ACTH (100,101). The effect of ACTH provided a clue to the biochemical function of the B-50 acceptor when it was found in separate experiments that similar concentrations of the same ACTH fragments stimulated in membrane preparations the conversion of the lipid diphosphoinositide (DPI) to triphosphosphoinositide (TPI). Further work showed that the B-50 polypeptide copurified with DPI kinase activity and that the rate of TPI formation catalysed by this enzyme was inversely related to the state of phosphorylation of B-50 (33). This suggested that the B-50 polypeptide is either a subunit or a regulatory factor associated with the DPI kinase, the activity of which is inhibited by phosphorylation. It is of interest to note that the polyphosphoinositides are potent chelators of Ca^{2+}, and, by virtue of their phosphate groups, carry a high proportion of the negative charge of membranes. Thus, as pointed out by Jolles et al. (33), changes in the relative amounts of the three phosphoinositides in membranes (MPI, DPI, and TPI) may affect both the conformation of membrane proteins and the quantity of Ca^{2+} bound to the membrane. Moreover, it appears that the B-50 polypeptide is phosphorylated by the "C" kinase of Takai et al. (83, *personal communication* from W. H. Gispen and co-workers), which is also stimulated in a Ca^{2+}-dependent fashion by diacylglycerols derived from the hydrolysis of phosphoinositide. The significance of these observations for the well known receptor-mediated phosphoinositide response in cell membranes remains to be elucidated.

ACKNOWLEDGMENT

We are grateful to the Medical Research Council of the UK for support for part of this work.

REFERENCES

1. Aghajanian, G. K., and Bloom, F. E. (1967): The formation of synaptic junctions in developing rat brains: A quantitative electron microscopic study. *Brain Res.*, 6:716–727.
2. Babitch, J. A., and Benavides, L. A. (1979): Comparison of synaptic plasma membrane and synaptic vesicle polypeptides by two-dimensional polyacrylamide gel electrophoresis. *Neuroscience*, 4:603–613.
3. Bloom, F. E., Ueda, T., Battenberg, E., and Greengard, P. (1979): Immunocytochemical localisation in synapses of protein I, an endogenous substrate for protein kinases in mammalian brain. *Proc. Natl. Acad. Sci. USA*, 76:5982–5986.
4. Browning, M., Baudry, M., Bennett, W. F., and Lynch, G. (1981): Phosphorylation mediated changes in pyruvate dehydrogenase activity influence pyruvate-supported calcium accumulation in brain mitochondria. *J. Neurochem.*, 36:1932–1940.
5. Browning, M., Bennett, W. F., Kelly, P., and Lynch, G. (1981): The 40000 M_r phosphoprotein influenced by high frequency synaptic stimulation is the alpha-subunit of pyruvate dehydrogenase. *Brain Res.*, 218:255–266.
6. Browning, M., Dunwiddie, T., Bennett, W. F., Gispen, W. H., and Lynch, G. (1979): Synaptic phosphoproteins: Specific changes after repetitive stimulation of the hippocampal slice. *Science*, 203:60–62.
7. Brunner, G., Bauer, H. C., Sater, D., and Speth, V. (1978): Artefacts produced during plasma membrane isolation. I. Cell disruption causes alteration in the structure of the plasma membrane of thymocytes. *Biochim. Biophys. Acta*, 507:419–424.
8. Carlin, R. K., Grab, D. J., and Siekevitz, P. (1980): Isolation and characterization of postsynaptic densities from various brain regions: Enrichment of different types of postsynaptic densities. *J. Cell Biol.*, 86:831–843.
9. Castellucci, V. F., Kandel, E. R., Schwartz, J. H., Wilson, F. D., Nairn, A. C., and Greengard, P. (1980): Intracellular injection of the catalytic subunit of cyclic AMP-dependent protein kinase stimulates facilitation of transmitter release underlying behavioral sensitization in *Aplysia*. *Proc. Natl. Acad. Sci. USA*, 77:7492–7496.
10. Cheung, W. Y. (1980): Calmodulin plays a pivotal role in cellular regulation. *Science*, 207:19–27.
11. Cohen, P. (ed.) (1980): *Recently Discovered Systems of Enzyme Regulation by Reversible Phosphorylation*. Elsevier/North Holland, Amsterdam.
12. DeCamilli, P., Ueda, T., Bloom, F. E., Battenberg, E., and Greengard, P. (1979): Widespread distribution of protein I in the central and peripheral nervous system. *Proc. Natl. Acad. Sci. USA*, 76:5977–5981.
13. DeLorenzo, R. J. (1981): Calcium, calmodulin and synaptic function: Modulation of neurotransmitter release, nerve terminal protein phosphorylation and synaptic vesicle morphology by calcium and calmodulin. In: *Regulatory Mechanisms of Synaptic Transmission*, edited by R. Tapia and C. W. Cotman, pp. 205–239. Plenum Press, New York.

14. DeLorenzo, R. J., and Freedman, S. D. (1977): Calcium-dependent phosphorylation of synaptic vesicle proteins and its possible role in mediating neurotransmitter release and vesicle function. *Biochem. Biophys. Res. Commun.*, 77:1036–1043.

15. DeLorenzo, R. J., Freedman, S. D., Yohe, W. B., and Maurer, S. C. (1979): Stimulation of Ca²⁺-dependent neurotransmitter release and presynaptic nerve terminal protein phosphorylation by calmodulin and a calmodulin-like protein isolated from synaptic vesicles. *Proc. Natl. Acad. Sci. USA*, 76:1838–1842.

16. Dolphin, A. C., and Greengard, P. (1981): Presence of protein I, a phosphoprotein associated with synaptic vesicles, in cerebellar granule cells. *J. Neurochem.*, 36:1627–1631.

17. Downes, P., and Michell, R. H. (1981): Human erythrocyte membranes exhibit a co-operative calmodulin-dependent Ca²⁺-ATPase of high calcium sensitivity. *Nature (Lond.)*, 290:270–271.

18. Dunkley, P. R. (1981): Phosphorylation of synaptosomal membrane proteins and evaluation of nerve cell function. In: *New Approaches to Nerve and Muscle Disorders. Basic and Applied Contributions*, edited by A. D. Kidman, J. K. Tomkins, and R. A. Westerman, pp. 38–51. Excerpta Medica, Amsterdam.

19. England, P. J. (1980): Protein phosphorylation in the regulation of muscle contraction. In: *Recently Discovered Systems of Enzyme Regulation by Reversible Phosphorylation*, edited by P. Cohen, pp. 153–173. Elsevier/North-Holland, Amsterdam.

20. Ehrlich, Y. H., Davis, L. G., Gilfoil, T., and Brunngraber, E. G. (1977): Distribution of endogenously phosphorylated proteins in subcellular fractions of rat cerebral cortex. *Neurochem. Res.*, 2:533–548.

21. Finn, R., Browning, M., and Lynch, G. (1980): Trifluoperazine inhibits hippocampal long-term potentiation and the phosphorylation of a 40000 dalton protein. *Neurosci. Lett.*, 19:103–108.

22. Forn, J., and Greengard, P. (1978): Depolarizing agents and cyclic nucleotides regulate the phosphorylation of specific neuronal proteins in rat cerebral cortex slices. *Proc. Natl. Acad. Sci. USA*, 75:5195–5199.

22a. Gower, H., and Rodnight, R. (1982): Intrinsic protein phosphorylation in synapic plasma membrane fragments from the rat. General characteristics and migration behaviour on polyacrylamide gels of the main phosphate acceptors. *Biochem. Biophys. Acta*, 716:45–52.

23. Grab, D. J., Berzins, R. J., Cohen, R. S., and Siekevitz, P. (1979): Presence of calmodulin in postsynaptic densities isolated from canine cerebral cortex. *J. Biol. Chem.*, 254:8690–8696.

24. Grab, D. J., Carlin, R. K., and Siekevitz, P. (1981): Function of calmodulin in postsynaptic densities. II. Presence of calmodulin-activatable protein kinase activity. *J. Cell Biol.*, 89:440–448.

25. Greengard, P. (1978): *Cyclic Nucleotides, Phosphorylated Proteins and Neuronal Function*. Raven Press, New York.

26. Hattori, T., and McGeer, E. G. (1977): Fine structural changes in the rat striatum after local injection of kainic acid. *Brain Res.*, 129:174–180.

27. Hershkowitz, M. (1978): Influence of calcium on phosphorylation of a synaptosomal protein. *Biochim. Biophys. Acta*, 542:274–283.

28. Hitzemann, R. J., and Loh, H. H. (1978): High affinity GABA and glutamate transport in developing nerve ending particles. *Brain Res.*, 159:29–40.

29. Hofstein, R., Hershkowitz, M., Gozes, I., and Samuel, D. (1980): The characterization and phosphorylation of an actin-like protein in synaptosomal membranes. *Biochim. Biophys. Acta*, 624:153–162.

30. Holmes, H., and Rodnight, R. (1981): Ontogeny of membrane bound protein phosphorylating systems in the rat. *Dev. Neurosci.*, 4:79–88.

31. Huttner, W. B., DeGennaro, L. J., and Greengard, P. (1981): Differential phosphorylation of multiple sites in purified protein I by cyclic AMP-dependent and calcium-dependent protein kinases. *J. Biol. Chem.*, 256:1482–1491.

32. Huttner, W. B., and Greengard, P. (1979): Multiple phosphorylation sites in protein I and their differential regulation by cyclic AMP and calcium. *Proc. Natl. Acad. Sci. USA*, 76:5402–5406.

33. Jolles, J., Zwiers, H., van Dongen, J. J., Schotman, P., Wirtz, K. W. A., and Gispen, W. H. (1980): Modulation of brain phosphoinositide metabolism by ACTH-sensitive protein phosphorylation. *Nature (Lond.)*, 286:623–626.

34. Jones, D. H., and Matus, A. I. (1974): Isolation of synaptic plasma membrane from brain by combined flotation-sedimentation density gradient centrifugation. *Biochim. Biophys. Acta*, 356:276–287.

35. Kaczmarek, L. K., Jennings, K. R., Strummwasser, F., Nairn, A. C., Walter, U., Wilson, F. D., and Greengard, P. (1980): Microinjection of catalytic subunit of cyclic AMP-dependent protein kinase enhances calcium action potentials of bag cell neurons in cell culture. *Proc. Natl. Acad. Sci. USA*, 77:7487–7491.

36. Kennedy, M. B., and Greengard, P. (1981): Two calcium/calmodulin dependent protein kinases which are highly concentrated in brain phosphorylate protein I at distinct sites. *Proc. Natl. Acad. Sci. USA*, 78:1293–1297.

37. Klee, C. B., Crouch, T. H., and Richman, P. G. (1980): Calmodulin. *Annu. Rev. Biochem.*, 49:489–515.

38. Krueger, B. K., Forn, J., and Greengard, P. (1977): Depolarization-induced phosphorylation of specific proteins mediated by calcium ion flux, in rat brain synaptosomes. *J. Biol. Chem.*, 252:2764–2773.

39. Kuhn, D. M., O'Callaghan, J. P., Juskevich, J., and Lovenberg, W. (1980): Activation of brain tryptophan hydroxylase by ATP-Mg²⁺: Dependence on calmodulin. *Proc. Natl. Acad. Sci. USA*, 77:4688–4691.

40. Kuo, C.-H., Ichida, S., Matsuda, T., Kakiuchi, S., and Yoshida, H. (1979): Regulation of ATP-dependent Ca-uptake of synaptic plasma membranes by Ca-dependent modulator protein. *Life Sci.*, 25:235–240.

41. Kuo, J. F., Andersson, R. G. G., Wise, B. C., Mackerlova, L., Salomonsson, I., Brackett, N. L., Katoh, N., Shoji, M., and Wrenn, R. W. (1980): Calcium-dependent protein kinase: Widespread occurrence in various tissues and phyla of the animal kingdom and comparison of effects of phospholipid, calmodulin and trifluoperazine. *Proc. Natl. Acad. Sci. USA*, 77:7039–7043.

42. Landt, M., and McDonald, J. M. (1980): Calmodulin-activated protein kinase activity of adipocyte microsomes. *Biochem. Biophys. Res. Commun.*, 93:881–888.

43. LePeuch, C. J., Haiech, J., and Demaille, J. G. (1979): Concerted regulation of cardiac sarcoplasmic reticulum calcium transport by cyclic adenosine monophosphate-dependent and calcium-dependent phosphorylations. *Biochemistry*, 18:5150–5157.

44. Lin, C.-T., Dedman, J. R., Brinkley, B. R., and Means, A. R. (1980): Localization of calmodulin in rat cerebellum by immuno-electron microscopy. *J. Cell Biol.*, 85:473–480.

45. Llinas, R. (1979): The role of calcium in neuronal function. In: *The Neurosciences. Fourth Study Program*, edited by F. O. Schmitt and F. G. Worden, pp. 555–571. MIT Press, Cambridge, Massachusetts.

46. Llinas, R., Steinberg, I. Z., and Walton, K. (1976): Presynaptic calcium currents and their relation to synaptic transmission; voltage clamp study in squid giant axon and theoretical model for calcium gate. *Proc. Natl. Acad. Sci. USA*, 73:2918–2922.

47. Lohmann, S. M., Ueda, T., and Greengard, P. (1978): Ontogeny of synaptic phosphoproteins in brain. *Proc. Natl. Acad. Sci. USA*, 75:4037–4041.

48. Lohmann, S. M., Walter, U., and Greengard, P. (1978): Protein kinases in developing rat brain. *J. Cyclic Nucleotide Res.*, 4:445–452.

49. Lohmann, S. M., Walter, U., and Greengard, P. (1980): Identification of endogenous substrate proteins for cAMP-dependent protein kinase in bovine brain. *J. Biol. Chem.*, 255:9985–9992.

50. Magilen, G., Gordon, A., Au, A., and Diamond, I. (1981): Identification of mitochondrial phosphoprotein in brain synaptic membrane preparations. *J. Neurochem.*, 36:1861–1864.

51. Marchbanks, R. M. (1979): Role of storage vesicles in synaptic transmission. In: *Society for Experimental Biology Symposium XXXIII. Secretory Mechanisms*, edited by C. R. Hopkins and C. J. Duncan, pp. 251–276. CUP, Cambridge, U.K.

52. Matus, A., Pehling, G., Ackermann, M., and Maeder, J. (1980): Brain postsynaptic densities: Their relationship to glial and neuronal filaments. *J. Cell. Biol.*, 87:346–359.

53. Meyer, E. M., and Cooper, J. R. (1981): Correlations between Na⁺, K⁺-ATPase activity and acetylcholine release in rat cortical synaptosomes. *J. Neurochem.*, 36:467–475.

54. Michaelson, D. M., and Avissar, S. (1979): Ca²⁺-dependent protein phosphorylation of purely cholinergic Torpedo synaptosomes. *J. Biol. Chem.*, 254:12542–12546.

55. Morgan, D. G., and Routtenberg, A. (1980): Evidence that a 41000 dalton brain phosphoprotein is pyruvate dehydrogenase. *Biochem. Biophys. Res. Commun.*, 95:569–576.

56. Nairn, A. C., and Perry, S. V. (1979): Role of calmodulin in the myosin light chain kinase systems. *Biochem. Soc. Trans.*, 7:966–967.

57. Niggli, V., Adunyah, E. S., Penniston, J. T., and Carofoli, E. (1981): Purified (Ca²⁺, Mg²⁺)ATPase of the erythrocyte membrane. Reconstitution and effects of calmodulin and phospholipids. *J. Biol. Chem.*, 256:395–401.

58. Nishida, E., Kumagai, Y., Ohtsuki, I., and Sakai, H. (1979): The interaction between calcium-dependent regulatory protein of cyclic nucleotide phosphodiesterase and microtubule proteins. I. Effect of calcium-dependent regulatory protein on the calcium-sensitivity of microtubule assembly. *J. Biochem. (Jpn.)*, 85:1257–1266.

59. O'Callaghan, J. P., Dunn, L. A., and Lovenberg, W. (1980): Calcium-regulated phosphorylation in synaptosomal cytosol: Dependence on calmodulin. *Proc. Natl. Acad. Sci. USA*, 77:5812–5816.

60. Oestreicher, A. B., Zwiers, H., Schotman, P., and Gispen, W. H. (1981): Immunohistochemical localisation of a phosphoprotein (B-50) isolated from rat brain synaptosomal plasma membranes. *Brain Res. Bull.*, 6:145–153.

61. Perrin, D. D., and Sayce, I. G. (1967): Computer calculation of equilibrium concentrations in mixtures of metal ions and complexing species. *Talanta*, 14:833–842.

62. Pershadsingh, H. A., Landt, M., and McDonald, M. (1980): Calmodulin-sensitive ATP-dependent Ca²⁺ transport across adipocyte membranes. *J. Biol. Chem.*, 255:8983–8986.

63. Potter, P., and White, T. D. (1980): Release of adenosine triphosphate from synaptosomes from different regions of rat brain. *Neuroscience*, 5:1351–1356.

64. Rahaminoff, R. (1974): Modulation of transmitter release at the neuromuscular junction. In: *The Neurosciences. Third Study Program*, edited by F. O. Schmitt and F. G. Worden, pp. 943–952. MIT Press, Cambridge, Massachusetts.

65. Rodnight, R. (1979): Cyclic nucleotides as second messengers in synaptic transmission. *Int. Rev. Biochem.*, 26:1–80.

66. Rodnight, R. (1980): Cyclic nucleotides, calcium ions and protein phosphorylation in synaptic transmission. In: *Synaptic Constituents in Health and Disease*, edited by M. Brzin, D. Sket, and H. Bachelard, pp. 81–96. Pergamon Press, Oxford.

67. Rodnight, R. (1980): Molecular aspects of the actions of cyclic nucleotides at synapses. *Neurochem. Int.*, 2:113–122.

68. Rodnight, R. (1981): Molecular aspects of brain function. In: *Investigations of Brain Function*, edited by A. W. Wilkinson, pp. 197–215. Plenum Press, New York.

69. Roufogalis, B. D. (1980): Calmodulin: Its role in synaptic transmission. *Trends Neurosci.*, 3:238–241.

70. Rubin, R. P. (1974): *Calcium and the Secretory Process.* Plenum Press, New York.

71. Scholey, J. M., Taylor, K. A., and Kendrick-Jones, J. (1980): Regulation of non-muscle assembly by calmodulin-dependent light chain kinase. *Nature (Lond.)*, 287:233–235.

72. Schubart, U. K., Fleischer, N., and Erlichman, J. (1980): Ca²⁺-dependent protein phosphorylation and insulin release in intact hamster insuloma cells. *J. Biol. Chem.*, 255:11063–11066.

73. Schulman, H., and Greengard, P. (1978): Ca²⁺-dependent protein phosphorylation system in membranes from various tissues, and its activation by "calcium-dependent regulator." *Proc. Natl. Acad. Sci. USA*, 75:5432–5436.

74. Schwarcz, R., and Coyle, J. T. (1978): Striatal lesions with kainic acid: Neurochemical characteristics. *Brain Res.*, 127:235–249.

75. Sieghart, W., Forn, J., Schwarcz, R., Coyle, J. T., and Greengard, P. (1978): Neuronal localisation of specific brain phosphoproteins. *Brain Res.*, 156:345–350.

76. Sieghart, W., Schulman, H., and Greengard, P. (1980): Neuronal localisation of Ca²⁺-dependent protein phosphorylation in brain. *J. Neurochem.*, 34:548–553.

77. Sieghart, W., Theoharides, T. C., Alpen, S. L., Douglas, W. W., and Greengard, P. (1978): Ca²⁺-dependent protein phosphorylation during secretion by exocytosis in the mast cell. *Nature (Lond.)*, 275:329–331.

78. Sobue, K., Ichida, S., Yoshida, H., Yamazaki, R., and Kakiuchi, S. (1979): Occurrence of a Ca²⁺- and modulator protein-activatable ATPase in the synaptic plasma membranes of brain. *FEBS Lett.*, 99:199–202.

79. Sorenson, R. G., Kleine, L. P., and Mahler, H. R. (1981): Presynaptic localisation of phosphoprotein B-50. *Brain Res. Bull.*, 7:57–61.

80. Stadler, H., and Tashiro, T. (1979): Isolation of synaptosomal plasma membrane from cholinergic nerve terminals and a comparison of their proteins with those of synaptic vesicles. *Eur. J. Biochem.*, 101:171–178.

81. Steiner, A. W., and Smith, R. A. (1981): Endogenous protein phosphorylation in rat brain mitochondria: Occurrence of a novel ATP-dependent form of the autophosphorylated enzyme succinyl CoA synthetase. *J. Neurochem.*, 37:582–590.

82. Sulakhe, P. V., Petrali, E. H., Davis, E. R., and Thiessen, B. J. (1980): Calcium-ion stimulated endogenous protein kinase catalyzed phosphorylation of basic proteins in myelin subfractions and myelin-like membrane fraction from rat brain. *Biochemistry*, 19:5363–5371.

83. Takai, Y., Kishimoto, A., Iwasa, Y., Kawahara, Y., Mori, T., and Nishizuka, Y. (1979): Calcium-dependent activation of a multifunctional protein kinase by membrane phospholipids. *J. Biol. Chem.*, 254:3692–3695.
84. Ueda, T. (1981): Attachment of the synapse-specific phosphoprotein I to the synaptic membrane: A possible role of the collagenase-sensitive region of protein I. *J. Neurochem.*, 36:297–300.
85. Ueda, T., and Greengard, P. (1977): Adenosine 3′:5′-monophosphate regulated phosphoprotein system of neuronal membranes. I. Solubilization, purification and some properties of an endogenous phosphoprotein. *J. Biol. Chem.*, 252:5155–5163.
86. Ueda, T., Greengard, P., Berzins, K., Cohen, R. S., Blomberg, F., Grab, D. J., and Siekevitz, P. (1979): Subcellular distribution in cerebral cortex of two proteins phosphorylated by a cyclic AMP-dependent protein kinase. *J. Cell. Biol.*, 83:308–319.
87. Uno, I., Ueda, T., and Greengard, P. (1977): Adenosine 3′:5′-monophosphate regulated phosphoprotein system of neuronal membranes. II. Solubilization, purification and some properties of an endogenous 3′:5′-monophosphate-dependent protein kinase. *J. Biol. Chem.*, 252:5164–5174.
88. Waisman, D. M., Gimble, J. M., Goodman, D. B. P., and Rasmussen, H. (1981): Studies of the Ca²⁺-transport mechanism of human erythrocyte inside-out plasma membrane vesicles. I. Regulation of the pump by calmodulin. *J. Biol. Chem.*, 256:409–414.
89. Waisman, D. M., Singh, T. J., and Wang, J. H. (1978): The modulator-dependent protein kinase. A multifunctional protein kinase activatable by the calcium dependent modulator protein of the cyclic nucleotide system. *J. Biol. Chem.*, 253:3387–3390.
90. Wallace, R. W., Tallant, E. A., and Cheung, W. Y. (1980): High levels of a heat-labile calmodulin binding protein in bovine neostriatum. *Biochemistry*, 19:1831–1837.
91. Walsh, M., and Stevens, F. C. (1978): Preparation, characteristics and properties of a novel triple-modified derivative of the Ca²⁺-dependent protein modulator. *Can. J. Biochem.*, 56:420–429.
92. Walter, U., Kanof, P., Schulman, H., and Greengard, P. (1978): Adenosine 3′:5′-monophosphate receptor proteins in mammalian brain. *J. Biol. Chem.*, 253:6275–6280.
93. Walter, U., Lohmann, S. M., Sieghart, W., and Greengard, P. (1979): Identification of the cyclic AMP-dependent protein kinase responsible for the endogenous phosphorylation of substrate proteins in synaptic membrane fraction from rat brain. *J. Biol. Chem.*, 254:12235–12239.
94. Weller, M. (1977): Evidence for the presynaptic location of adenylate cyclase and cyclic AMP-stimulated protein kinase which is bound to synaptic membranes. *Biochim. Biophys. Acta*, 469:350–354.
95. Weller, M. (1979): *Protein Phosphorylation*. Pion Ltd., London.
96. Williams, M., and Rodnight, R. (1977): Protein phosphorylation in nervous tissue: Possible involvement in nervous tissue function and relationship to cyclic nucleotide metabolism. *Prog. Neurobiol.*, 8:183–250.
97. Wolff, D. J., Poirier, P. G., Brostrom, C. O., and Brostrom, M. A. (1977): Divalent cation binding properties of bovine brain Ca²⁺-dependent regulator protein. *J. Biol. Chem.*, 252:4108–4117.
98. Wood, J. G., Wallace, R. W., Whitaker, J. N., and Cheung, W. Y. (1980): Immunocytochemical localization of calmodulin and a heat-labile calmodulin binding protein (CaM-BP₈₀) in basal ganglia of mouse brain. *J. Cell. Biol.*, 84:66–76.
99. Yamauchi, T., and Fusijawa, H. (1979): Activation of tryptophan-5-monooxygenase by calcium dependent regulatory protein. *Biochem. Biophys. Res. Commun.*, 90:28–35.
100. Zwiers, H., Schotman, P., and Gispen, W. H. (1980): Purification and characteristics of an ACTH-sensitive protein kinase and its substrate protein in rat brain membranes. *J. Neurochem.*, 34:1689–1699.
101. Zwiers, H., Tonnaer, J., Wiegant, V. M., Schotman, P., and Gispen, W. H. (1979): ACTH-sensitive protein kinase from rat brain membranes. *J. Neurochem.*, 33:247–256.

Neural Transmission, Learning and Memory,
edited by R. Caputto and C. Ajmone Marsan.
Raven Press, New York © 1983.

Neuronal Na^+,K^+-ATPase and Its Regulation by Catecholamines

G. Rodríguez de Lores Arnaiz

Instituto de Biología Celular, Facultad de Medicina, Universidad de Buenos Aires, Paraguay, 2155, 1121 Buenos Aires, Argentina

The existence of a Na^+,K^+-activated ATPase (EC 3.6.1.3) in animal tissues was first described by Skou (24). This enzyme activity is Mg^{2+}-dependent and sensitive to ouabain. Different experimental evidences have demonstrated the participation of Na^+,K^+-ATPase on the transport of alcali cations across the membranes (see 23,25).

In this laboratory the subcellular distribution of cation-stimulated ATPases in brain was studied (1). It was observed that Na^+,K^+-ATPase was preferentially particulated; by differential centrifugation it was found that it appeared concentrated in microsomal and crude mitochondrial fractions, the latter containing the intact nerve endings (synaptosomes). The use of a sucrose density gradient led to show that the highest concentration of Na^+,K^+-ATPase activity was associated with the nerve ending fractions. A special concentration of Na^+,K^+-ATPase in the nerve endings was also reported by other authors (11,14).

It is known that the isolated nerve endings are able to carry out numerous metabolic reactions, which suggested that these structures behave as small whole cells. In fact they are able to produce high-energy compounds through glycolysis and oxidative phosphorylation; they synthesize different types of small and also larger molecules such as proteins, lipids, and glycolipids when incubated in the presence of the corresponding precursors. Further, the isolated nerve endings have the ability to accumulate or extrude ions, to transport different types of molecules by facilitated, passive, or active mechanisms, some of them being precursors of neurotransmitters or neurotransmitters themselves. It is interesting to mention that many of those reactions may be blocked by ouabain, which inhibits Na^+,K^+-ATPase activity (see 20 for original references). These facts suggest that Na^+,K^+-ATPase may play a central role in metabolic activity of the synaptic region and in processes directly related to neurotransmission.

The function of the limiting membrane of the nerve ending is the regulation of the passage of ions, metabolites, and other small molecules, thus maintaining a particular milieu for the metabolic activity of this compartment. To isolate and purify the external membrane of the nerve endings a subcellular fractionation technique was developed (18). Our starting point has been the crude mitochondrial fraction of the cerebral cortex; this fraction was shocked by hypotonic treatment. With the use of a sucrose gradient the nerve ending membranes were separated from myelin fragments and free mitochondria. In this way it was possible to separate the limiting membrane of the nerve endings to which some of the postsynaptic structures are attached. Since Na+,K+-ATPase appeared mainly associated to the nerve ending membranes (18), this fraction was employed to study its activity in the presence of catecholamines and other neurotransmitter substances.

EFFECTS OF NOREPINEPHRINE ON ATPases ACTIVITIES

To study the effect of norepinephrine on ATPases, nerve ending membranes were preincubated in the presence or absence of brain soluble fraction and norepinephrine. With the membranes alone, 10^{-4} M norepinephrine produced a decrease of 43% of Na+,K+-ATPase activity and no change in Mg^{2+}-ATPase (Fig. 1). In the presence of the brain soluble fraction norepinephrine produced a stimulatory effect on Na+,K+-ATPase activity. The increase was about 140% in relation to normal membranes

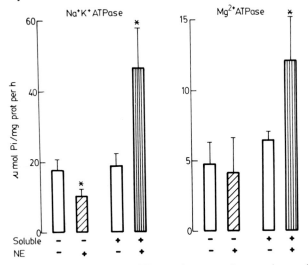

FIG. 1. Activities of Na+,K+- and Mg^{2+}-ATPases of nerve ending membranes in the presence and the absence of brain soluble fraction and norepinephrine. In each experiment the cerebral cortices of three rats were pooled and submitted to subcellular fractionation to separate the nerve ending membranes (18). The soluble fraction was prepared by homogenization of the cerebral cortex in water and centrifugation for 30 min at 100,000 × *g*; the nonsedimentable portion was used 30 min after. Samples of the nerve ending membranes were mixed with water or soluble fraction and were preincubated for 10 min at 37°C in the presence or absence of 10^{-4} M norepinephrine or other drugs; samples of these preparations were transferred in triplicate into microtubes containing the buffer substrate mixtures to assay ATPases according to Albers et al. (1). Mg^{2+}-, Na+, K+, and Mg^{2+}-ATPases were determined and the difference between the two was taken as the Na+,K+-ATPase activity. The substrate was Sigma muscle Tris-ATP. The results are the means of six experiments ± SD. NE, norepinephrine; *$p < 0.01$. (From ref. 21, with permission.)

and 350% if the membranes with norepinephrine are taken as controls. Mg^{2+}-ATPase activity was increased by the presence of the soluble fraction, and the addition of norepinephrine produced a further stimulation (86%) (Fig. 1).

STUDIES OF THE POSSIBLE PARTICIPATION OF ADRENERGIC RECEPTORS AND ADENYLATE CYCLASE

The activity of ATPases of nerve ending membranes with addition of the brain soluble fraction was assayed in the presence of several concentrations of phenoxybenzamine. By itself this drug produced a stimulation of Na^+,K^+-ATPase activity of about 100% at 10^{-4} M concentration but it did not decrease significantly maximal activity achieved with norepinephrine. Phenoxybenzamine produced no change on Mg^{2+}-ATPase or on the activation by norepinephrine (Fig. 2). Similar results were obtained with phentolamine.

Propranolol also stimulated Na^+,K^+-ATPase activity but it did not decrease the effect of norepinephrine. Propranolol slightly simulated Mg^{2+}-ATPase but less than norepinephrine (Fig. 3).

These results suggest that the stimulatory action of norepinephrine on Na^+,K^+-ATPase activity seems to be a direct effect on the enzyme not mediated by the adrenergic receptors.

To determine whether the effect of norepinephrine could be related to adenylate cyclase, experiments with cyclic AMP instead of norepinephrine were performed. In nerve ending membranes alone essentially negative results were obtained with

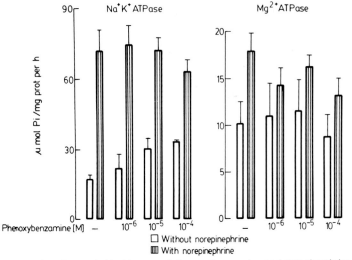

FIG. 2. Effect of α-adrenergic blocking agent phenoxybenzamine and norepinephrine on nerve ending membrane ATPases. The experimental schedule was similar to that described in the legend to Fig. 1 except that the brain soluble fraction was present in all cases. Samples of the nerve ending membranes were preincubated with the brain soluble fraction for 5 min at 37°C in the presence of phenoxybenzamine, then norepinephrine was added to achieve 10^{-4} M and the incubation continued for another 5 min; samples of these preparations were used to assay ATPases. Values are means ± SD of three experiments. (From ref. 21, with permission.)

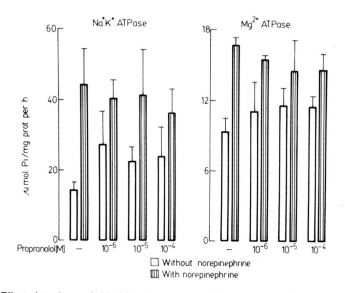

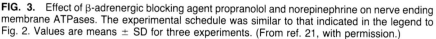

FIG. 3. Effect of β-adrenergic blocking agent propranolol and norepinephrine on nerve ending membrane ATPases. The experimental schedule was similar to that indicated in the legend to Fig. 2. Values are means ± SD for three experiments. (From ref. 21, with permission.)

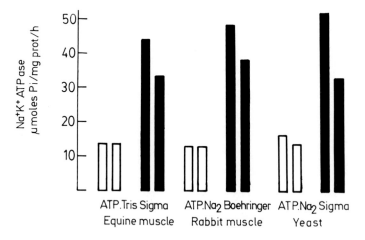

FIG. 4. Stimulation of Na⁺,K⁺-ATPase by norepinephrine with different types of ATP. The experimental schedule was the same as indicated in the legend to Fig. 1. The soluble fraction was always present. The substrate was Sigma Tris-ATP from muscle, Boehringer disodium ATP from muscle, and Sigma disodium ATP from yeast, obtained by phosphorylation of adenosine. For each type of ATP the results for Na⁺,K⁺-ATPase from two separate experiments are presented. White bars, without norepinephrine; black bars, with norepinephrine. (From ref. 21, with permission.)

10^{-7} to 10^{-3} M cyclic AMP; in nerve ending membranes plus soluble fraction, 10^{-4} M cyclic AMP produced only a small increase in Na+,K+-ATPase activity (about 15% of that obtained with 10^{-4} M norepinephrine). These findings suggest that catecholamine stimulatory effect is probably not mediated by cyclic AMP, a result that is in line with those of Yoshimura (28) and Wu and Phillis (27).

STIMULATION OF NA+,K+ATPase BY NOREPINEPHRINE WITH DIFFERENT TYPES OF ATP

The presence of contaminants in some ATP preparations that inhibit Na+,K+-ATPase has been reported (3,12,13). Further, it was observed that the inhibition could be reversed by norepinephrine (8), the contaminant being identified as vanadate (5). By using ATP of different origin, including yeast ATP which is free of vanadate, a similar stimulation of Na+,K+-ATPase by norepinephrine was found (Fig. 4). The stimulation of ATPase by dopamine was also obtained with the different types of ATP (see Fig. 5 and Tables 1 and 2). These findings indicate the independence of catecholamines effect with vanadate present in the substrate ATP.

ACTION OF SEVERAL NEUROTRANSMITTER SUBSTANCES ON NERVE ENDING MEMBRANE ATPases

In Fig. 5 it may be observed that Na+,K+-ATPase activity of nerve ending membranes in the presence of the soluble fraction increased about 200% by the addition of 10^{-4} M norepinephrine, dopamine, or 5-hydroxytryptamine. Mg^{2+}-ATPase activity also increased with catecholamines and 5-hydroxytryptamine but to a lesser extent (35–90%). On the other hand, histamine, acetylcholine, GABA, and glutamate did not change Na+,K+- and Mg^{2+}-ATPases.

TABLE 1. *Total ATPase activity in cerebral cortex, kidney, and heart preparations in the presence of brain soluble fraction and dopamine*

Soluble fraction	Dopamine	Mg^{2+},Na+,K+-ATPase μmoles P_i/mg protein/hr		
		Cerebral cortex	Kidney	Heart
−	−	32.4 ± 5.9 (7)	18.3 ± 1.7 (4)	46.7 ± 0.1 (2)
−	+	16.2 ± 5.2 (3)[a]	18.2 ± 5.5 (4)	44.2 ± 1.1 (2)
+	−	26.4 ± 2.6 (3)	18.3 ± 2.4 (4)	40.8 ± 3.6 (3)
+	+	77.7 ± 7.1 (3)[a]	23.5 ± 4.2 (4)	42.3 ± 2.1 (3)

Nerve ending membranes isolated from rat cerebral cortex, a commercial dog kidney preparation, and heart microsomes were used. Samples of these preparations were preincubated in the presence or absence of brain soluble fraction and/or 10^{-4} M dopamine. The general schedule was similar to that indicated in Fig. 1; the substrate was Sigma yeast disodium ATP. The number of experiments appears between parentheses. Values are expressed as mean ± SD.
[a]$p < 0.001$ with respect to the control without dopamine.
(From ref. 2, with permission.)

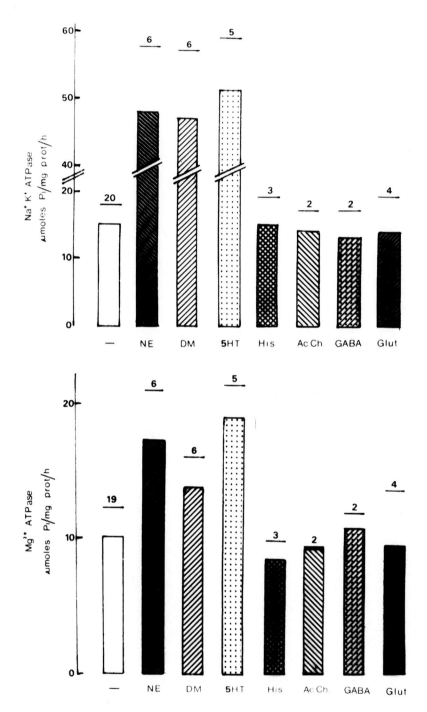

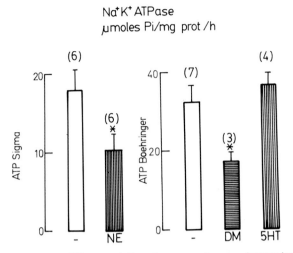

Na⁺K⁺ ATPase
μmoles Pi/mg prot /h

FIG. 6. Na+,K+- and Mg²⁺-ATPase activities of nerve ending membranes in the presence of catecholamines and 5-hydroxytryptamine. The experimental schedule was similar to that described in Fig. 1; the brain soluble fraction was not present. The substrate was Sigma Tris-ATP or Boehringer disodium ATP. Values are means ± SD; the number of experiments appears between parentheses. *$p < 0.001$. NE, norepinephrine; DM, dopamine; 5-HT, 5-hydroxytryptamine. (From ref. 19, with permission.)

   In the absence of the soluble fraction, dopamine produced a pattern of changes similar to that shown with norepinephrine in Fig. 1, that is, about 40% inhibition on Na+,K+-ATPase but no effect on Mg²⁺-ATPase; 5-hydroxytryptamine did not change ATPases in this condition (Fig. 6).

   The concentration of neurotransmitters used is not within the range usually referred to as physiological. It is worth mentioning some effects described with neurotransmitters *in vitro* at concentrations around 10^{-4} M. For example, in slices of the nervous tissue the stimulation of cyclic AMP accumulation was achieved with 10^{-5}–10^{-4} M neurotransmitters (see 17) and the stimulation of endogenous biosynthesis of prostaglandins was obtained with 10^{-3} M norepinephrine (26). Moreover, the maximal pharmacological response in peripheral adrenergic nerve endings was achieved with 10^{-4}–10^{-3} M norepinephrine (4).

   The stimulation of ATPases by catecholamines in whole brain and certain subcellular fractions has also been studied by several authors (6,7,9,10,15,16,22,28).

FIG. 5. Activities of nerve ending membrane ATPases in presence of the soluble fraction and several neurotransmitter substances. The experimental schedule was similar to that reported in Fig. 1; samples of the nerve ending membranes were preincubated with the brain soluble fraction and various neurotransmitters (10^{-4}M concentration); samples of these preparations were used to assay ATPases. The SD and the number of experiments are indicated above the bars. *$p < 0.001$ for norepinephrine (NE), dopamine (DM), and 5-hydroxytryptamine (5-HT). The differences were not significant for histamine (HIS), acetylcholine (AcCh), GABA, and glutamate (Glut.). (From ref. 19, with permission.)

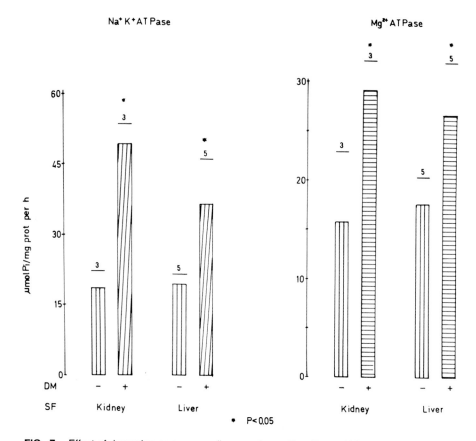

FIG. 7. Effect of dopamine on nerve ending membrane Na⁺,K⁺, and Mg²⁺-ATPases in presence of kidney or liver soluble fractions. The general schedule was similar to that described in the legend to Fig. 1. Above the bars the SD and the number of experiments are indicated. SF, soluble fraction; DM, dopamine. Asterisks denote statistical difference with respect to the control without dopamine. (From ref. 2, with permission.)

The results were essentially coincident for the stimulation of Na⁺,K⁺-ATPase by norepinephrine but some discrepancies account for some of the other neurotransmitters; they are probably due to the differences in experimental conditions, as previously discussed (19,21).

TISSUE SPECIFICITY OF DOPAMINE EFFECTS ON Mg²⁺, Na⁺,K⁺-ATPase

Tissue specificity of catecholamine effects on brain ATPase regarding the soluble fraction and enzyme source was investigated (2). It was observed that the stimulation of nerve ending membrane Na⁺,K⁺- and Mg²⁺-ATPases by dopamine may also be achieved when the brain soluble was replaced by the soluble fractions obtained from either kidney or liver (Fig. 7).

TABLE 2. *Effect of NEM on dopamine action on nerve ending membrane ATPases in presence and absence of brain soluble fraction*

Soluble fraction	NEM	Na$^+$,K$^+$-ATPase μmoles P$_i$/mg protein/hr		Mg^{2+}-ATPase μmoles P$_i$/mg protein/hr	
		Without dopamine	With dopamine	Without dopamine	With dopamine
−	−	27.6 ± 5.9 (10)	10.4 ± 2.9 (5)[a]	6.6 ± 1.5 (10)	6.9 ± 1.5 (10)
−	+	30.3 ± 5.7 (6)	22.5 ± 7.6 (6)	5.4 ± 2.1 (6)	4.1 ± 0.9 (6)
+	−	34.5 ± 11.0 (9)	55.6 ± 13.9 (4)[a]	14.1 ± 5.0 (9)	21.4 ± 5.4 (9)[a]
+	+	33.5 ± 7.4 (5)	32.6 ± 6.4 (5)	8.9 ± 1.1 (5)	9.9 ± 0.9 (5)

The experimental schedule was similar to that reported in the legend to Fig. 1. The concentration of NEM and dopamine was 5×10^{-5} M and 10^{-4} M, respectively; the substrate was Boehringer muscle disodium ATP. The number of experiments appears between parentheses. Values are expressed as mean ± SD.

[a] $p < 0.05$ with respect to the corresponding control without dopamine.

NEM, N-etylmaleimide. Data from Rodríguez de Lores Arnaiz and Antonelli de Gómez de Lima *(unpublished observations)*.

Table 1 shows that total ATPase activity of nerve ending membranes was inhibited by dopamine in the absence of the brain soluble fraction; in the presence of the soluble fraction, a significant stimulation was found. In contrast, the addition of dopamine or dopamine plus soluble brain fraction did not produce significant changes on total ATPase activity in commercial kidney or cardiac microsomal preparations.

These studies show that there is no tissue specificity with regard to the origin of the soluble fraction to achieve the stimulation of nerve ending membrane ATPases by dopamine. On the other hand, there might be a particular sensitivity of neural ATPase to dopamine that is not found in kidney and heart ATPases.

BLOCKING ACTION OF N-ETHYLMALEIMIDE ON DOPAMINE EFFECTS ON Na^+,K^+-ATPase

The possible involvement of thiol groups in catecholamine effects on Na^+,K^+-ATPases was studied by using N-ethylmaleimide (NEM) (Table 2). Basal activity of nerve ending membrane Na^+,K^+-ATPase was not changed by the addition of 5×10^{-5} M NEM; the inhibition produced by 10^{-4} M dopamine was decreased by the presence of NEM. The statistical analysis of the data has shown that the inhibition achieved with dopamine in presence of NEM was not significant with respect to the control without dopamine. The addition of NEM did not modify basal activity of Na^+,K^+-ATPase of nerve ending membranes in presence of the brain soluble fraction; in this condition NEM abolished dopamine effect. Mg^{2+}-ATPase activity was reduced by NEM in absence and presence of the brain soluble fraction, with or without dopamine (Table 2).

These findings could be interpreted as a consequence of an interaction between NEM and Na^+,K^+-ATPase at some thiol groups located outside the catalytic site where dopamine might act (Rodríguez de Lores Arnaiz and Antonelli de Gómez de Lima, *unpublished observations*).

CONCLUSIONS

1. Neuronal Na^+,K^+-ATPase is sensitive to catecholamines noradrenaline and dopamine and to 5-hydroxytryptamine.
2. In the presence of the soluble brain fraction, catecholamines and 5-hydroxytryptamine stimulate the enzyme (kidney or liver soluble fractions may substitute the brain soluble fraction).
3. The activation of Na^+,K^+-ATPase by norepinephrine is not reproduced by cyclic AMP and it is not antagonized by either α- or β-adrenergic blocking agents.
4. In the absence of the soluble fraction, catecholamines inhibit Na^+,K^+-ATPase but 5-hydroxytryptamine has no effect.
5. Kidney or heart membrane ATPases (with or without the soluble) are insensitive to dopamine.
6. It is suggested that some thiol groups located outside the catalytic site could be involved in dopamine effects on Na^+,K^+-ATPase.

7. Neuronal Na$^+$,K$^+$-ATPase could be regulated by catecholamines and 5-hydroxytryptamine; a factor present in the soluble fraction could modulate the action of such neurotransmitters on the enzyme.

SUMMARY

Na$^+$,K$^+$-ATPase is an enzyme firmly associated with the nerve ending (synaptosomal) membranes. Different experimental evidences have demonstrated the participation of Na$^+$,K$^+$-ATPase in the transport of alcali cations across the membranes. Its inhibition by ouabain blocks numerous metabolic reactions occurring in the isolated nerve endings. These facts give a special interest to the study of the regulatory mechanisms involved in neuronal Na$^+$,K$^+$-ATPase activity.

We have studied the effect of catecholamines on ATPase activity of nerve ending membranes isolated from rat cerebral cortex. It was found that norepinephrine and dopamine stimulated Na$^+$,K$^+$-ATPase when in presence of the brain soluble fraction but produced its inhibition in the absence of the soluble fraction.

The activation of Na$^+$,K$^+$-ATPase by norepinephrine was not reproduced by cyclic AMP and was not antagonized by either α- or β-adrenergic blocking agents.

5-Hydroxytryptamine stimulated Na$^+$,K$^+$-ATPase in the presence of the brain soluble fraction but it has no effect in the absence of the soluble fraction. Acetylcholine, histamine, GABA and glutamate produced no effect on ATPase.

Dopamine stimulation was achieved irrespective of whether brain, kidney or liver soluble fractions were used. On the other hand, dopamine effects were not observed on kidney or heart ATPase preparations.

The use of N-ethylmaleimide suggested that some thiol groups located outside the catalytic site could be involved in dopamine effects.

It is suggested that neuronal Na$^+$,K$^+$-ATPase could be regulated by catecholamines and 5-hydroxytryptamine. A soluble factor might modulate the effect of such neurotransmitters on the enzyme.

ACKNOWLEDGMENT

This research was supported by grants from the Consejo Nacional de Investigaciones Científicas y Técnicas and Secretaría de Estado de Ciencia y Tecnología, Argentina.

REFERENCES

1. Albers, R. W., Rodríguez de Lores Arnaiz, G., and De Robertis, E. (1965): Sodium-potassium-activated ATPase and potassium activated p-nitrophenylphosphatase: A comparison of their subcellular localizations in rat brain. *Proc. Natl. Acad. Sci. USA*, 53:557–564.
2. Antonelli de Gómez de Lima, M., and Rodríguez de Lores Arnaiz, G. (1981): Tissue specificity of dopamine effects on brain ATPases. *Neurochem. Res.*, 6:969–977.
3. Beaugé, L. A., and Glynn, I. M. (1977): A modifier of (Na$^+$-K$^+$) ATPase in commercial ATP. *Nature*, 268:355–356.
4. Brimijoin, S., Pluchino, S., and Trendelenburg, U. (1970): On the mechanism of supersensitivity to norepinephrine in the denervated cat spleen. *J. Pharmacol. Exp. Ther.*, 175:503–513.

5. Cantley, L. C., Jr., Josephson, L., Warner, R., Yanagisawa, M., Lechene, C., and Guidotti, G. (1977): Vanadate is a potent (Na+-K+)-ATPase inhibitor found in ATP derived from muscle. *J. Biol. Chem.*, 252:7421–7423.

6. Chappuis, A., Enz, A., and Iwangoff, P. (1975): Some comments on the adrenergic regulation of the Na+K+ATPase system in the brain. *Triangle*, 14:96–98.

7. Desaiah, D., and Ho, T. K. (1977): Kinetics of catecholamine sensitive Na+K+ATPase activity in mouse brain synaptosomes. *Biochem. Pharmacol.*, 26:2029–2035.

8. Fagan, J. B., and Racker, E. (1977): Reversible inhibition of (Na+,K+)ATPase by Mg2+, adenosinetriphosphate, and K+. *Biochemistry*, 16:152–158.

9. Gilbert, J. C., Wyllie, M. G., and Davison, D. V. (1975): Nerve terminal ATPase as possible trigger for neurotransmitter release. *Nature*, 255:237–238.

10. Godfraind, T., Kock, M. C., and Verbeke, N. (1974): The action of EGTA on the catecholamines stimulation of rat brain Na-K-ATPase. *Biochem. Pharmacol.*, 23:3505–3511.

11. Hosie, R. J. A. (1965): The localization of adenosine triphosphatases in morphologically characterized subcellular fractions of guinea pig brain. *Biochem. J.*, 96:404–412.

12. Hudgins, P. M., and Bond, G. H. (1977): (Mg2+-K+) dependent inhibition of Na+K+ATPase due to a contaminant in equine muscle ATP. *Biochem. Biophys. Commun.*, 77:1024–1029.

13. Josephson, L., and Cantley, C., Jr. (1977): Isolation of a potent (Na+K+)ATPase inhibitor from striated muscle. *Biochemistry*, 16:4572–4578.

14. Kurokawa, M., Sakamoto, T., and Kato, M. (1965): Distribution of sodium-plus-potassium stimulated adenosine-triphosphatase activity in isolated nerve ending particles. *Biochem. J.*, 97:833–844.

15. Lee, S. L., and Phillis, J. W. (1977): Stimulation of cerebral cortical synaptosomal Na-K-ATPase by biogenic amines. *Can. J. Physiol. Pharmacol.*, 55:961–964.

16. Logan, J. G., and O'Donovan, D. J. O. (1976): The effects of ouabain and the activation of neural membrane ATPase by biogenic amines. *J. Neurochem.*, 27:185–189.

17. Nathanson, J. A., and Greengard, P. (1976): Cyclic nucleotides and synaptic transmission. In: *Basic Neurochemistry*, 2nd ed., edited by G. Siegel, R. W. Albers, K. Katzman, and B. Agranoff, pp. 246–262. Little Brown and Co., Boston.

18. Rodríguez de Lores Arnaiz, G., Alberici, M., and De Robertis, E. (1967): Ultrastructural and enzymic studies of cholinergic and noncholinergic synaptic membranes isolated from brain cortex. *J. Neurochem.*, 14:215–225.

19. Rodríguez de Lores Arnaiz, G., and Antonelli de Gómez de Lima, M. (1981): The effect of several neurotransmitter substances on nerve ending membrane ATPases. *Acta Physiol. Latinoam.*, 31:39–44.

20. Rodríguez de Lores Arnaiz, G., and De Robertis, E. (1972): Properties of the isolated nerve endings. In: *Current Topics in Membranes and Transport, Vol. 3*, edited by F. Bronner and A. Kleinzeller, pp. 237–272. Academic Press, New York.

21. Rodríguez de Lores Arnaiz, G., and Mistrorigo de Pacheco, M. (1978): Regulation of (Na+,K+) adenosinetriphosphatase of nerve ending membranes. Action of norepinephrine and a soluble factor. *Neurochem. Res.*, 3:733–744.

22. Schaefer, A., Seregi, A., and Komlos, M. (1974): Ascorbic acid-like effect of the soluble fraction of rat brain on adenosine triphosphatases and its relation to catecholamines and chelating agents. *Biochem. Pharmacol.*, 23:2257–2271.

23. Swanson, P. D., and Stahl, W. L. (1976): Ion transport. In: *Basic Neurochemistry*, 2nd ed., edited by G. Siegel, R. W. Albers, K. Katzman, and B. Agranoff, pp. 125–147. Little Brown and Co., Boston.

24. Skou, J. C. (1957): The influence of some cations on an adenosine triphosphatase from peripheral nerves. *Biochim. Biophys. Acta*, 23:394–401.

25. Skou, J. C. (1971): Sequence of steps in the (Na+ + K+)-activated enzyme system in relation to sodium and potassium transport. In: *Current Topics in Bioenergetics, Vol. 4*, edited by D. R. Sanadi, pp. 357–398. Academic Press, New York.

26. Wolfe, L. S. (1976): Prostaglandines and synaptic transmission. In: *Basic Neurochemistry*, 2nd ed., edited by G. Siegel, R. W. Albers, K. Katzman, and B. Agranoff, pp. 263–275. Little Brown and Co., Boston.

27. Wu, P. H., and Phillis, J. W. (1980): Characterization of receptor-mediated catecholamine activation of rat brain cortical Na+-K+-ATPase. *Int. J. Biochem.*, 12:353–359.

28. Yoshimura, K. (1973): Activation of Na-K activated ATPase in rat brain by catecholamine. *J. Biochem.*, 74:389–391.

Neural Transmission, Learning and Memory,
edited by R. Caputto and C. Ajmone Marsan.
Raven Press, New York © 1983.

Possible Functional Role of Brain Gangliosides in Adaptive Neuronal Processes

H. Rahmann

*Zoological Institute, University of Stuttgart-Hohenheim,
Stuttgart (Hohenheim), West Germany*

The ability of vertebrates to adapt to fluctuations in their environment is based mainly upon adaptive changes within the central nervous system (CNS). On the basis of electrophysiological investigations, the synapses had been shown to be the most sensitive areas of the nervous system (17). Therefore it was assumed that changes in the physicochemical properties of the neuronal membrane probably are responsible for the processes of nervous stimulation, transmission, and learning. Special emphasis was focused on those molecular adaptive processes that might occur in the synaptic terminal itself. With regard to this, many investigations had been carried out, for example, with phospholipids. It had been shown that the degree of unsaturation of their fatty acids changes depending on altered environmental parameters (20,42). Since phospholipids are not highly specific compounds of synapses, but are ubiquitously distributed in all biological membranes, the interest of research became focused on those compounds that are particularly enriched in synaptic terminals.

In this regard gangliosides seem to be very suitable candidates. Although providing only a small portion of the complex carbohydrate content of all vertebrate cell surfaces (43), these sialic acid (-neuraminic acid, NeuAc)-containing glycosphingolipids are known to be highly concentrated in synaptic membranes (18). They are assumed to be anchored with their nonpolar ceramide moiety in the outer lipid layer of the membrane, while exposing the polar carbohydrate portion including different numbers of negatively charged sialic acids into the extracellular space (Fig. 1). Later gangliosides are submitted to significant changes in amount as well as complexity during ontogenetic and phylogenetic development (3,11–13,15,26,36–38,41). Cell contact-depending variations emphasize their importance for synapse-formation (7). Further, gangliosides show receptor associated binding capacities for neurotropic substances such as, for example, tetanus toxin (9), serotonin (47), and tubocurarine (40).

As a result of their great capacity to complex with calcium ions (23) these sialoglycolipids are assumed to play an important functional role in the process of synaptic transmission (25,33) and consequently in adaptive neuronal functions (27–29).

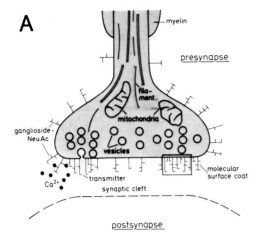

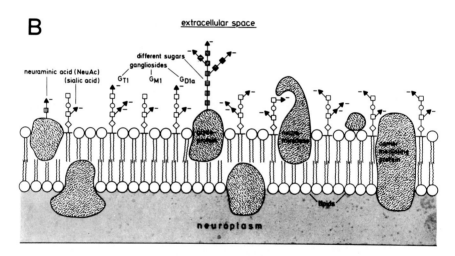

FIG. 1. Model of a synapse **(A)** including localization of different gangliosides (G_{M1}, G_{D1a}, G_{T1}) and sialoglycoproteins in the neuronal membrane **(B)**.

To obtain further information concerning the biological role of gangliosides in the CNS three sets of experimental approaches are reported demonstrating various phenomenological lines of evidence for the possible functional participation of gangliosides in neuronal processes. The first aspect is concerned with the involvement of gangliosides in the long-term process of thermal adaptation in vertebrates, which is of utmost significance for their survival in cold. The second deals with some *in vitro* interactions between calcium ions and various gangliosides with regard to the involvement of these complexes in the process of synaptic transmission. Thirdly, changes in the ganglioside metabolism of the CNS in relation to sensory stimulations are reported.

MATERIALS AND METHODS

The neuronal gangliosides of more than 60 vertebrate species belonging to the classes of agnathe fish, elasmobranch fish, teleost fish, amphibians, reptiles, birds, and mammals were analyzed. Total ganglioside extracts from whole brains as well as individual brain regions (subtectum, brainstem, cerebellum, pons, and medulla oblongata) were prepared according to the method of Svennerholm and Fredman (46). Quantitative estimations of ganglioside-bound neuraminic acid (NeuAc) were carried out according to the method of Svennerholm (45). Single ganglioside fractions were separated by high-performance thin-layer chromatography on precoated silica gel plates (HPTLC, 0.2 mm; Merck; solvent system: chloroform-methanol-water containing 12 mM $MgCl_2$ concentrated ammonia $= 60:35.5:7.5:0.4$; Fig. 2), visualized with resorcinol reagent (45), and quantified by spectralphotometric

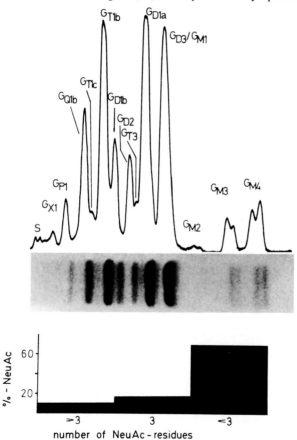

FIG. 2. Densitogram and chromatogram of brain gangliosides from adult chick (silica gel 60 HP-TLC; chloroform-methanol-water containing 0.02% $MgCl_2$ conc. ammonia $= 60:30:7.5:0.4$; by vol.). **Below:** relative proportion of different gangliosides containing either more or less NeuAc residues than three per molecule.

scanning at 580 nm (chromatogramspectralphotometer KM3, Zeiss). From the identified peak areas the percent distribution and concentration of the single ganglioside fractions were calculated (MOP II, Kontron; 9825 calculator, Hewlett Packard). For comparative calculations the gangliosides were classified into three groups according to their increase of NeuAc residues and therefore polarity (3 NeuAc residues, respectively more or less than 3). The ganglioside fractions were named according to Svennerholm's nomenclature (45).

In addition, ganglioside concentration and composition had been analyzed in various brain structures of the weak electric tapirfish *Gnathonemus petersi* following artificial electric stimulation or deprivation according to Bässler et al. (1,2). Further, the influence of temperature changes on the capacity of various brain gangliosides to form complexes with calcium ions were investigated by means of potentiometry (22,23) and equilibrium dialysis using $^{45}Ca^{2+}$ (21).

RESULTS

Neuronal Gangliosides and Thermal Adaptation Phenomena

Comparative investigations of more than 60 vertebrate species reveal an extraordinary variability in concentration and composition of brain gangliosides between ecto- and homeothermic vertebrates. The concentration obviously correlates to the level of nervous organization (Fig. 3): about 110 to 700 μg ganglioside-bound NeuAc/g fresh weight in lower ectothermic vertebrates (agnathe fish to reptiles), about 500 to 1000 μg/g in homeothermic birds and mammals. The brain gangliosides of the homeotherms constitute only a relatively small number (7–10) of less polar ganglioside fractions (mainly G_{D1a} and G_{T1b}). In contrast, in ectotherms up to 17 different fractions can be distinguished from which polar tetra- and even higher sialylated polar gangliosides prevail (12). In addition, in contrast with the ectotherms, in which all three pathways of ganglioside-biosynthesis (48) are present, a reduction of the c-pathway had occurred (32) in homeotherms.

Because no clear correlations between the ganglioside composition and the systematical position of the investigated vertebrate species could be shown until recently, the question was raised whether the great differences, especially in the ganglioside pattern, indeed could be correlated with the ecofactor temperature, which has particular significance for the survival of vertebrates in the cold.

Therefore, the brain gangliosides of various representatives from different classes of vertebrates, having developed special strategies for survival in the cold, were investigated (Table 1).

In a first approach the brain gangliosides of species that were adapted phylogenetically to extremely different temperature biotopes, as, for example, the antarctic icefish *Tematomus hansoni* or the tropic cichlid fish *Tilapia mariae* were analyzed (Fig. 4). In the icefish brain more than 45% of all ganglioside fractions are sialylated to a higher degree than the tetrasialoganglioside G_{Q1b}, whereas in the tropic fish less polar di-, tri-, and tetrasialogangliosides dominate. As a whole the

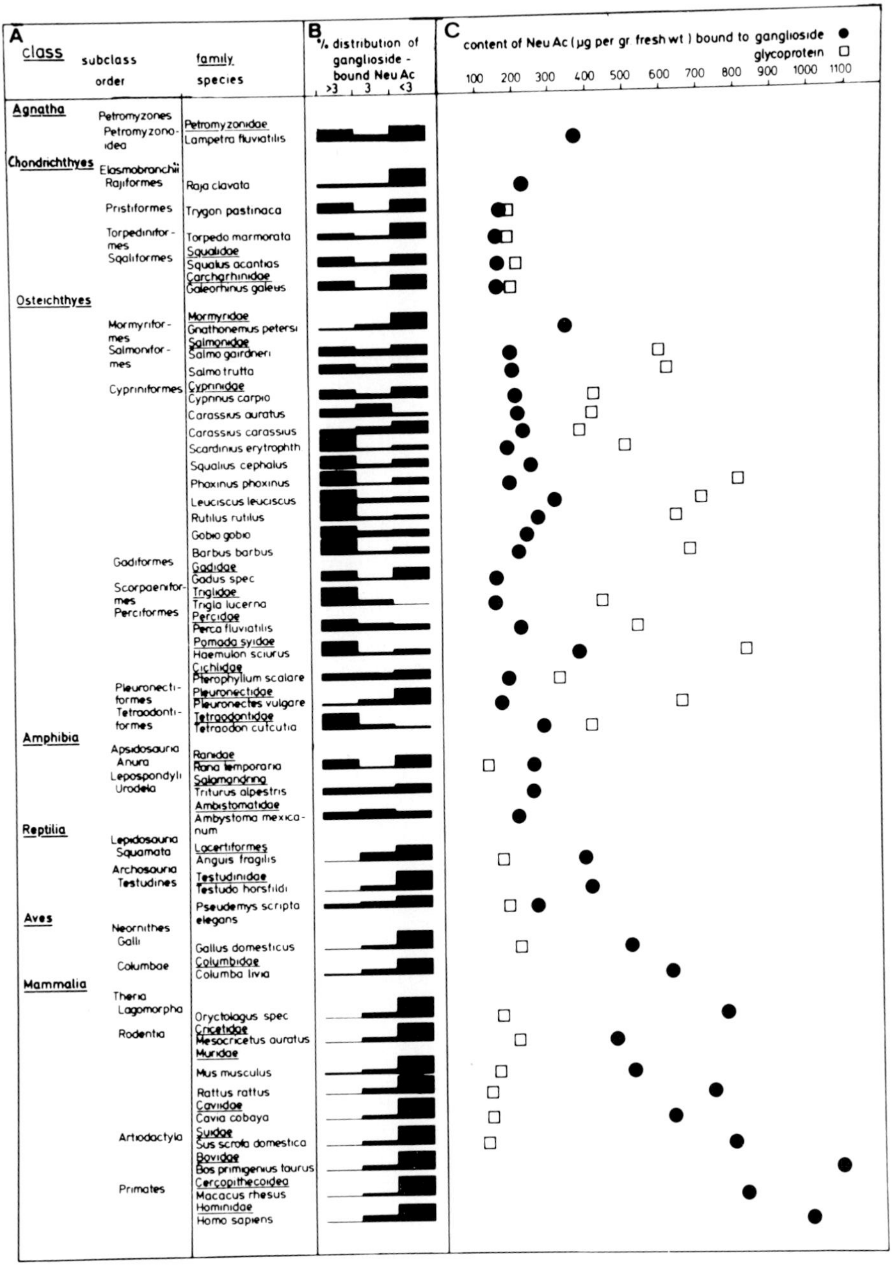

A
class subclass family
order species

B % distribution of ganglioside - bound Neu Ac
>3 3 <3

C content of Neu Ac (µg per gr fresh wt) bound to ganglioside ●
glycoprotein □
100 200 300 400 500 600 700 800 900 1000 1100

Agnatha
  Petromyzones
  Petromyzono-   Petromyzonidae
  idea   Lampetra fluviatilis
Chondrichthyes
  Elasmobranchii
  Rajiformes   Raja clavata
  Pristiformes   Trygon pastinaca
  Torpedinifor- Torpedo marmorata
  mes   Squalidae
  Squaliformes   Squalus acantias
                 Carcharhinidae
                 Galeorhinus galeus
Osteichthyes
  Mormyrifor-   Mormyridae
  mes   Gnathonemus petersi
  Salmonifor-   Salmonidae
  mes   Salmo gairdneri
                 Salmo trutta
  Cypriniformes Cyprinidae
                 Cyprinus carpio
                 Carassius auratus
                 Carassius carassius
                 Scardinus erytrophth
                 Squalius cephalus
                 Phoxinus phoxinus
                 Leuciscus leuciscus
                 Rutilus rutilus
                 Gobio gobio
                 Barbus barbus
  Gadiformes   Gadidae
                 Gadus spec
  Scorpaenifor- Triglidae
  mes   Trigla lucerna
  Perciformes   Percidae
                 Perca fluviatilis
                 Pomadasyidae
                 Haemulon sciurus
                 Cichlidae
                 Pterophyllum scalare
  Pleuronecti-   Pleuronectidae
  formes   Pleuronectes vulgare
  Tetraodonti-   Tetraodontidae
  formes   Tetraodon cutcutia
Amphibia
  Apsidosauria
  Anura   Ranidae
  Lepospondyli   Rana temporaria
  Urodela   Salamandrina
                 Triturus alpestris
                 Ambystomatidae
                 Ambystoma mexica-
                 num
Reptilia
  Lepidosauria
  Squamata   Lacertiformes
                 Anguis fragilis
  Archosauria   Testudinidae
  Testudines   Testudo horsfildi
                 Pseudemys scripta
Aves   elegans
  Neornithes
  Galli   Gallus domesticus
  Columbae   Columbidae
                 Columba livia
Mammalia
  Theria
  Lagomorpha   Oryctolagus spec
  Rodentia   Cricetidae
                 Mesocricetus auratus
                 Muridae
                 Mus musculus
                 Rattus rattus
                 Caviidae
                 Cavia cobaya
  Artiodactyla   Suidae
                 Sus scrofa domestica
                 Bovidae
                 Bos primigenius taurus
  Primates   Cercopithecoidea
                 Macacus rhesus
                 Hominidae
                 Homo sapiens

FIG. 3. Brain gangliosides of vertebrates including taxonomic classification of species **(A)**, relative proportion of main ganglioside fraction groups migrating slower or faster than trisialo-gangliosides **(B)**, and content of ganglioside- and glycoprotein-bound NeuAc/g fresh weight **(C)**.

TABLE 1.   *Strategies of temperature adaptation in vertebrates*

I.   Poikilo- or ectothermic: body temperature is directly correlated with ambient temperature; compensatory adaptation only within distinct range of thermotolerance
   1. Cold-stenothermic (antarctic icefish *Trematomus hansoni*, $-2°$ to $+4°C$)
   2. Warm-stenothermic (tropic fish *Pseudotrophaeus zebra*, $25°-28°C$)
   3. Eurythermic (goldfish *Carassius auratus*, $4°-28°C$)
II. Homeothermic: constant body temperature by means of thermoregulation (adult rat *Rattus Lorwegicus*, $38°C$)
III. Heterothermic: variable body temperature
   1. Ontogenetic: nonstable thermoregulation (neonatal rat *Rattus Lorwegicus*, $4°-38°C$)
   2. Phylogenetic: thermoregulation not yet well developed (monotremes, marsupials)
   3. Hibernation: by means of thermoregulation (fat dormouse *Glis glis*, $4°-38°C$)

---

icefish pattern of brain gangliosides exhibited the highest polarity among all vertebrates that have been investigated to date (31).

In adaptation to seasonally or experimentally induced fluctuations of the environmental temperature the composition of brain gangliosides had been examined in several species (carp, goldfish, trout, plaice, and tilapia; 14,32). A reorganization dependent on long-term adaptations to lowered temperatures of the ganglioside pattern occurred, which resulted in a more polar neuronal membrane configuration (compare, for example, Fig. 5, acclimatization of rainbow trout). Quite similar results were obtained in hibernating mammals (golden hamster: 10; fat dormouse: 8), and in chicken, mice, and rats during their early neonatal developmental phase, when the capacity of temperature regulation is not yet developed (29,41).

From all these data, schematically summarized in Fig. 6, it can be concluded, that the neuronal membranes of the vertebrates investigated to date become equipped with higher sialylated gangliosides during the process of adaptation to lowered temperatures, by which they become more polar. All results that have been reported here are based on whole brain investigations. Consequently, an open question remained: whether the temperature-dependent sialylation phenomena were due to reactions that simultaneously had occurred in all brain regions in the same way or whether there might be structure-dependent differences, thus indicating specific molecular mechanisms.

Therefore in another experimental approach the influence of changes in the environmental temperature on content and composition of gangliosides from various brain regions of the cichlid fish *Tilapia mariae* were investigated. Following a decrease of temperature from $32°$ to $16°C$ the concentration of ganglioside-bound NeuAc was reduced in the cerebellum from about 800 to 600 µg/g fresh weight. The content was increased in the subtectum from about 410 to 570 µg but it remained on a constant level in the medulla (about 500 µg each, Table 2).

Quite similar data were obtained from hibernating fat dormice *(Glis glis)* as compared with normothermic controls (8). In this species only in the pons region,

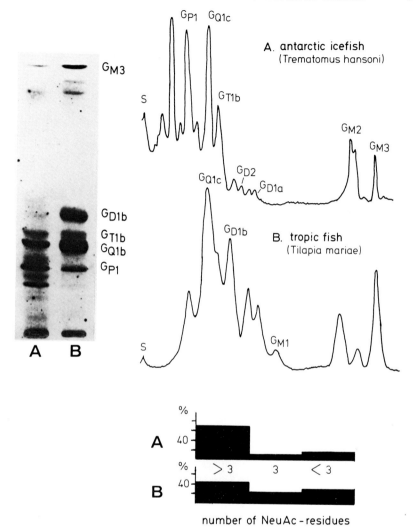

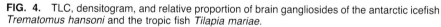

FIG. 4. TLC, densitogram, and relative proportion of brain gangliosides of the antarctic icefish *Trematomus hansoni* and the tropic fish *Tilapia mariae*.

the olfactory bulb and the midbrain significant decreases in the concentration of gangliosides were found, whereas all other structures (cortex, brainstem, cerebellum) remained constant. Both in the cichlid fish and in the hibernator those changes were shown to be due to significant alterations in the composition of the individual ganglioside fractions (Fig. 7). Generally in adaptation to cold the amount of polar sialoganglioside fractions in the affected structures significantly increased (10–30%), whereas the less polar mono- and disialogangliosides decreased (>20%).

In summary, the data on long-term molecular adaptations of brain gangliosides in homeotherms during their heterothermic phases (hibernation, neonatal devel-

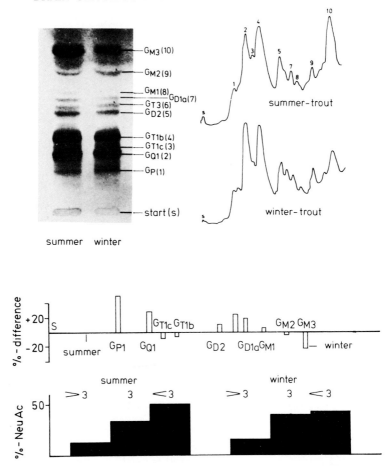

FIG. 5. TLC, densitogram, and relative proportion of brain gangliosides from rainbow trout acclimatized to summer and winter conditions, respectively. **Below:** Different percentages of single fractions of winter trout in comparison with summer fish.

opment) and in poikilotherms during acclimatization, acclimation, and adaptation to their natural habitat demonstrate (Fig. 6) that the molecular mechanism of thermal adaptation in the CNS of these vertebrates obviously is based on similar principles: The lower the ambient temperature (and consequently the body temperature), the higher the degree of sialylation of neuronal membranes and by this of the polarity. These results permit the following conclusions:

During several hundred millions of years the vertebrates in general have adapted to various temperature habitats. Obviously it had been of great evolutionary advantage to develop a large variety of gangliosides in order to adapt to alterations in the environmental temperature. This occurred by means of changes of the neuronal ganglioside composition, which probably enabled the transmission process to proceed more effectively under changed temperature conditions. Only adult birds and

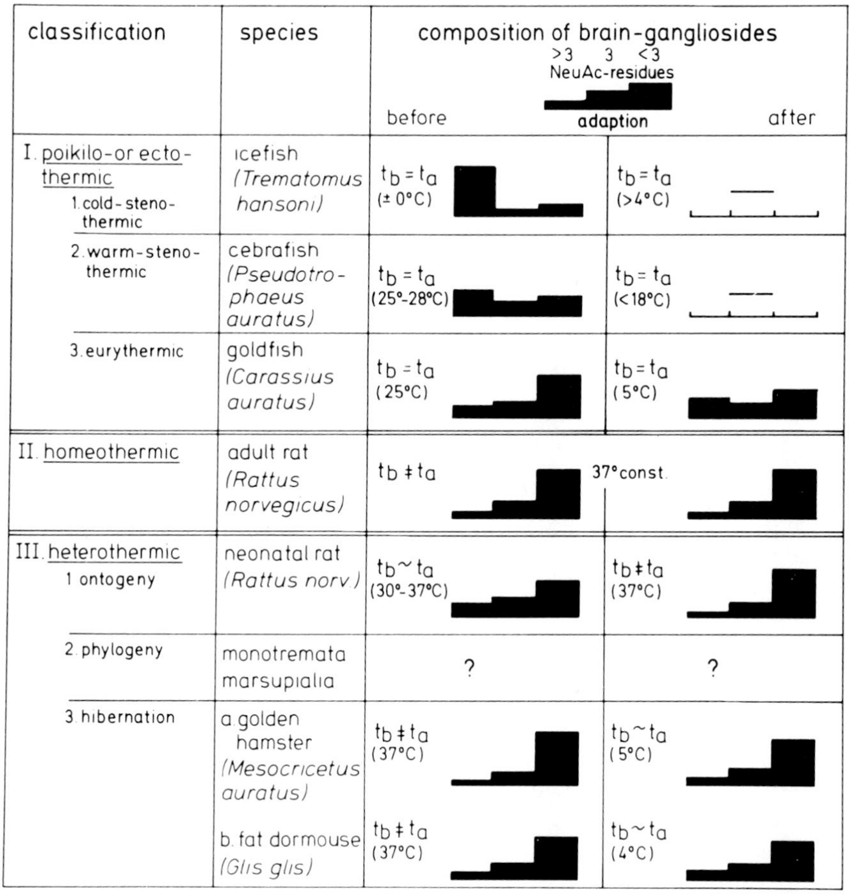

classification	species	composition of brain-gangliosides		
		before	>3 3 <3 NeuAc-residues / adaption	after
I. poikilo- or ecto-thermic 1. cold-steno-thermic	icefish (*Trematomus hansoni*)	$t_b = t_a$ ($\pm$ 0°C)		$t_b = t_a$ (>4°C)
2. warm-steno-thermic	cebrafish (*Pseudotrophaeus auratus*)	$t_b = t_a$ (25°-28°C)		$t_b = t_a$ (<18°C)
3. eurythermic	goldfish (*Carassius auratus*)	$t_b = t_a$ (25°C)		$t_b = t_a$ (5°C)
II. homeothermic	adult rat (*Rattus norvegicus*)	$t_b \neq t_a$	37° const.	
III. heterothermic 1. ontogeny	neonatal rat (*Rattus norv.*)	$t_b \sim t_a$ (30°-37°C)		$t_b \neq t_a$ (37°C)
2. phylogeny	monotremata marsupialia	?		?
3. hibernation	a. golden hamster (*Mesocricetus auratus*)	$t_b \neq t_a$ (37°C)		$t_b \sim t_a$ (5°C)
	b. fat dormouse (*Glis glis*)	$t_b \neq t_a$ (37°C)		$t_b \sim t_a$ (4°C)

FIG. 6. Relative proportion of the three different polar groups of ganglioside fractions (compare Fig. 2) of several vertebrates according to their thermal classification and adaptation properties to changes in the ambient temperature.

TABLE 2. *Adaptation of concentration of gangliosides in the CNS of* Tilapia mariae *to various temperatures*

CNS region	Ganglioside-bound NeuAc (μg/g fresh weight) after adaptation to various temperatures		
	16°C	25°C	32°C
Subtectal region	565 $\pm$ 72.3 $\leftarrow$	440 $\pm$ 56.1 $\leftarrow$	410 $\pm$ 52.5
Medulla oblongata	500 $\pm$ 64.0 —	465 $\pm$ 59.5 —	490 $\pm$ 63.7
Cerebellum	600 $\pm$ 76.8 —	590 $\pm$ 75.5 $\rightarrow$	800 $\pm$ 100.5

mammals succeeded in acquiring the thermoregulatory capacity, thus being able to keep their body temperature at a constant level. In the brains of these homeotherms the composition of the brain gangliosides in comparison with the ectotherms had become reduced to the well-known less polar pattern. It may be assumed that during

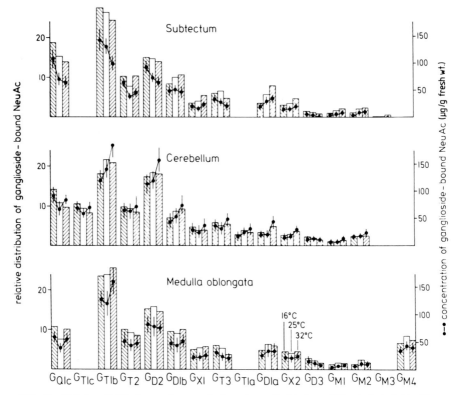

FIG. 7.   Relative distribution and concentration of ganglioside-bound NeuAc in individual fractions of subtectum, cerebellum, and medulla of *Tilapia* fish following long-term acclimation to 16°, 25°, and 32°, respectively.

phylogeny of the higher vertebrates the acquisition of thermoregulation simultaneously induced the loss of thermal adaption.

In Vitro Investigations on the Influence of Temperature Changes on the Ability of Gangliosides to Complex with Ca^{2+}

On one hand Ca^{2+} is known to be essentially involved in all neuronal functional processes, especially in transmission (24); further, gangliosides were shown to possess a pronounced capacity to bind Ca^{2+} (21,23). To elucidate the phenomenological data on the formation of more polar, polysialylated brain gangliosides in adaptation to lowered environmental temperatures, the influence of temperature changes on the binding capacities of differently composed brain gangliosides and single ganglioside species to Ca^{2+} were investigated. The investigations were carried out by means of potentiometrical procedures using Ca^{2+}-selective electrodes (22). Some binding characteristics of the various gangliosides to Ca^{2+} are given in Table 3.

TABLE 3. Ca^{2+} binding to gangliosides

	Ligand				
	G_{M1}	G_{D1a}	G_{T1b}	Adult chicken	1-Day-old chicken
Ca^{2+} binding positions/NeuAc = n_1	0.16	1.73	0.19	0.78	0.22
1. Binding dissociation constant (pK_{D1})	6.25	3.99	4.64	5.43	5.72
Upper limit of available range of n_1 and pK_{D1} mM Ca^{2+}	0.02	0.4	0.06	0.04	0.04
Ca^{2+} binding positions/NeuAc = n_2	0.28	—	0.24	0.84	1.82
2. Binding dissociation constant (pK_{D2})	5.03	—	4.02	5.14	4.47
Upper limit of available range of n_2 and pK_{D2} mM Ca^{2+}	0.2	—	0.4	0.2	0.4

Ganglioside-NeuAc, 0.1 mM, 5 mM triethanolamine-HCl buffer, pH 7.3, 37°C.
Data derived from graphical evaluation by plotting reciprocal values of free Ca^{2+} versus bound Ca^{2+}. (From ref. 22.)

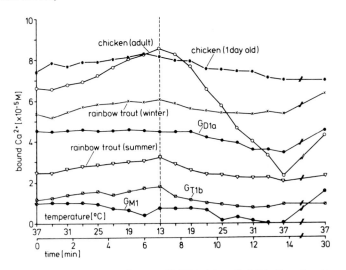

FIG. 8. Influence of temperature changes (3.5°C/min) on Ca^{2+} binding of various ganglioside fractions (G_{M1}, G_{D1a}, and G_{T1b}) and ganglioside mixtures of differing composition (0.1 mM ganglioside-NeuAc; 0.1 mM Ca^{2+} in triethanolamine-HCl buffer; pH 7.3).

At 37°C the highly polar brain ganglioside mixture of 1-day-old chicken showed the greatest binding ability for Ca^{2+} (NeuAc-Ca^{2+} isomolar at 0.1 mM), followed by the less polar mixture of near-adult chicken, then followed by that of a winter-acclimated rainbow trout, and finally summer trout. Among single gangliosides G_{D1a} was found to bind most Ca^{2+}, followed by G_{T1b} and G_{M1} (Fig. 8). Following cooling (3.5°C/min) from 37° to 13°C the Ca^{2+}-binding, especially to the brain ganglioside mixtures, was increased (7–30%). Subsequent rewarming resulted in up to 100% release of previously bound Ca^{2+}. Here especially the ganglioside-mixture from adult chicken, which contains more than 60% G_{D1a}, showed the highest thermosensitivity. In the meantime similar results were obtained by equilibrium dialysis using ^{45}Ca (21).

From these results it can be concluded that an increase in the polarity of gangliosides leads to a decrease in the thermal sensitivity of Ca^{2+} binding to these molecules. Accordingly it may be considered that the polysialylation of neuronal membranes of ectothermic vertebrates in adaptation to lowered ambient temperature, and also in homeotherms during their heterothermic phase, may be part of a molecular adaptation mechanism in the CNS of the vertebrates in the course of phylogeny. This may be particularly important in regulating Ca^{2+}-related processes at synapses as, for example, the process of neuronal transmission.

Neuronal Gangliosides in Relation to Poststimulation Processes

Since gangliosides were assumed to play an essential role in neuronal adaptive functions the question was raised whether they also might be involved in poststimulation reactions of the nerve cells. At present, there are only few and partly contradictory reports regarding the dependence on short-term stimulation of the neuronal ganglioside metabolism (4,6,16,44). To elucidate this aspect it was of utmost interest to find a specific neuronal system where quantitatively defined stimulation parameters could be correlated distinctly with correspondent brain structures. The weak electric tapirfish *Gnathonemus petersi* (Fig. 9A) living in Central Africa represents an ideal experimental system because it shows definite neuronal connection between different organs, e.g., the peripheral electric organ in the tail, centers of primary perception on the linear lobe for the signal derived from the mormyroblasts, centers of signal reception in the midbrain, and finally integration centers in the extremely enlarged valvula cerebelli (Fig. 9B). The telencephalon represents a control structure, as it is not involved in the process of electroperception.

After a 2-day habituation period 30 tapirfish were stimulated (each fish in a single trial) for 2 days with a so-called "threatening frequency" of 40 Hz (2V), which was conducted into the test aquarium by means of an artificial tapirfish dummy (1). In addition, corresponding numbers of nonstimulated, socially isolated fish ("deprived") and normal controls living in swarms of 5 to 10 fish under almost natural habitat conditions were investigated. In the stimulated test group the mean daily rate of electrical organ discharges (EOD) was in the range of $9.6 \pm 0.25 \times 10^5$ impulses ($= 11.1$ Hz), in the controls $8.1 \pm 0.02 \times 10^5$ ($= 9.4$ Hz), and in the deprived fish only $6.8 \pm 0.2 \times 10^5$ ($= 7.9$ Hz) ($\pm$ indicates SEM).

The ganglioside concentration of the four brain structures and the electric organ of the three test groups was determined. In addition, the incorporation of intracranially injected 2 μCi N-acetyl-D-[U-^{14}C]mannosamine (specific activity 254 mCi/mole; Amersham) into gangliosides of all structures was investigated.

Following electric stimulation the concentration of total gangliosides increased slightly only within the mesencephalon ($+ 10\%; p < 0.05$), while all other structures did not show significant changes (Fig. 9C). After social and stimulatory deprivation no differences could be registered either. Nevertheless, when analyzing

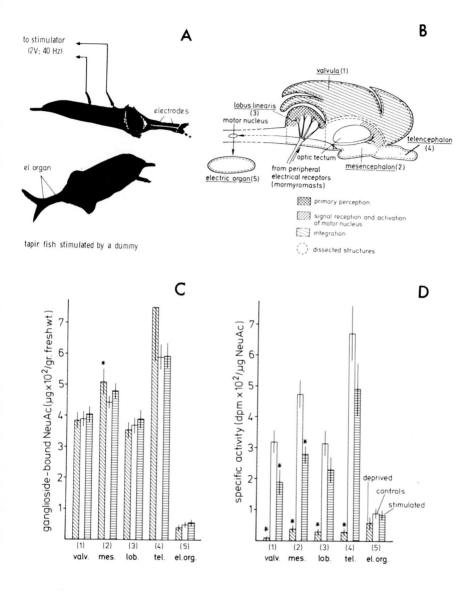

FIG. 9. Influence of electric stimulation (2 d, 40 Hz, 2 V) or deprivation (16 months social isolation) on ganglioside concentration **(C)** and specific activity (*N*-acetyl-[14C]mannosamine incorporation, 4 d); **(D)** in valvula cerebelli, mesencephalon, linear lobe, telencephalon, and electric organ of the electric tapir fish *Gnathonemus petersi*. Artificial stimulation of tapirfish by means of a dummy **(A)**. Schematic diagram of longitudinal section of tapirfish brain **(B)**.

the composition (pattern constellation) of the individual ganglioside fractions of the various structures, significant changes had been observed. Following stimulation increases in the amount of the end-products of the a- and b-pathways of ganglioside biosynthesis (48) occurred in the electro-perceiving structures, which mainly were due to corresponding decreases in the amount of their intermediate compounds. The corresponding values of the electrically deprived fish, on the other hand, deviated in quite other directions (30).

The specific NeuAc-radioactivity (d.p.m./μg NeuAc, after 4 days incorporation of *N*-acetyl-D-mannosamine) of total gangliosides was decreased in all neuronal structures as well following stimulation or deprivation, but not in the electric organ (Fig. 9D). After stimulus deprivation the specific activity was extremely low, obviously as a result of a generally lowered metabolic rate.

The specific radioactivity in all brain structures, but not in the electric organ of the stimulated tapirfish after the 4-day incorporation period, was significantly higher than that of the deprived animals. In comparison with the controls it was generally reduced. This can be interpreted as a higher turnover rate in the stimulated animals insofar as the amount of soluble precursor following the 4-day incorporation period already was diminished.

In summary, the data presented demonstrate that there are structure-dependent differences in amount and specific radioactivity of the brain gangliosides of the electric tapirfish following electrical stimulation or deprivation. These results are considered as evidence for the hypothesis that these molecular changes reflect an important mechanism of modulating the sensitivity of the membrane-mediated process of transmission, in which the membrane-bound ganglicsides are highly involved (33).

DISCUSSION

The above-mentioned data relative to changes in concentration and especially in composition of brain gangliosides dependent on long-term thermal adaptation phenomena and in relation to poststimulation processes provide evidence for the assumption that these compounds are indeed functionally involved in the process of neuronal transmission. This assumption is supported by the *in vitro* experiments concerning the complexation capacity of gangliosides with calcium ions. From these data it can be concluded that those changes in the molecular composition of the neuronal membrane-bound gangliosides may reflect an important and more general mechanism of modulating the sensitivity of membrane-mediated processes, as, e.g., transmission. With regard to the long-term adaptive changes of gangliosides following alterations in the environmental temperature, this assumption is supported by some recent physiologically relevant findings in teleost fish in which various long-term compensatory events had been observed (29). Goldfish when rapidly transferred from warm to cold water show typical behavioral and physiological changes: After a short initial phase of hyperexcitability they remain apparently dead for about 2 weeks. Then a compensatory regaining of mobility occurs step by step within a few days which, of course, remains on a lower level according to the temperature coefficient, but which enables the fish to react normally again (Fig. 10a). In addition, the rapid transfer of goldfish within 6 min to warmth or coldness also caused initial changes in the field potential amplitudes of photic evoked potentials in the optic tectum, especially in the postsynaptic amplitude, changes that reflect the high thermal sensitivity of this system (Fig. 10b and c). These effects lasted for about 1 to 2 weeks. Then slow compensatory reactions became evident: The previously reduced postsynaptic amplitude regained its 100% control level within 5 to 6 weeks after the transfer (35).

Further, the conditionability of fish was tested after long-term acclimation to water temperatures of 5° to 28°C by means of electrical avoidance conditioning in a shuttle tank (34). After acclimation to 5°, 9°, 16°, 21°, and 28°C a significant dependence of the learning rate on acclimation temperature was shown: the lower

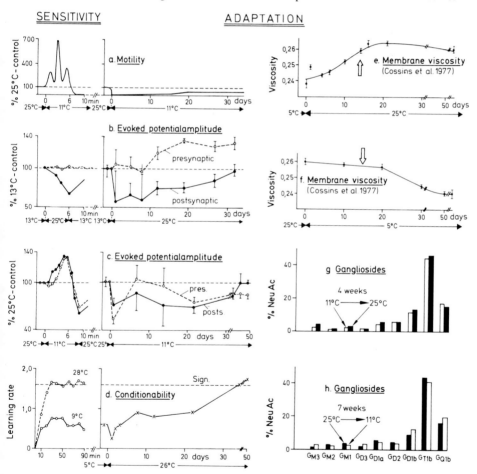

FIG. 10. Correlations between long-term thermal adaptations of regained motor activity (a), bioelectrical activity (photic evoked potential amplitudes; b, c), avoidance conditionability (d), membrane viscosity of synaptosomes (e, f), and degree of neuronal ganglioside-sialylation (g, h) of fish (e and f: values according to Cossins et al., ref. 5).

the environmental temperature, the poorer was the conditioning response. Following a transfer from cold to warm water the length of acclimation is most important for regaining full learning ability: Between 0 and 22 days after transfer no successful avoidance responses were observed. First correct responses were obtained 34 days after the transfer. Full conditionability, comparable with that of long-term warmth-adapted fish, was attained for the first time 50 days after the transfer (Fig. 10d).

These long-lasting compensatory phenomena in their course of time are in full agreement with changes in the composition of fatty acids and especially in the viscosity of synaptic membranes of the goldfish brain after alterations of temperature (5). Following transfer of goldfish from 5° to 25°C or the reverse long-lasting changes in the viscosity of synaptosomal membranes occurred until about 50 days after the transfer (Fig. 10e and f). In our hypothesis (33) these physicochemical adaptations of the synaptosomal membrane constituents in accordance with concomitant changes in the composition of the brain gangliosides (Fig. 10g and h) are assumed to be due to configurational changes in the degree of sialylation (and thus polarity) of the neuronal gangliosides.

In summary, all results concerning the various long-term thermal adaptation phenomena in vertebrates and changes in the brain ganglioside metabolism following short-term sensory stimulation are taken as evidence for the hypothesis that these molecular changes may reflect an important general mechanism with regard to a participation of gangliosides in modulating the sensitivity of the membrane-mediated process of transmission. These modulatory effects probably might be also essentially involved in the process of learning and memory formation. It seems to be likely that memory formation to an essential extent is related with configurational changes in the synaptic membrane, which might be due to changes in the composition and the capacity of membrane-bound gangliosides to complex with calcium ions.

SUMMARY

Neuronal gangliosides (sialoglycolipids with different numbers of sialic-neuraminic acid; NeuAc), which are highly enriched in synaptic membranes, are shown to play a prominent role in neuronal functions of the vertebrates.
1. The concentration and composition of ganglioside-bound NeuAc obviously are correlated with the level of evolutionary organization.
2. There are distinct correlations between the brain ganglioside composition and the state of thermal adaptation (adaptation to habitats with extreme temperature conditions, seasonal acclimatization, experimentally induced acclimation, hibernation, heterothermia during neonatal development).
3. The individual brain structures show significant differences in content and composition of gangliosides following thermal adaptation.
4. The capacity of neuronal gangliosides to form *in vitro* complexes with calcium ions is influenced by temperature changes.
5. There are distinct correlations between temperature-dependent changes in the brain ganglioside composition and other neurophysiologically relevant phenom-

ena (membrane viscosity, bioelectric activity, motor activity, and degree of conditioning response).

6. Following artificial electric stimulations (40 Hz, 2 V, 2 days) of the weak electric tapirfish *(Gnathonemus petersi)* structure-specific changes in amount and complexity of brain gangliosides were found, which were mostly due to changes in their more polar end-products of biosynthesis.

These results are considered as evidence for the hypothesis that variations in the composition of synaptic membrane-bound gangliosides reflect a mechanism of modulating the sensitivity of the membrane-mediated process of transmission.

ACKNOWLEDGMENTS

This work was supported by the Deutsche Forschungsgemeinschaft.

REFERENCES

1. Bässler, G., Hilbig, R., and Rahmann, H. (1978): Elektrische und motorische Aktivität von *Gnathonemus petersi* nach künstlicher elektrischer Stimulation. *Zool. Physiol*, 82:493–504.
2. Bässler, G., Hilbig, R., and Rahmann, H. (1979): Untersuchungen zur circadianen Rhythmik der elecktrischen und motorischen Aktivität von *Gnathonemus petersi* (Mormyridae, Pisces). *Z. Tierpsychol.*, 49:156–163.
3. Breer, H., and Rahmann, H. (1977): Cholinesterase-Aktivität und Hirnganglioside während der Fisch-Entwicklung. *Roux's Arch. Dev. Biol.*, 181:65–72.
4. Caputto, R., Maccioni, H. J., Arce, A., and Cumar, F. A. (1976): Biosynthesis of brain gangliosides. *Adv. Exp. Med. Biol.*, 71:27–43.
5. Cossins, A. R., Friedlander, M. M., and Prosser, C. L. (1977): Correlations between behavioral temperature adaptations of goldfish and the viscosity and fatty acid composition of their synaptic membranes. *J. Comp. Physiol.*, 120:109–121.
6. Dreyfus, H., Harth, S., Urban, P. F., and Mandel, P. (1976): Stimulation of chick retinal ganglioside synthesis by light. *Vision Res.*, 16:1365–1369.
7. Fishman, P. H., and Brady, R. O. (1976): Biosynthesis and function of gangliosides. *Science (NY)* 194:906–915.
8. Geiser, F., Hilbig, R., and Rahmann, H. (1981): Hibernation-induced changes in the ganglioside composition of fat dormice *(Glis glis)*. *J. Therm. Biol.*, 6:145–151.
9. Van Heyningen, W. E., and Mellanby, J. (1971): Tetanustoxin. In: *Microbiological Toxins, Vol. 2A: Bacterial Protein Toxins*, edited by S. Kadis, T. C. Montie, and S. J. Ajl, pp. 69–108. Academic Press, New York.
10. Hilbig, R., and Rahmann, H. (1979): Changes in brain ganglioside composition of normothermic and hibernating golden hamsters. *Comp. Biochem. Physiol.*, 62B:527–531.
11. Hilbig, R., and Rahmann, H. (1979): Comparative phylogenetical investigations of brain gangliosides in vertebrates. In: *Glycoconjugates*, edited by R. Schauer, P. Boer, E. Buddecke, M. F. Kramer, J. F. G. Vliegenthart, and H. Wiegandt, pp. 708–709. G. Thieme Publishers, Stuttgart.
12. Hilbig, R., and Rahmann, H. (1980): Variability in brain gangliosides of fishes. *J. Neurochem.*, 34:236–240.
13. Hilbig, R., and Rahmann, H. (1980): Phylogenetic differences in concentration and composition of brain gangliosides. *Hoppe-Seyler's Physiol. Chem.*, 361:268.
14. Hilbig, R., Rahmann, H., and Rösner, H. (1979): Brain gangliosides and temperature adaptation in eury- and stenothermic teleost fish (carp and rainbow trout). *J. Therm. Biol.*, 4:29–34.
15. Hilbig, R., Rösner, H., and Rahmann, H. (1981): Phylogenetic recapitulation of brain ganglioside composition during ontogenetic development. *Comp. Biochem. Physiol.*, 68B:301–305.
16. Irwin, L. N. (1974): Glycolipids and glycoproteins in brain function. *Rev. Neurosci.*, 1:137–179.
17. Katz, B., and Miledi, R. (1970): Further study of the role of calcium in synaptic transmission. *J. Physiol. (Lond.)*, 207:789–801.
18. Ledeen, R. W. (1979): Structure and distribution of gangliosides. In: *Complex Carbohydrates of Nervous Tissue*, edited by U. Margolis and K. Marsolls, pp. 1–23. Plenum Press, New York/London.

19. Maggio, B., Cumar, F. A., and Caputto, R. (1980): Configuration and interactions of the polar head group in gangliosides. *Biochem. J.*, 189:435–440.
20. Matheson, D. F., Oel, F., and Roots, B. I. (1980): Changes in the fatty acyl composition of phospholipids in the optic tectum and optic nerve of temperature-acclimated goldfish. *Physiol. Zool.*, 53:57–69.
21. Mühleisen, M., Probst, W., Wiegandt, H., and Rahmann, H. (1979): *In vitro* studies on the influence of cations, neurotransmitters and tubocurarine on calcium-ganglioside-interactions. *Life Sci.*, 25:791–796.
22. Probst, W., and Rahmann, H. (1980): Influence of temperature changes on the ability of gangliosides to complex with Ca^{2+}. *J. Therm. Biol.*, 5:243–247.
23. Probst, W., Rösner, H., Wiegandt, H., and Rahmann, H. (1979): Das Komlexationsvermögen von Gangliosiden für Ca^{2+}. *Hoppe-Seyler's Z. Physiol. Chem.*, 360:979–986.
24. Rahamimoff, R., Eulkar, S. D., Alnaes, E., Mairi, H., Rotshenker, S., and Rahamimoff, H. (1976): Modulation of transmitter release by calcium ions and nerve impulses. *Cold Spring Harbor Symp. Quant. Biol.*, 40:107–116.
25. Rahmann, H. (1976): *Neurobiologie.* UTB Verlag Eugen Ulmer, Stuttgart, 273 pp.
26. Rahmann, H. (1977): Synaptogenese und Gangliosid-Synthese im Zentralnervensystem von Teleosteern während der Ontogenese. *Hoppe-Seyler's Z. Physiol. Chem.*, 358:290.
27. Rahmann, H. (1978): Gangliosides and thermal adaptation in vertebrates. Review. *Jpn. J. Exp. Med.*, 48:85–96.
28. Rahmann, H. (1980): Gangliosides and thermal adaptation. In: *Structure and Function of Gangliosides*, edited by L. Svennerholm, H. Dreyfus, and P. F. Urban. Plenum Press, New York.
29. Rahmann, H. (1981): Die Bedeutung der Hirnganglioside bei der Temperaturadaptation der Vertebraten. *Zool. Physiol.*, 85:209–248.
30. Rahmann, H., Bässler, G., and Hilbig, R. (1981): Changes in the ganglioside metabolism in relation to sensory stimulation of the electric tapirfish (Gnathonemus petersi). *Hoppe-Seyler's Z. Physiol. Chem.*, 362:229.
31. Rahmann, H., and Hilbig, R. (1980): Brain gangliosides are involved in the adaptation of antarctic fish to extreme low temperatures. *Naturwiss.*, 67:259.
32. Rahmann, H., and Hilbig, R. (1981): Involvement of neuronal gangliosides and thermal adaptation. In: *Survival in Cold; Hibernation and Other Adaptations*, edited by X. J. Musacchia and L. Jansky, pp. 177–189, Elsevier, North-Holland, Amsterdam.
33. Rahmann, H., Rösner, H., and Breer, H. (1976): A functional model of sialo-macromolecules in synaptic transmission and memory formation. *J. Theor. Biol.*, 57:231–237.
34. Rahmann, H., Schmidt, W., and Schmidt, B. (1980): Influence of longterm thermal acclimation on the conditionability of fish. *J. Therm. Biol.*, 5:11–16.
35. Reckhaus, W., and Rahmann, H. (1979): Long-term thermal adaptation of evoked potentials in the optic tectum of goldfish. *IRCS Med. Sci.*, 7:290.
36. Rösner, H. (1975): Changes in the contents of gangliosides and in the ganglioside pattern of the chicken brain. *J. Neurochem.*, 24:815–816.
37. Rösner, H. (1977): Gangliosides, sialoglycoproteins and acetylcholinesterase of the developing mouse brain. *Wilhelm Roux Arch.*, 183:325–335.
38. Rösner, H. (1981): Ganglioside changes in the chicken optic lobes as biochemical indicators of brain development and maturation. *Brain. Res.*, 236:49–61.
39. Rösner, H., Breer, H., Hilbig, R., and Rahmann, H. (1979): Temperature effects on the incorporation of sialic acid into gangliosides and glycoproteins of fish brain. *J. Therm. Biol.*, 4:69–73.
40. Rösner, H., Merz, G., and Rahmann, H. (1979): Binding of *d*-tubocurarine by gangliosides. *Hoppe-Seyler's Z. Physiol. Chem.*, 260:413–420.
41. Rösner, H., Segler, K., and Rahmann, H. (1979): Changes of brain gangliosides in chicken and mice during heterothermic development. *J. Therm. Biol.*, 4:121–124.
42. Roots, B. I. (1968): Phospholipids of goldfish *(Carassius auratus L.)* brain: The influence of environmental temperature. *Comp. Biochem. Physiol.*, 25:457–466.
43. Sato, S., Kawamura, N., and Taketomi, T. (1979): Brain glycolipids of a wild Japanese adult bear. *Jpn. J. Exp. Med.*, 49:139–146.
44. Savaki, H. E., and Levis, G. M. (1977): Changes in rat brain gangliosides following active avoidance conditioning. *Pharmacol. Biochem. Behav.*, 7:7–12.
45. Svennerholm, L. (1957): Quantitative estimation of sialic acis. A colorimetric resorcinol-hydrochloric acid method. *Biochim. Biophys. Acta*, 24:604–611.

46. Svennerholm, L., and Fredman, P. (1980): A procedure for the quantitative isolation of brain gangliosides. *Biochim. Biophys. Acta*, 617:97–100.
47. Wolley, D. W., and Gommi, B. W. (1965): Activities of various pure gangliosides as the receptors, serotonin receptors. *Proc. Natl. Acad. Sci. USA*, 53:959–963.
48. Yu, R. K., and Ando, S. (1980): Structures of some new complex gangliosides of fish brain. *Adv. Exp. Med. Biol.*, 125:33–45.

Neural Transmission, Learning and Memory,
edited by R. Caputto and C. Ajmone Marsan.
Raven Press, New York © 1983.

Effect of Light on the Labeling of Gangliosides and Glycoproteins of Individually Caged Chickens

R. Caputto, B. L. Caputto, G. A. Nores, and B. N. Cemborain

Departamento de Química Biológica, Facultad de Ciencias Químicas, Universidad Nacional de Córdoba, Ciudad Universitaria, Córdoba, R. Argentina

It is noteworthy that among the many studies on the chemical correlates of memory and learning relatively little attention has been given the constituents of membranes. It is somehat contradictory that in spite of the fact that the importance of the membrane constituents has frequently been stressed in the establishment of connections and in the recognition between cells—mechanisms that appear of fundamental importance in establishing nervous pathways—most correlates studied to date are proteins or nucleic acids, without regard to whether or not they are membrane constituents.

It is conceivable that in man an important part of learned and memorized concepts is obtained without participation of the sensory organs by retrieval and combination of previous knowledge, but in all forms of memory and learning in animals, the processes are either genetic or a consequence of sensory stimulation. The underlying reason for the little attention paid to the sensory organs in the study of the higher functions of the brain may be the assumption that they serve only as instruments for the transduction of the physical stimulus. The nerve waves that they originate are transmitted to the brain as transient ionic changes that are responsible for the subsequent events from which memory and learning arise.

However, other types of materials may be sent by the sensory organs to the brain. The carbohydrate chain of gangliosides and glycoproteins is synthesized in the Golgi apparatus located in the perikaryon of the neuronal cell. Some of the evidence for this statement was obtained working with the optical tract of chickens, rabbits, and goldfish (3–5,7). In these animals the axons of the ganglion cells of the inner layer of the retina end in the contralateral optic tectum in the brain. Through these axons some of the material synthesized in the retina is transported to the brain by the process known as axonal transport. It is a fortunate situation that most if not all of the axons originated in one eye end in the contralateral tectum. By taking advantage of this disposition it is possible to know after an intraocular injection of a labeled precursor how much of a product synthesized in the retina was taken to the tectum by axonal transport. This can be obtained by subtracting the labeling of one and the same product in the ipsilateral tectum from that in the contralateral tectum, since the amount of labeling due to arrival of either precursor or product through systemic transport should be identical for both tecta (Fig. 1).

EFFECT OF LIGHT ON THE LABELING IN RETINA

The various types of cells in the chick retina of singly housed chickens apparently react in different ways to the light stimulus. Because of the difficulties of separation of some cell layers only two of them have been isolated and their labeling studied after an intraocular injection of [³H]N-acetylmannosamine ([³H]ManNAc), a specific sialic acid precursor. The layers studied are those of the rod outer segment (ROS) and the ganglion cells. Both have been found with increased labeling in their gangliosides and glycoproteins after being subjected to light stimulus. The ROS was increased by just 15% whereas the ganglion cell layer was increased by about 20–45% with respect to the animals that remained in complete darkness (Fig. 2). However, determinations in the labeling of the total retina showed no significant changes. Moreover, it had been previously found that when labeled glucosamine (instead of [³H]ManNAc) was given subcutaneously the labeling of the total retina diminished under the effect of light (1). Another indication that different reactions occur in different layers was found in the observation that the increase of labeling of both gangliosides and glycoproteins is more marked in the optic tectum than in

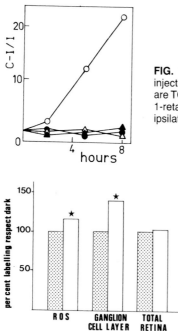

FIG. 1. Radioactivity of gangliosides (○) after an intraocular injection of [³H]ManNAc. Other materials shown in the figure are TCA–PTA-soluble: evaporable (●); nonevaporable: Dowex-1-retained (△) and nonretained (▲). C, Contralateral tectum; I, ipsilateral tectum. (From ref. 5.)

FIG. 2. Labeling of gangliosides of rod outer segment (ROS), ganglion cells, and total retina from chicks in light or dark. Ganglioside labeling from chickens in dark was considered as 100%. Differences were significant when $p < 0.025$ as indicated by a star. Values are the means of 15 determinations.

the ganglion cell layer (2). This indicated that in this layer only (or mostly) those cells that send their axons to the tectum increase their labeling or else that other synapses that can be present in the layer of ganglion cells do not have gangliosides or glycoproteins with increased labeling.

EFFECT OF LIGHT ON THE LABELING OF THE OPTIC TECTUM

Three hours after an intraocular injection of labeled [³H]ManNAc the gangliosides and glycoproteins of the optic tectum of singly housed chickens exposed to light are more highly labeled than those of the chickens that remained in darkness (Fig. 3). That the difference is due to the effect of light and not to the switching from dark to light was shown by two different experiments. Animals in continuous light for 3 hr were compared with animals that during the same total period were changed from dark to light and vice versa every 15 min or with animals that remained the 3 hr in darkness. The chickens with the highest labeling were those in continuous light, followed by those that were changed every 15 min and lastly, those that remained in darkness (Fig. 3). In another type of experiment groups of 40 chickens were kept in light or dark for 48 hr. At the end of this period all the animals received an injection of [³H]ManNAc and immediately one-half of each group was taken to darkness while the other half was put in light. The labeling of the tectum gangliosides of the animals that changed from dark to light increased whereas those of the animals that passed from light to dark decreased (Fig. 4).

EFFECT OF ANESTHETICS

Chickens anesthetized with either urethane or chloral hydrate did not show the effect of light on the labeling of optic tectum gangliosides. The effect of these anesthetics was, however, different for both of them. Whereas urethane inhibited the additional labeling obtained in the light-exposed chickens leaving unchanged the labeling in darkness, anesthesia with chloral hydrate resulted in a strong inhibition of all labeling, whether in light or dark. The effects obtained in the optic tectum were very similar to those in retina but the ratio of labeling between tectum and retina in anesthetized and control animals indicated that in the chloral hydrate-

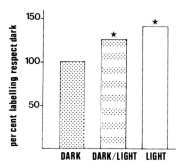

FIG. 3. Labeling of optic tectum gangliosides from chickens exposed to dark, light, or intermittent illumination. Animals were decapitated 3 hr after an intraocular injection of [³H]ManNAc. Dark/light cycles were 15 min each. Labeling of gangliosides from animals in dark was considered as 100%. Differences were significant when $p < 0.025$, as indicated by a star.

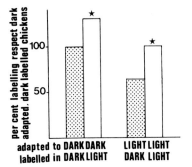

FIG. 4. Five-hour labeling of optic tectum gangliosides in chickens previously adapted to light or dark. Animals subjected to 48 hr of continuous light or continuous darkness were given an intraocular injection of [³H]ManNAc and then exposed to light or dark. Five hours later animals were decapitated and the labeling of the contralateral optic tectum gangliosides determined. Incorporation values in dark adapted, dark labeled chickens were considered as 100%. Statistical differences were calculated for those dark and light groups that had been submitted to the same adaptation condition. Differences were significant when $p < 0.005$, as indicated by a star.

treated chickens there was impairment in the axonal transport of the gangliosides (V. Allende and B. Caputto, *unpublished results*).

LACK OF EFFECT OF LIGHT ON THE LABELING OF PROTEINS BY [³H]PROLINE

The effect of light on the labeling of gangliosides and glycoproteins is apparently not a general one. The effect has not been extensively investigated but it has been established that the labeling of the tectum proteins after an intraocular injection of [³H]proline does not change by exposing the singly housed animals to light. Similar results were obtained whether the precursors — [³H]proline or [³H]ManNAc — for the synthesis of proteins and gangliosides, respectively, were injected separately, one into each eye of the chicken or together, in the same solution, into one eye (6).

NATURE AND FATE OF THE ADDITIONAL LABELING

Methods currently available to study the nature and the subcellular disposition of gangliosides and glycoproteins are probably not accurate enough to determine subtle variations in case that one of these variations had taken place. In any case, both studies have been carried out with negative results. We could not detect qualitative differences in the thin-layer chromatographic patterns of the gangliosides of chicks that had been in the dark or exposed to light. The differences were purely quantitative, the three peaks of labeling usually seen in retina and optic tectum being increased in the same proportions in the animals subjected to light.

The distribution of labeled glycoproteins and gangliosides in the subcellular fractions of the optic tectum, obtained after a hypoosmotic shock and centrifugal preparation, was practically identical in both groups of animals. The fractions with the highest labeling were in both cases those enriched in plasma membranes.

A difference was, however, found in the percent of radioactivity released from the gangliosides of the tectum of animals exposed to light or remaining in the dark, under the effect of neuraminidase. At 5 hr after the intraocular injection of the precursor a higher percent of releasable labeling from gangliosides was found in the chicks exposed to light (Fig. 5). The complete information for the interpretation of these results is not available but if it is assumed that eventually all of the gangliosides synthesized in the neuronal perikarya find a position in the plasma membrane where they are exposed to neuraminidase, these results indicate that in the light the gangliosides reach their position in the tecta in less time than in the dark.

POSSIBLE MECHANISMS

We feel inclined to disregard the possibility of a direct effect of the light on retina as the responsible factor for the increased labeling of gangliosides and glycoproteins because of the continuous failure to produce the phenomenon on the isolated eye retina. Exposure *in vitro* of retina to light has not brought about an increase in either the uptake of precursors or an increase of labeling of gangliosides and glycoproteins in either the total retina or the ganglion cell layer.

Recent experiments in our laboratory (S. Quiroga, et al., *unpublished observations*) showed that the uptake of precursors by the layer of ganglion cells is rather diminished than increased under the influence of light and so is the activity of the glycosyl (sialyl, galactosyl, and galactosaminyl) transferases in the same layer (G. Nores, S. Quiroga, and R. Caputto, *unpublished observations*).

In vivo, chicks whose optic nerve had been cut showed no light effect in the ganglion cells of the corresponding eye (B. Caputto and N. Cemborain, *unpublished observations*). These observations indicate that the effect is not confined to the eye or in other words, the nerve wave that originates in the photoreceptors of the retina is not directly or solely responsible for the increase of ganglioside labeling in the ganglion cells.

Provided that an effect limited to the retina could be disregarded there are several possible mechanisms by which the effect may be brought about. Since it has been convincingly shown (5) that the main, if not the only, site of synthesis of gangliosides is in the neuronal perikarya and that they are translated from there to the plasma membrane of the nerve ending, it is possible that an increased demand for gangliosides from the nerve ending triggers an increase in the synthesis of gangliosides. In agreement with this possibility is the finding that the concentration of gangliosides

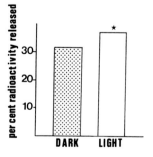

FIG. 5. Radioactivity (in percent) released from optic tectum gangliosides by treatment with neuraminidase. Animals were decapitated 5 hr after an intraocular injection of [³H]ManNAc. Tectum homogenates were incubated with 0.4 units of neuraminidase per optic tectum during 90 min. Reactions were stopped by the addition of TCA-PTA (10%–1%) and the remaining ganglioside labeling determined. Results are given as percent of the total initial labeling of the samples. Star indicates $p < 0.025$.

in a synthetic system regulates their own rate of synthesis (G. Nores et al., *unpublished results*).

Another possible mechanism is through an endocrinological effect. It is known that exposure to light produces the inhibition of the secretion of pineal hormones (8). It is conceivable that the secretion of those hormones in darkness regulates the activity of the transferring enzymes that synthesize the carbohydrate chain of the gangliosides and glycoproteins.

An endocrine effect could come also through the situation of stress that is apparent in singly housed chickens in light.

IMPLICATIONS

Besides the acts of memory and learning that must be attributed to genetic mechanisms we know of no other mechanism for acquiring memory or learning in lower than primate animals than perception of sensory stimulus. It is, consequently, possible that through the modification of pathways that start in the retina as an organ of perception and diversify in the tectum, the formation of membrane constituents such as gangliosides and glycoproteins plays a role in the acquisition of memory and learning. It is realized that there are difficulties in verification of this hypothesis because of the necessary small effect that nonstressing stimulus should have on the brain chemistry and because of certain self-denial conditions for verification of the hypothesis, since any interruption of the perception should cut not only the one suggested by the experiments reported above but all the possible mechanisms for the development of memory and learning.

SUMMARY

The study of the effects of any sensory stimulus on the chemical responses of the brain produced diverse results in different parts of the nervous system, including the sensory organs, and in the same organ in different species of animals. In an attempt to localize the effects of light on the optic tectum, the labeling of some membrane components—such as gangliosides—was studied in the ganglion cellular body and axon terminals after an intraocular injection in individually housed chickens. An increase in the labeling of gangliosides and glycoproteins was found, which did not affect either the distribution or the relative concentration of the gangliosides formed. The only difference that could be detected was that a higher percentage labeling of the animals in the light became susceptible to neuraminidase 5 hr after the intraocular injection.

ACKNOWLEDGMENTS

This investigation was supported in part by grants from the Secretaría de Ciencia y Tecnología, the Consejo Nacional de Investigaciones Científicas y Técnicas, and the Foundation Lucio Cherny, of Argentina.

REFERENCES

1. Caputto, B. L., Maccioni, A. H. R., and Caputto, R. (1975): Light inhibits the labeling of gangliosides in chicken retina. *Nature (Lond.)*, 257:492–493.
2. Caputto, B. L., Nores, G. A., Cemborain, B. N., and Caputto, R. (1982): The effect of light, exposure following an intraocular injection of N-^{3}H-acetylmannosamine on the labeling of gangliosides and glycoproteins. *Brain Res.*, 245:231–238.
3. Forman, D. S., and Ledeen, R. W. (1972): Axonal transport of gangliosides in the goldfish optic nerve. *Science*, 177:630–633.
4. Holm, M. (1972): Gangliosides of the optic pathway; biosynthesis and biodegradation studied *in vivo*. *J. Neurochem.*, 19:623–629.
5. Landa, C. A., Maccioni, H. J. F., and Caputto, R. (1979): The site of synthesis of gangliosides in the chick optic system. *J. Neurochem.*, 33:825–838.
6. Marchionatti, A. M. (1981): Thesis, Facultad de Ciencias Exactas, Físicas y Naturales, Universidad Nacional de Córdoba.
7. Rosner, H. (1975): Incorporation of sialic acid into gangliosides and glycoproteins of the optic pathway following an intraocular injection of N-^{3}H acetylmannosamine in the chicken. *Brain Res.*, 97:107–116.
8. Smith, J. A. (1981): The transduction of environmental lighting cues into biochemical rhythms via mammalian pineal gland. *Neurochem. Int.*, 3:21–25.

Neural Transmission, Learning and Memory,
edited by R. Caputto and C. Ajmone Marsan.
Raven Press, New York © 1983.

Seizures Promote Breakdown of Membrane Phospholipids in the Brain

**N. G. Bazan and *E. B. Rodriguez de Turco

**Instituto de Investigaciones Bioquimicas, Universidad Nacional del Sur-Consejo
Nacional de Investigaciones Cientificas y Tecnicas, Bahia Blanca, Argentina; and **LSU
Eye Center, Louisiana State University Medical Center School of Medicine,
New Orleans, Louisiana*

Excitation, inhibition, and other membrane-mediated information transfers are intimately related to biochemical events taking place within the neuronal plasma membrane. Moreover, at the synapse, which is the main locus of cell-to-cell communication in the neural tissue, membrane constituents may be subtly changed by the experiences of learning, memory, and epilepsy (15). This, in fact, is one of the reasons why researchers have focused on seaching for membrane modifications in abnormal experiences such as epilepsy (15,25). Although information is available on membrane-bound enzymes that translocate ions (15), little is known about the chemical components of membranes during epileptogenesis, largely because of the technical difficulties involved in the quantitative measurements of endogenous components of membranes and because of the rapidity with which biochemical events take place during seizures.

Phospholipids are present in relatively large quantities in a wide variety of classes and molecular species in neuronal membranes. These molecules are composed of head groups with different charges and, in addition, contain several acyl groups with varying carbon chain lengths and numbers of double bonds. The combination of the different varieties of phospholipids results in several hundred kinds of individual molecules interacting among themselves and also with other membrane components, such as proteins. Phospholipids are arranged in a bilayer, and the phospholipid classes seem to be asymmetrically distributed (26a).

The highly unsaturated long acyl chains facing away from the membrane surfaces create a fluid environment in the membrane. Different regions of the same membrane may actually vary in chemical composition. Lipid molecules and proteins can move both laterally and in the transverse plane of the membrane. Thus, the fluid mosaic structure (12) is a highly dynamic organization to which metabolic transformation of membrane components provides increased plasticity and additional means of retailoring modifications in chemical structure.

These chemical components and their interactions affect membrane functioning. However, the role of phospholipids in the reading and interpretation of intercellular signals and the resulting intracellular functions or the modulation of membrane-bound enzymes is not understood. There are at least four groups of biochemical observations that may have a bearing on "in-membrane" events in the nervous system: (a) the drug and hormonally enhanced [^{32}P] turnover of phospholipids (18,19), including the receptor-stimulated phosphatidylinositol breakdown (23); (b) the methylation pathway of phospholipids coupled to a phospholipase A_2 (18a); (c) the unsaturated diacylglyceride stimulation of Ca^{2+}-dependent, phospholipid-dependent protein kinase (20); and (d) the production of free arachidonic acid (3a,16,17, 22) and diacylglycerides (3,3a,19) in the brain in response to brief ischemia (1,4,7,16,17,20,22,23), drug-induced convulsions (4,6,10), and electroshock (2,3a,6,8).

This chapter summarizes our recent studies on the action of bicuculline-induced status epilepticus on the lipid effect mentioned above in (d).

Bicuculline is a γ-aminobutyric acid (GABA) antagonist more potent and selective than the picrotoxin that sets off a status epilepticus condition after intraperitoneal injection (13,26,29).

FREE ARACHIDONIC ACID PRODUCTION

The onset of ischemia (23), certain drug-induced convulsions (10), and electro-convulsive shock (3a,4,8) trigger the release of brain free fatty acids at a rate of the same order of magnitude as occurs in adipose tissue under maximal stimulation by lipolytic hormones. Arachidonic acid is the main component liberated, and the convulsion-induced change in this fatty acid is the first change seen in an endogenous component of membranes stimulated within physiological limits *in vivo*.

BICUCULLINE STIMULATES THE RELEASE OF BRAIN FREE FATTY ACIDS

When bicuculline was given intraperitoneally to rats, status epilepticus was generated; during the first tonic-clonic seizure, a greatly increased amount of brain free fatty acid was found (Fig. 1). The animals were decapitated immediately, and the heads were frozen in liquid N_2 with vigorous stirring for rapid fixation. Lipid extracts were made from frozen, pulverized tissue. Thus, pool size estimates were close to those of the *in vivo* situation. Bicuculline-induced convulsions produced predominantly arachidonic acid and stearic acid, both in cerebrum and cerebellum. In the cerebrum, a more than 12-fold increase in free arachidonic acid was observed; in the cerebellum, much smaller changes took place (Fig. 1). In the cerebrum, stearic acid increased fourfold, whereas free palmitic, docosahexaenoic, and oleic acid did not quite double. Similar changes were seen in the cerebellum; however, proportionally more free docosahexaenoic acid was released.

INCREASED CONTENT OF DIACYLGLYCEROLS DURING BICUCULLINE-INDUCED SEIZURES

Bicuculline-induced seizures also stimulated the accumulation of diacylglycerols in the cerebrum and cerebellum. The fatty acid composition of this neutral lipid

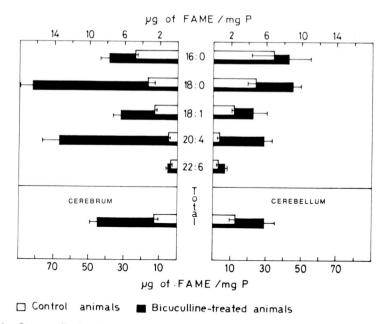

FIG. 1. Status epilepticus induced by bicuculline increases the pool size of free fatty acid pool in the cerebrum and cerebellum in the rat. FAME, fatty acid methyl esters; P, total phospholipid P. Total includes minor fatty acids not shown in the upper portion of the figure. *White bars*, controls; *black bars*, bicuculline-treated animals. Lipid extraction, free fatty acid isolation, and quantification were carried out as described elsewhere (2,3a).

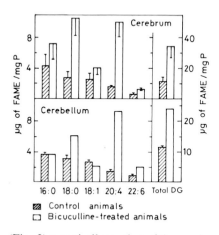

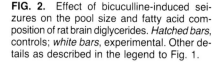

FIG. 2. Effect of bicuculline-induced seizures on the pool size and fatty acid composition of rat brain diglycerides. *Hatched bars*, controls; *white bars*, experimental. Other details as described in the legend to Fig. 1.

(Fig. 2) was similar to that of the produced free fatty acids (Fig. 1). The predominant acyl group in the accumulated diacylglycerols in the cerebrum was arachidonate, followed by stearate and docosahexaenoate. In the cerebellum, a much larger accumulation of arachidonoyl-diglycerides was seen, and there was no increase in palmitate or oleate. Moreover, total diglyceride accumulation was greater in the cerebrum than in the cerebellum.

Two features of the lipids accumulated during bicuculline-induced seizures deserve further comment. First, the fatty acid profiles in both parts of the central nervous system were very similar in terms of free fatty acids and diacylglycerols. Second, striking differences were seen in the magnitude of the lipid effect produced by bicuculline in the cerebrum and the cerebellum. Of the acyl groups in cerebellar diglycerides, only palmitate and oleate did not change; all others increased. The predominant molecular species was stearoyl-arachidonyl; these two fatty acids were also the main free components found. Hence, it is likely that there may be a metabolic relationship between the diacylglycerols and the free fatty acids produced.

These results led to the question of the origin of these molecules from a membrane phospholipid rich in these fatty acids. Phosphatidylinositol and/or phosphatidylcholine degradation may be involved either by a sequential phospholipase C-diglyceride lipase-monoglyceride lipase mechanism or by two enzymatic mechanisms: phospholipase C, on the one hand, and phospholipases A_1-A_2, on the other. In any event, the process is rapid and transient when electroshock is the stimulus (3a,6,8). Although the increase was severalfold in relation to the resting pool sizes, it was extremely small in comparison with the membrane phospholipid concentration in the brain. Thus, a highly specific pathway for the degradation of a selective membrane phospholipid is involved. It may be that a synaptic membrane phospholipid is involved in inner membrane events during epileptogenesis.

Since the pool sizes involved are small, the measurement of these endogenous pools in isolated synaptosomes from convulsing animals may not yield clear-cut data due to the rapid changes taking place in these lipids during preparation of the fractions (24). However, with the use of labeled fatty acids, a high turnover rate of arachidonoyl groups of phosphatidylinositol in synaptosomes was observed (28).

The results obtained from the measuring of endogenous membrane-related pools in the brain were extended by pretreating the animals with drugs to modify the neural content of neurotransmitters. The hypothesis was that seizures trigger a chain of events wherein selective membrane breakdown occurs as a result of the action of a modulator. Hence, neural depletion of catecholamines by α-methyl-*p*-tyrosine and of serotonin by *p*-chlorophenylalanine was explored. The question was asked whether the accumulation of free fatty acids and diacylglycerol is affected by bicuculline under these conditions.

α-METHYL-*p*-TYROSINE AND THE EFFECT OF BICUCULLINE ON BRAIN LIPIDS

Although pretreatment with the competitive inhibitor of tyrosine hydrolase, α-methyl-*p*-tyrosine, depletes the brain of catecholamines, it does not modify the resting levels of free fatty acids and does not alter the stimulated increase in free fatty acids caused by bicuculline (Table 1). However, a potentiation of the bicuculline effect was seen in the cerebellum (Table 2).

TABLE 1. *Changes in cerebral free fatty acids in rats undergoing status epilepticus by bicuculline. Effect of α-methyl-p-tyrosine*

Free fatty acid	Control			α-Methyl-*p*-tyrosine		
	Basal[a]	Bicuculline[a]	Δ%	Basal[a]	Bicuculline[a]	Δ%
16:0	4.97	7.83	(164)	2.79	5.9	(212)
18:0	3.35	16.49	(492)	3.97	13.37	(337)
18:1	2.68	6.38	(238)	2.41	4.62	(192)
20:4 n-6	1.00	13.54	(1354)	1.00	10.35	(1035)
22:6 n-3	0.74	1.11	(150)	0.46	0.34	(74)
Total	12.96	45.35	(350)	10.63	34.42	(324)

α-Methyl-*p*-tyrosine was given intraperitoneally during the 24 hr prior to injecting bicuculline (80 mg/kg body weight four times every 6 hr).
[a] μg of fatty acid methyl esters/mg of lipid P.

TABLE 2. *Free fatty acids in the cerebellum from rats treated with bicuculline, α-methyl-p-tyrosine, or α-methyl-p-tyrosine plus bicuculline*

Fatty acid	Control			α-Methyl-*p*-tyrosine		
	Basal[a]	Bicuculline[a]	Δ%	Basal[a]	Bicuculline[a]	Δ%
16:0	6.76	8.44	(125)	7.16	11.84	(165)
18:0	4.74	9.13	(193)	3.51	14.19	(404)
18:1	2.41	4.57	(190)	2.42	6.25	(258)
20:4 n-6	0.72	5.87	(825)	1.08	9.01	(834)
22:6 n-3	0.65	1.35	(207)	0.53	1.40	(264)
Total	13.44	29.36	(218)	14.69	42.68	(290)

[a] μg of fatty acid methyl esters/mg of lipid P.

A similar experimental outline employing electroshock instead of bicuculline to induce seizures resulted in an inhibition of the convulsion-stimulated free fatty acid production (2). Hence, different mechanisms may operate to accumulate free fatty acids according to the stimulating agent used.

p-CHLOROPHENYLALANINE AND THE EFFECT OF BICUCULLINE ON BRAIN LIPIDS

We found that *p*-chlorophenylalanine pretreatment stimulated the production of all free fatty acids except docosahexaenoic acid in the cerebrum and the cerebellum (only data for cerebellum are shown, see Table 3). Since the resulting free fatty acid levels are high, the bicuculline effect on the release of palmitic and oleic acids is masked and does not affect the accumulation of arachidonic and stearic acids. In cerebral hemispheres, a 50% reduction in the release of these two fatty acids was found (data not shown).

SEIZURES, EPILEPTIC BRAIN DAMAGE, AND STATUS EPILEPTICUS

Our data indicate that membrane phospholipids and their acyl chains in the brain are affected during convulsions induced by bicuculline. How the changes are brought

TABLE 3. *Bicuculline-induced status epilepticus. Free fatty acids in cerebellum and effects of p-chlorophenylalanine*

	Control			p-Chlorophenylalanine		
Fatty acid	Basal[a]	Bicuculline[a]	Δ%	Basal[a]	Bicuculline[a]	Δ%
16:0	6.76	8.44	(125)	8.48	6.47	(76)
18:0	4.74	9.13	(193)	6.18	14.43	(233)
18:1	2.41	4.57	(190)	8.23	10.50	(128)
20:4 n-6	0.72	5.87	(825)	2.47	8.35	(338)
22:6 n-3	0.65	1.35	(207)	0.93	1.38	(148)
Total	13.44	29.36	(218)	26.29	41.12	(156)

[a] μg of fatty acid methyl esters/mg of lipid P.

about is not yet known; however, it may be that a hydrolytic enzyme is activated and, in turn, a specific pool of membrane phospholipid is degraded. Whether the initiation, maintenance, or propagation of seizures gives rise to such changes is not certain. It seems likely that the effect occurs at the onset of the seizure, since a single electroconvulsive shock produced a transient increase in brain free fatty acids (3a,8) and because only at the time of the first tonic-clonic seizure induced by bicuculline was an effect seen (10). Thereafter, increased production of free fatty acids indicated that the hydrolytic system was still functioning. It is interesting that, even after several minutes of status epilepticus induced by bicuculline, the same fatty acid profile was seen, that is, arachidonic and stearic acids were still predominant, indicating that other acyl groups of phospholipids were not split off during repeated seizures. However, the amount of diacylglycerols enriched in arachidonate and stearate tends to decrease as a function of time after bicuculline injection (11), indicating that perhaps the diacylglycerols formed are being degraded and are releasing free fatty acids. As discussed above, the type of enzymes involved is not yet known, but it is likely that phospholipases C, diglyceride lipases, and phospholipases A are involved. How are they activated, where they are located, what is the sequence of their action, and what kind of membrane changes their activation produces all remain questions for the future.

During status epilepticus, the repeated seizures may unbalance the reacylation pathway by overstimulation of the deacylation reactions. As a result, the increasingly larger free fatty acid pool may be a factor in the pathogenesis of epileptic brain damage, as suggested for brain edema (9). Therapeutic ways to limit the degradative pathway or to remove the accumulated products may help to ameliorate brain damage, since free fatty acids are harmful to cellular membranes at relatively low concentrations (5). Prostaglandins and thromboxane are also produced during seizures, and their production is linked to increased central nervous system activity (21,27).

Bicuculline antagonizes GABA receptors and neuronally evoked presynaptic and strychnine-insensitive postsynaptic inhibition (29). Thus, the lipid effect seen in seizures induced by this drug suggests the involvement of components of synaptic membranes. Other effects of bicuculline also support this idea. It is known that bicuculline exerts a direct excitatory effect on neurons by blocking the activation of Cl^- channels at postsynaptic junctions. Bicuculline also elicits a direct excitatory action on neuronal plasma membranes, in addition to the above effects (29). The blockade of inhibitor systems by bicuculline, as well as the enhancement of excitatory mechanisms by pentylenetetrazol or electroshock, stimulates arachidonic acid production in the brain. Since other convulsive states such as those produced by blocking the energy metabolism by methionine sulfoximine (4) or by intraventricular injections of 3'-5'adenosine monophosphate (4) do not produce a similar effect, a specific mechanism may be involved in this phenomenon.

REFERENCES

1. Aveldano, M. I., and Bazan, N. G. (1975): Differential lipid deacylation during brain ischemia in a homeotherm and a poikilotherm. Content and composition of free fatty acids and triacylglycerols. *Brain Res.*, 100:99–110.
2. Aveldano de Caldironi, M. I., and Bazan, N. G. (1979): α-Methyl-*p*-tyrosine inhibits the production of free arachidonic acid and diacylglycerols in brain after a single electroconvulsive shock. *Neurochem. Res.*, 4:213–221.
3. Banshbach, M. W., and Geison, R. L. (1974): Postmortem increase in rat cerebral hemisphere diglyceride pool size. *J. Neurochem.*, 23:875–877.
3a. Bazan, N.G. (1970): Effects of ischemia and electroconvulsive shock on free fatty acid pool in the brain. *Biochem. Biophys. Acta*, 218:1–10.
4. Bazan, N. G. (1971): Changes in free fatty acids of brain by drug-induced convulsions, electroshock and anesthesia. *J. Neurochem.*, 18:1379–1385.
5. Bazan, N. G. (1976): Free arachidonic acid and other lipids in the nervous system during early ischemia and after electroshock. In: *Function and Metabolism of Phospholipids in the Central and Peripheral Nervous Systems*, edited by R. Paoletti, G. Porcellati, and G. Jacini, pp. 89–97, Raven Press, New York.
6. Bazan, N. G., Aveldano de Caldironi, M. I., Cascone de Suarez, G. D., and Rodriguez de Turco, E. B. (1980): Transient modifications in brain free arachidonic acid in experimental animals during convulsions. In: *Neurochemistry and Clinical Neurology*, edited by L. Batistin, G. Hashim, and A. Lajtha, pp. 167–169. Alan R. Liss, New York.
7. Bazan, N. G., Pascual de Bazan, H. E., Kennedy W. G., and Joel, C. D. (1971): Regional distribution and rate of production of free fatty acids in rat brain. *J. Neurochem.*, 18:1387–1393.
8. Bazan, N. G., and Rakowski, H. (1970): Increased levels of brain free fatty acids after electroconvulsive shock. *Life Sci. Part I*, 9:501–507.
9. Bazan, N. G., and Rodriguez de Turco, E. B. (1980): Membrane lipids in the pathogenesis of brain edema: Phospholipids and arachidonic acid, the earliest membrane components changed at the onset of ischemia. In: *Advances in Neurology, Vol. 28: Brain Edema*, edited by J. Cervos Navarro, and R. Freyszt, pp. 197–205, Raven Press, New York.
10. Bazan, N. G., Rodriguez de Turco, E. B., and Morelli de Liberti, S. A. (1982): Free arachidonic acid and membrane lipids in the central nervous system during status epilepticus by bicuculline. In: *Advances in Neurology*, 34:302–310.
11. Bazan, N. G., Rodriguez de Turco, E. B., and Morelli de Liberti, S. M. (1982): Arachidonic acid and arachidonoyl-diglycerols increase in rat cerebrum in bicuculline-induced status epilepticus. *Neurochem. Res.*, 7:839–843.
12. Bell, R. M., and Coleman, R. A. (1980): Enzymes of glycerolipid synthesis in eukaryotes. *Annu. Rev. Biochem.*, 49:459–487.
13. Chapman, A. G., Meldrum, B. S., and Siesjo, B. K. (1977): Cerebral metabolic changes during prolonged epileptic seizures in rats. *J. Neurochem.*, 28:1025–1035.
14. Reference deleted in proof.
15. Delgado-Escueta, A. V. (1980): Brain synaptosomes in epilepsy: Organization of ionic channels and the Na^+-K^+ pump. In: *Neurobiology. General Principles Related to Epilepsy*, edited by G. H. Glaser, J. K. Penry, and D. M. Woodbury, pp. 85–125. Raven Press, New York.

16. DeMedio, G. E., Goracci, G., Horrocks, L. A., Lazarewicz, J. W., Mazzari, S., Porcellati, G., Strosznajder, J., and Trovarelli, G. (1980): The effect of transient ischemia on fatty acid and lipid metabolism in the gerbil brain. *Italian J. Biochem.*, 29:412–432.
17. Galli, C., and Spagnuolo, C. (1976): The release of brain free fatty acids during ischaemia in essential fatty acid-deficient rats. *J. Neurochem.*, 26:401–404.
18. Hawthorne, J. N., and Pickard, M. R. (1979): Phospholipids in synaptic function. *J. Neurochem.*, 32:5–14.
18a. Hirata, F., and Axelrod, J. (1980): Phospholipid methylation and biological signal transmission. *Science*, 209:1082–1090.
19. Hokin-Neaverson, M. R. (1977): Metabolism and role of phosphatidylinositol in acetylcholine-stimulated membrane function. *Adv. Exp. Med. Biol.*, 83:429–446.
20. Kishimoto, A., Takai, Y., Mori, T., Kikkawa, U., and Nishuzuka, Y. (1980): Activation of calcium and phospholipid-dependent protein kinase by diacylglycerol, its possible relation to phosphatidylinositol turnover. *J. Biol. Chem.*, 215:2273–2276.
21. Marion, J., and Wolfe, L. S. (1978): Increase *in vivo* of unesterified fatty acids, prostaglandin $F_{2\alpha}$ but not thromboxane B_2 in rat brain during drug-induced convulsions. *Prostaglandins*, 16:99–110.
22. Marion, J., and Wolfe, L. S. (1979): Origin of the arachidonic-acid released postmortem in rat forebrain. *Biochim. Biophys. Acta*, 574:25–32.
23. Michell, R. H. (1975): Inositol phospholipids and cell surface receptor function. *Biochim. Biophys. Acta*, 415:81–147.
24. Pediconi, M. F., Rodriguez de Turco, E. B., and Bazan, N. G. (1981): Changes in free fatty acids and acyl groups of phospholipids during subcellular fractionation of cerebral cortex and cerebellum. In: *Abstracts, Eighth Meeting of the International Society for Neurochemistry*, Nottingham, England.
25. Prince, D. A. (1969): Electrophysiology of "epileptic" neurons: Spike generation. *Electroencephalogr. Clin. Neurophysiol.*, 26:476–487.
26. Rehncrona, S., Siesjo, B. K., and Westerberg, E. (1978): Adenosine and cyclic AMP in cerebral cortex of rats in hypoxia, status epilepticus and hypercapnia. *Acta Physiol. Scand.*, 104:453–463.
26a. Rhotman, J. E., and Lenard, J. (1977): Membrane asymmetry. *Science*, 195:743–753.
27. Steinhauer, H. B., Anhut, H., and Hertting, G. (1979): The synthesis of prostaglandins and thromboxane in the mouse brain in vivo. Influence of drug-induced convulsions, hypoxia and the anticonvulsants trimethadione and diazepam. *Naunyn Schmiedeberg's Arch. Pharmacol.*, 310:53–58.
28. Sun, G. Y., Su, K. L., Der, O. M., and Tang, W. (1979): Enzymatic regulation of arachidonate metabolism in brain membrane phosphoglycerides. *Lipids*, 14:229–235.
29. Woodbury, D. M. (1980): Convulsant drugs: mechanisms of action. In: *Antiepileptic Drugs: Mechanisms of Action*, edited by G. H. Glaser, J. K. Penry, and D. M. Woodbury, pp. 249–303. Raven Press, New York.

Neural Transmission, Learning and Memory,
edited by R. Caputto and C. Ajmone Marsan.
Raven Press, New York © 1983.

Molecular Aspects of Neuroendocrine Integrative Processes in the Brain

D. P. Cardinali, M. N. Ritta, and M. I. Vacas

*Centro de Estudios Farmacológicos y de Principios Naturales (CEFAPRIN),
Buenos Aires, Argentina*

Balanced interaction and timing of biological processes in living organisms depend upon effective means of communication. Two types of chemical signals, neurotransmitters and hormones, mediate such a communication in mammals; we will briefly discuss the major differences and the ways of interaction between both categories of signals (4).

The transmission of a neuronal signal across a synapse is mediated by a specific neurotransmitter substance released into the synaptic cleft from the presynaptic cell. The neurotransmitter then diffuses across a short distance to reach a specialized receptor zone on the postsynaptic cell, where it alters the flux of specific ions and/or the activity of specific enzymes, such as, for example, adenylate cyclase. The "privacy" of this communication is achieved by rapid deactivation of the neurotransmitter either by specific enzymes or by physical processes such as its reuptake into the neuron of origin. Therefore only a small number of cells with which a neuron makes direct synaptic contact or which lie within a few hundred Å of its terminal endings is activated, the circulating concentrations of neurotransmitter tending to be very low.

Hormone signals are transmitted via the bloodstream or the cerebrospinal fluid (CSF). Theoretically at least a given signal may be distributed to every cell in the body. In this case the privacy of the communication is attained biochemically, i.e., only those cells able to recognize the message by having the appropriate receptor are activated.

Although neurotransmitters and hormones operate through specific networks, the nervous and the endocrine systems, interaction arises at many organizational levels; the scope of neuroendocrinology is the study of these interactions (4). In the brain specialized cells known as "neuroendocrine transducers" translate an input of neural activity into a hormonal output, e.g., the hypothalamic magnocellular and parvicellular systems which produce neurohypophysial and hypophysiotropic hormones. Other, more typical neurons make the reverse conversion by transforming hormonal signals into changes in their firing rate; to follow the same nomenclature they should be called "endocrine-neural transducers." In addition, an increasing body of evidence now suggests that hypothalamic neurons initially considered as neuroendo-crine transducers have chemoreceptive properties that allow them to monitor changes in plasma hormone concentrations and to translate the information carried out by the hormonal signal into another, different, hormonal output (thus exhibiting "en-docrine-endocrine transducing" properties) (Fig. 1). The net balance between these three processes should be considered when analyzing the primary mechanisms underlying the action of a hormone on any central neuroendocrine process. However, the manner in which these mechanisms operate to give the integrative response is poorly understood at present. For example, responsiveness of the cells to a hormone may be controlled by the neuronal input arriving at the cell (Fig. 2), or the interaction of the neurotransmitter with its receptors (or any of the metabolic events that follow neurotransmitter-receptor interaction) may be affected by the concentration of the hormone at the biophase (Fig. 3). A still more complex interrelationship can be visualized, e.g., hormone levels may modulate neurotransmitter release while at the same time synaptic signals may control hormone action; this type of division

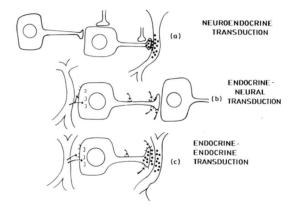

FIG. 1. Basic mechanisms of neuroendocrine integration. *Arrows:* Hormone signals interacting with their receptors.

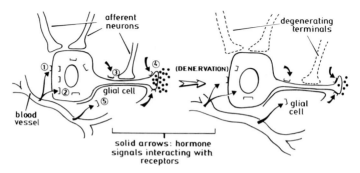

FIG. 2. Modulation of hormone response by the neural input. Hormones can interact with receptors located in the surface (1,3,4) or cytoplasm (2) of neurons; they also may act on glial cells (5). Hormone receptors can be under partial control of afferent neurons.

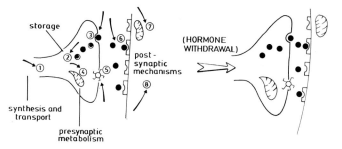

FIG. 3. Modulation of neural activity by hormones. Hormones may affect synthesis and transport of neurotransmitter (1), storage (2), release (3), or presynaptic metabolism (4). They also may affect transmitter uptake (5), transmitter interaction with receptor (6), or its postsynaptic metabolism (7). Other postsynaptic mechanisms can be also under hormone control (8).

of labor might operate for example through subsensitivity and supersensitivity changes at hormone or transmitter receptor sites.

All these phenomena representing the central dogma of hypothalamic neuroendocrine function are poorly understood at present. Although there is considerable information on the dynamic fluctuations of the different components of the reproductive system, for example, variations in plasma levels of steroids and gonadotropins, the mechanisms and intracellular sites involved in hormone action on central neuroendocrine structures are largely undefined. The description of these mechanisms may be a fundamental step towards the understanding of the integrative neuroendocrine processes.

This chapter discusses the molecular aspects of neuroendocrine, endocrine-neural, and endocrine-endocrine transducing events in the pineal gland, and their possible implication for the understanding of those mechanisms in the neuroendocrine hypothalamus. The major assumption of the present work is that what is true for relatively simple neuroendocrine structures like the pineal gland and its innervating sympathetic neurons is also true for anatomically and functionally more complicated and heterogenous neuroendocrine structures like the hypothalamus (4). The anatomical similarities between the pineal gland and other circumventricular organs such as the median eminence have already been pointed out (30).

PHYSIOLOGICAL SIGNIFICANCE OF THE PINEAL GLAND

Probably no other organ in the body has suffered so long from a lack of its true functional recognition as the pineal gland. For more than 2 centuries the pineal was thought to be the seat of soul or a vestigial remnant of the parietal eye. However, pineal research over the last 20 years has contributed significantly to unravelling the functional meaning of this endocrine gland. Today the mammalian pineal is recognized as an active functioning neuroendocrine organ that responds primarily to photic stimuli attaining the gland via its sympathetic nerves (and secondarily to hormonal signals originating in target tissues), exhibits circadian rhythms and influences the metabolic activity of a host of endocrine glands (22,23). Secretions from the pineal gland participate in several neural and neuroendocrine mechanisms, including control of gonadal, adrenal, and thyroid functions; sleep; and various biological rhythms. The pineal is an essential component of the neuroendocrine system regulating circannual rhythms in endocrine activity, remarkably reproduction (33). Most species that inhabit the temperate and polar regions of the earth are seasonal breeders in their natural habitat. The variable that keeps their reproduction behavior in synchrony with the environment is the length of the photoperiod. Such a synchronization requires the presence of an intact pineal gland; studies conducted in hamsters, ferrets, voles, deer, goats, and rams indicate that photoperiod-related changes of the reproductive function can be modified by pineal ablation or denervation (5,22). For example, the exposure of hamsters to short photoperiods induces marked decreases in the weight of testes and accessory organs, the critical photoperiod length required to maintain normal testicular size and function in this species being 12.5 hr of light per day. The gonadal collapse induced by any daily light period less than this is prevented by the removal of the pineal gland or by disconnecting it from its central sympathetic innervation (22).

Two families of endocrine-active compounds, indoles and polypeptides, have been isolated from the pineal gland. The production of the best defined pineal hormone, i.e., melatonin (5-methoxy-*N*-acetyltryptamine) exhibits a circadian periodicity entrained by neural signals originating in the retina (5). A daily rhythm in melatonin secretion has been found to occur in all vertebrates tested to date, with high plasma, CSF, or urine levels during the dark period regardless of whether the animal is nocturnally or diurnally active. Melatonin is capable of reproducing the effects of darkness, or short days on the neuroendocrine reproductive axis (5). For example, in the hamster melatonin, when appropriately injected (i.e., at evening hours), induces a gonadal regression reminiscent of that seen in animals exposed to naturally short days of the autumn. Melatonin acts at specific receptor sites in the brain, particularly in the medial basal hypothalamus (MBH), to affect the hypothalamic-adenohypophysial function; its effect appears to involve the depression of prostaglandin (PG) and cAMP synthesis, and stimulation of guanylate cyclase (9,48).

Superimposed to the neural control of melatonin synthesis mediating the effects of environmental lighting, a feedback control by hormones takes place at the pineal level. In the adult female rat a number of pineal constituents change after ovariectomy or as a function of the stage of the estrous cycle. In general the obtained results are compatible with the view that melatonin synthesis and production, and probably the synthesis of antigonadal peptides, decrease at the time of the preovulatory peak of gonadotropins (11). A number of hormones can be implicated in these changes. Estradiol treatment affects melatonin release (50) as well as pineal serotonin and norepinephrine (NE) turnover rates (7,43), and NE-induced increase of adenylate cyclase and cAMP content (17). Progesterone treatment depresses melatonin synthesis and release (50); FSH, LH, or prolactin increase melatonin synthesis and modify the serotonin and NE turnover rates in castrated rats (11,43). In males, testosterone accelerates pineal serotonin and NE turnover rates and melatonin synthesis (7,43). Hence hormone activity in the pineal gland is best envisioned as the net balance of direct and neuronally mediated changes brought about by hormone administration (Fig. 4).

NEUROENDOCRINE-TRANSDUCING EVENTS

Like other neuroendocrine transducer cells the mammalian pinealocytes are able to convert a neuronal input, i.e., NE released at the synapse to an endocrine output: the secretion of melatonin. In addition to the magnocellular and parvicellular neurosecretory systems of the hypothalamus, other examples of neuroendocrine transducer cells include adrenomedullary chromaffin cells (which secrete epinephrine in response to acetylcholine released from the medulla's preganglionic neurons), the B-cells of the pancreatic islets, and renin-secreting juxtaglomerular and thyroidal

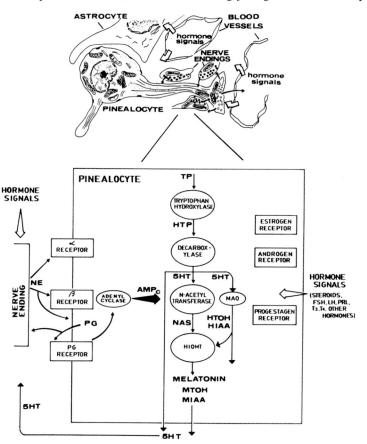

FIG. 4. Schematic representation of the mechanisms involved in neural and hormonal control of melatonin synthesis. TP, Tryptophan; HTP, 5-hydroxytryptophan; 5-HT, serotonin; NAS, *N*-acetylserotonin; HTOH, 5-hydroxytryptophol; HIAA, 5-hydroxyindoleacetic acid; MTOH, 5-methoxytryptophol; MIAA, 5-methoxyindoleacetic acid. (Reproduced with permission from ref. 5.)

follicular cells (the activity of which is affected by afferent sympathetic nerves). These cells all respond to humoral as well as to neuronal inputs; hence endocrine-endocrine transducing events may coexist with the neuroendocrine one in the same cell (4).

The rat pineal gland has provided an excellent model system for studying the control of cellular responses by sympathetic nerves. Pineal nerve endings contain the neurotransmitter NE as well as serotonin, the latter deriving from the pinealocyte compartment (Fig. 4). The pineal, which is a direct evagination from the diencephalic roof, receives not only vascular nerves but also adrenergic terminals innervating the pinealocytes; this sympathetic innervation is originated in the superior cervical ganglia (SCG). Through the peripheral sympathetic nerves environmental information originating in the retina is conveyed to the pineal gland (25). Photosensory information arrives at the pineal gland via a complex polyneuronal pathway which begins at the eye, synapses in the CNS, and leaves the CNS with the preganglionic fibers to the SCG. This pathway includes the retinohypothalamic projections to the suprachiasmatic nuclei and descending projections to the intermediolateral column of the spinal cord (25).

Shining a light into the rat's eyes diminishes the frequency of action potentials in the cervical sympathetic trunk. Likewise electrical stimulation of the suprachiasmatic nuclei greatly decreases neural activity in SCG (27). The reduced activity in the sympathetic trunk causes a decreased release of NE in the gland and as a consequence the organ remains in an inactive state. Conversely during darkness the pineal gland is activated due to the augmented release of NE.

When the rat pineal gland is stimulated by endogenous NE released from pineal nerves, or by exogenous catecholamines injected *in vivo* or added *in vitro* to the incubation medium of pineal organ cultures, a cascade of sequential events ensues culminating in melatonin synthesis and release (Fig. 4). β-Adrenergic stimulation by NE leads to the activation of the adenylcyclase-cAMP system, and some of the cAMP formed activates a protein kinase with concomitant phosphorylation of a specific nuclear protein and synthesis of messenger RNA (51). Newly synthesized enzyme proteins, e.g., serotonin-N-acetyltransferase (SNAT), contribute to the increase in melatonin biosynthesis and secretion that occurs in darkness as a consequence of catecholamine activation.

Recently a role for PGs has been proposed in the above mentioned metabolic cascade. Data suggesting such a role include (a) a dose-dependent release of PGs by NE in incubated bovine pineal glands (10); (b) blockade by indomethacin treatment of the nocturnal increase of pineal SNAT activity and melatonin content in rats (34); (c) occurrence of specific binding sites for PGs in 900 g supernatants from bovine pineal glands (10); (d) stimulation by nanomolar concentrations of PGE_2 of cAMP accumulation and SNAT activity in incubated rat pineals (35). It is generally acknowledged that the major role of cAMP in eukaryotic cells is to activate the catalytic subunit of protein kinase by binding with and dissociating the regulatory subunit from the holoenzyme. An assessment of the changes in occupancy of cAMP binding proteins in the pineal gland (an index of occupancy of protein kinase regulatory subunit) after PGE_2 incubation is shown in Fig. 5. Although cAMP-dependent protein kinase has 2 distinct binding sites for cAMP only one is detectable by the conventional membrane filtration method used in the experiments of Fig. 4 (28). Dissociation constants (K_D) found in the pineal gland (34 to 58 nM) are close to those reported for several diverse tissues (21,42). A 37% decrease in unoccupied cAMP binding sites of pineal homogenates was observed after exposure of explants to 50 nM PGE_2 suggesting that PGE_2 increased regulatory subunit occupancy probably as a direct consequence of the changes in tissue cAMP levels. Although pineal cAMP binding proteins were labile and decreased after the 16-hr incubation at 5°C used to measure total binding sites, depletion of unoccupied sites by PGE_2 was not accompanied by a significant reduction of the total binding site number (Fig. 5, right panel).

That the PG link is a complementary rather than a necessary step in the stimulation of melatonin synthesis brought about by NE is shown in Fig. 6. Addition of different PG synthesis inhibitors (indomethacin, acetylsalicylic acid, or mefenamic acid) in concentrations which totally prevented PG synthesis (20) only impaired the stimulation of melatonin release from rat pineal explants brought about by NE. At the pineal neuroeffector junction PGE_2 also influences the release of NE from sympathetic nerve endings (Table 1). Incubation of rat pineal glands with 0.1 μM PGE_2 impaired significantly the release of NE evoked by a 20 mM K^+. Therefore both pre- and postsynaptic effects of PGs occur in the pineal gland (Fig. 4).

Besides the well-characterized β-receptor-mediated effects on pineal cells, the NE released from pineal sympathetic nerve endings also interacts with postsynaptic

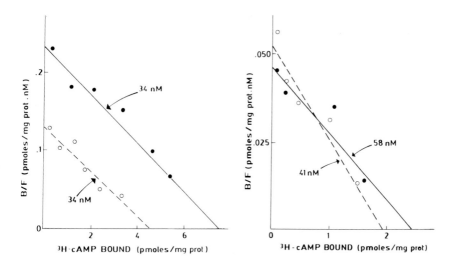

FIG. 5. Effect of PGE_2 on unoccupied **(left)** and total cAMP binding sites **(right)** in rat pineal gland. Pineal glands were incubated for 15 min with 50 nM PGE_2 (□----□) or vehicle (●——●) and cAMP binding was measured in 900 g supernatants (42). Data are presented as Scatchard plots. Each point is the mean of triplicate samples.

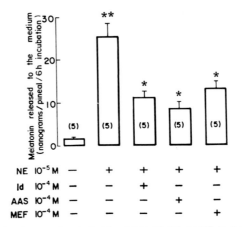

FIG. 6. Rat pineal glands were incubated for 6 hr with 10^{-5}M NE in the presence of one of the following 3 PG synthesis inhibitors (10^{-4}M): indomethacin (Id), acetylsalicylic acid (AAS), or mefenamic acid (MEF). Melatonin release to the medium was assessed by RIA. Shown are the means ± SEM. An analysis of variance followed by a Scheffé's test indicated significant differences between the glands incubated with NE alone and the remaining groups (**$p < 0.01$). Pineal glands incubated with NE plus inhibitor differed significantly from controls (*$p < 0.05$).

TABLE 1. *Effect of PGE_2 on [^3H]NE release elicited by K^+ in rat pineal gland*

	Fractional release ($\times 10^3$)		Ratio S_2/S_1
	S_1	S_2	
Control	20.9 ± 2.4	13.3 ± 2.2	0.64 ± 0.09
PGE_2, 10^{-7}M	20.9 ± 2.9	6.9 ± 1.4[a]	0.33 ± 0.05[a]

The endogenous NE stores were labelled *in vitro* by incubating rat pineal with 0.5 μM [^3H]NE for 30 min (31). At a time when the spontaneous efflux or radioactivity had levelled off, transmitter release was elicited by a 1-min exposure to 80 mM K^+. S_1 corresponds to the first exposure to K^+ and S_2 to the second one, 35 min after S_1. PGE_2 was added to the incubation medium 20 min before S_2. Results are expressed as mean ± SEM, $N = 6$ in each group.
[a]Significant differences with controls (Student's *t*-test. $p < 0.05$).

α-adrenoceptors (47) linked to stimulation of phosphatidylinositol turnover (38). There is also pharmacological evidence of α_2-adrenoceptors affecting NE release from pineal nerve endings (31).

It is of interest to compare information on pineal neuroendocrine events involving PGs with what is known about this phenomenon at the level of the hypothalamic LH-RH producing neurons. It is now firmly established that PGs, particularly those of the E series, can induce gonadotropin release in several species by acting on a neural rather than on a pituitary site (23,29). As for the induction of melatonin synthesis in the pinealocytes, PGE_2 was found to be most potent in inducing LH release, $PGF_{2\alpha}$ being only slightly effective. That endogenous PGs are involved in a physiological manner in the regulation of gonadotropin release is suggested by the experiments in which synthesis of PGs was inhibited by treatment with indomethacin. In the rat, indomethacin blocked the postcastration rise of LH (23); this finding is in remarkable agreement with the observation that this drug also impaired the nocturnal rise of pineal melatonin synthesis (34). Likewise, as in the pineal gland, NE added to the culture medium of rat MBH releases PGE_2, which in turn, when added to the same MBH preparation enhances LH-RH release (29).

In a neuroendocrine paradigm reportedly known to show a release of gonadotropins and prolactin that resembles that of proestrus, i.e., the ovariectomized rat injected with estradiol (3), we recently observed that at the time of high serum LH concentrations an increase in the spontaneous efflux of MBH PGE_2 but not of MBH $PGF_{2\alpha}$ took place (Fig. 7). Therefore these observations are compatible with the proposed role for PGE_2 in the LH-RH release mechanism at the hypothalamus. The changes in neuronal function after estradiol injection introduce the second basic neuroendocrine process: endocrine-neural transduction.

ENDOCRINE-NEURAL TRANSDUCING EVENTS

Considerable efforts have been devoted to elucidate the involvement of central catecholamine neurons in the regulation of the adenohypophyseal function, and the picture that has emerged supports a stimulatory role of the noradrenergic system in the mechanisms controlling LH release (49). Catecholaminergic pathways are also functionally linked to neuroendocrine activity in that amine turnover rates and the postsynaptic phenomena triggered by neurotransmitter release are modified by sex steroid or gonadotropin treatment.

Central noradrenergic neurons concentrate labeled estradiol after systemic injection (36). It has also become apparent that the effects of sex steroids on the CNS can be partly explained in terms of changing activity of central monoaminergic neurons (49). According to the current accepted view for the control of LH secretion in the rat, estradiol is the main ovarian signal for both cyclic and tonic LH release (26). The capacity of pharmacological estrogen antagonists or of estradiol antisera to block ovulation has firmly established that an increase in serum estradiol concentration is the signal for the preovulatory LH surge. Additionally estradiol injection readily depresses the postcastration rise of plasma LH, thereby constituting a major steroid inhibiting tonic LH secretion in female rats (1).

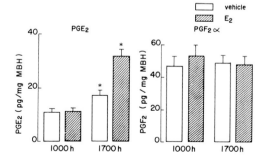

FIG. 7. Ovariectomized rats received 0.5 and 50 μg of estradiol (E_2) or vehicle on two consecutive days and were killed on the 3rd day at 1000 or 1700 h. PGE_2 and $PGF_{2\alpha}$ efflux from MBH explants was measured by RIA (9). Shown are the means ± SEM of eight determinations. PGE_2 efflux in vehicle or E_2-treated animals at 1700 h differed from their respective groups at 1000 h ($p < 0.01$, Student's t-test). PGE_2 efflux at 1700 h in E_2-treated animals was significantly greater than in vehicle ($p < 0.01$).

Estradiol treatment modifies hypothalamic NE content (19) as well as the activity of enzymes involved in catecholamine synthesis and metabolism (e.g., tyrosine hydroxylase, 2; catechol-O-methyl transferase, 37). Estrogen treatment also affects the density of β-adrenergic (45) and muscarinic receptors (32) in the hypothalamus.

A number of studies support the activation of catecholaminergic components in rat MBH preceding and during LH release in estradiol-primed spayed rats; NE uptake by MBH synaptosomes (6) and the [^{3}H]NE release from slices after a K$^+$-depolarizing stimulus *(unpublished results)* increase in steroid-treated rats during the morning hours. In agreement with these observations an increase in median eminence NE turnover rate was found in proestrous rats by the α-methyl-p-tyrosine method (18). Other central monoaminergic systems not strictly linked to neuroendocrine regulation are also affected by estradiol. For example, estrogen treatment modifies the basal firing rate and autoreceptor sensitivity of dopamine neurons in the substantia nigra (15).

The sympathetic pathway innervating the pineal gland is an appropriate model to examine endocrine-neural events because of the readiness of labeling NE stores in pineal nerves by intravenous injection of the isotope and due to the easiness of manipulation of the pre- and postganglionic components of the neural pathway.

Evidence concerning changes of sympathetic neuronal input to the pineal gland includes the modification of NE turnover in nerve endings following estradiol (7), testosterone (7), FSH (12), or LH (12) administration to castrated rats, and the changes in the synthesis and metabolism of NE in the SCG after estradiol (11,13), testosterone (11), gonadotropin (11,12), prolactin (11,12), or corticosteroid (16) treatment of rats. Some hormones also affect the postsynapsis at the pinealocyte level: for example, testosterone injection decreased significantly β-adrenoceptor density in the rat pineal gland (Fig. 8), as well as in MBH and cerebral cortex. The effects of testosterone on pineal β-adrenergic receptors were not mimicked by estradiol (45), FSH, or LH administration to castrated rats.

Theoretically the hormones may act on the pineal sympathetic pathway: (a) at the level of pineal nerve endings directly or through a local feedback loop involving the pinealocytes; (b) at the level of ganglionic perikarya; (c) at any point of the multisynaptic descending pathway connecting retinal photoreceptors with the SCG. Estrophilic receptors are detectable in SCG homogenates (13). In addition a cytosol glucocorticoid receptor exhibiting "transcortin-like" properties has been reported to occur in SCG (41). Conclusive proof of a link between hormone binding sites and effects on SCG is still lacking. However, in the case of estradiol several biochemical changes observed in SCG (e.g., stimulation of dopamine-β-hydroxylase activity) persist after decentralization (13), indicating that the hormone may act on the SCG themselves rather than through modification of the neuronal input to the SCG. The ganglionic target cell for the steroid hormones remains to be defined.

ENDOCRINE-ENDOCRINE TRANSDUCING EVENTS

Indication that this mechanism is operating in central neurosecretory neurons derives mainly from autoradiographic and immunohistochemical studies showing

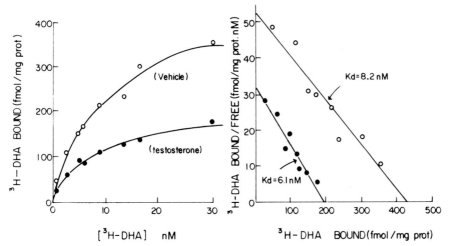

FIG. 8. Effect of testosterone treatment on pineal β-adrenoceptor density [assessed by [³H]dihydroalprenolol (DHA) binding] in pineal 900 *g* supernatants. Male rats castrated 72 hr earlier were treated for 3 days with two daily i.c. injections of 400 μg testosterone or vehicle. An additional injection of 400 μg was given on the day of sacrifice 3 hr before killing. [³H]DHA binding was determined as described elsewhere (45). Intercepts in Scatchard plots of testosterone- and vehicle-injected animals differed significantly ($p < 0.01$ analysis of covariance).

a similar distribution of steroid-concentrating and hypophysiotropic-containing cells in the anterior and basal hypothalamus (4,40). In the pineal the prerequisite for the occurrence of direct effects of hormones on cells, that is the existence of hormone binding to pineal tissue, has been investigated both *in vivo* and *in vitro*. Experiments carried out in animals injected with labeled steroids, or on subcellular fractions incubated with different radioactive hormones, indicate that the pineal gland of various species, i.e., rat, sheep, cow, rhesus monkey, exhibits protein components that bind the hormone with high affinity and specifically. To date putative receptors for estradiol (8,11), testosterone (8), 5α-dihydrotestosterone (8), and progesterone (46) have been detected in pineal subcellular fractions. Autoradiographic studies of rats injected with labeled estradiol or androgens have confirmed the biochemical indications of nuclear binding sites for these hormones in the pineal gland (40). Enzymatic activities that convert progesterone and testosterone to reduced metabolites, particularly to the functionally relevant 5α-reduced derivatives, are also present in the pinealocytes. In addition testosterone and androstenedione are aromatized to estrogens by pineal homogenates (11), a property that strongly supports the view that the pineal gland resembles other brain areas involved in gonadotropin regulation as far as the metabolism of steroids is concerned. That pineal hormone binding sites are operative in the absence of an intact sympathetic input has been demonstrated for two hormones to date: estradiol and progesterone. Estradiol added to the culture medium at physiological concentration (10^{-8}–10^{-9}M) induces the synthesis of a specific pineal protein resembling the estradiol-induced protein found in the uterus, and enhances the *O*-methylation of *N*-acetylserotonin to melatonin (24) (Fig. 9). At greater, pharmacological concentrations estradiol depressed mela-

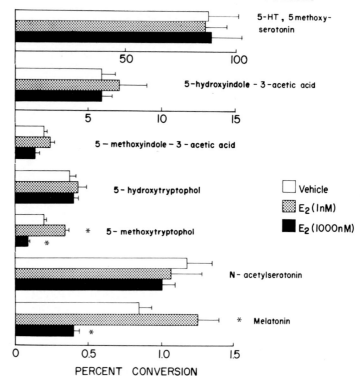

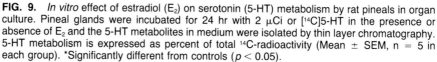

FIG. 9. *In vitro* effect of estradiol (E$_2$) on serotonin (5-HT) metabolism by rat pineals in organ culture. Pineal glands were incubated for 24 hr with 2 μCi or [^{14}C]5-HT in the presence or absence of E$_2$ and the 5-HT metabolites in medium were isolated by thin layer chromatography. 5-HT metabolism is expressed as percent of total ^{14}C-radioactivity (Mean $\pm$ SEM, n = 5 in each group). *Significantly different from controls ($p < 0.05$).

tonin synthesis probably by competitive inhibition of the *O*-methylating enzyme. Likewise progesterone added to the incubation medium of rat pineal glands depressed melatonin release (50). Other hormones, e.g., thyroxine, arginine vasotocin, melatonin, have been found to affect the pineal *in vitro*; for some of them (melatonin, 44) specific binding sites occur in the gland.

In general hormone effects on the pineal gland have been found to be subsidiary to the major circadian driving force coupled to activation by pineal sympathetic nerves. Evidence in this respect was provided by experiments demonstrating that the NE released from pineal nerve endings induces the synthesis of pineal receptor proteins for estrogens and androgens (8). *In vitro* experiments carried out on incubated pineal glands from chronically ganglionectomized rats revealed that high affinity specific hormone binding to cytoplasmic and nuclear components became severely depressed (11). Since hormone receptors were reinduced by NE interaction with pineal β-adrenoceptors (8,11) these data indicate that the trophic effects of the innervation in the pineal gland include the maintenance of appropriate hormone responsiveness. Moreover these studies offered the first indication as to the existence in the neuroendocrine apparatus of a hormone receptor which is controlled by a neurotransmitter. Recent data on depression of hypothalamic estrophilic receptors after complete deafferentation (14) or of depression of [^{3}H]dexamethasone binding in hypothalamus and hippocampus after reserpine treatment (39) indicate that such a phenomenon also occurs in other regions involved in neuroendocrine regulation.

A more physiological example of neuronal modulation of pineal responsiveness to circulating hormone signals is given by studies at different times of the day in rats (11). In these animals pineal response to androgens depends largely upon the time of day when the hormone is administered, e.g., the extent of stimulation of pineal protein synthesis brought about by testosterone parallels the daily rhythm in pineal hormone uptake, NE content and turnover, and pineal electrical activity, in that all these reach maximal values during the night. Thus the overall effects of sex steroids on the pinealocytes depend upon the level of activity of the innervating sympathetic neurons, probably through regulation of the number of hormone binding sites in target pineal cells.

CONCLUSIONS

From studies on neural and hormonal integrative mechanisms in the pineal gland it has become apparent that a number of biochemical sequelae may follow the manipulation of one or another input to the neuroendocrine cell. For example, the interruption of the neural input to the pineal can result in (a) abolished hormone effects, such as the stimulation of melatonin synthesis by FSH, LH or prolactin (43); (b) effects manifested only *after* denervation of the gland, such as the increase in serotonin levels following testosterone treatment (43); (c) effects unaffected by pineal denervation, like the changes in serotonin metabolism following gonadotropins (43). At least some of these effects appear to depend upon modulation by NE of hormone receptor sites.

The injection of several hormones affects neurotransmitter release and neurotransmitter-mediated mechanisms in the pineal gland. For example, testosterone treatment accelerates NE turnover rate in pineal nerves, depresses the density of pineal β-adrenoceptor sites and blocks postsynaptic β-agonist effects, like the increase in pineal protein synthesis brought about by isoproterenol. The occurrence of these and other neuroendocrine, endocrine-neural and endocrine-endocrine transducing events in the pineal gland supports the usefulness of the organ as a model for the study of basic mechanisms of neuroendocrine integration in the brain.

SUMMARY

In the brain specialized cells known as "neuroendocrine transducers" translate an input of neural activity into a hormonal output, e.g., oxytocin released to the bloodstream. Other more typical neurons make the reverse conversion, and constitute chemoreceptors that transform the hormonal "language" in changes in the neuronal firing rate ("endocrine-neural transducers"). "Endocrine-endocrine" transducing events occur at the level of the neurosecretory cells that translate a hormonal signal into another different hormonal output. The chapter discussed the molecular aspects of several neuroendocrine integrative processes in the hypothalamus and the pineal gland. The pineal gland and its innervating sympathetic neurons located in the superior cervical ganglia appear to be an easily manipulated system for the study of basic neuroendocrine mechanism because: (a) receptors for various hormones exist in the mammalian pineal and ganglia; (b) the pattern of pineal steroid metabolism resembles that in the neuroendocrine hypothalamus; (c) pineal estrophilic and androphilic receptors are modulated by the sympathetic nerves; (d) neuronal activity in the cervical sympathetic pathway is modified by hormone treatment at ganglionic and preganglionic sites.

ACKNOWLEDGMENTS

The technical assistance of Lic. M. I. Keller Sarmiento, Mrs. E. Pereyra, Mr. P. R. Lowenstein, and Mr. C. Gonzalez Solveyra is gratefully acknowledged.

These studies were supported by grant 6638 of the Consejo Nacional de Investigaciones Científicas y Técnicas (CONICET). D. P. Cardinali is an Established Investigator, CONICET. M. N. Ritta and M. I. Vacas are Research Fellows, CONICET.

REFERENCES

1. Advis, J. P., McCann, S. M., and Negro-Vilar, A. (1980): Evidence that catecholaminergic and peptidergic (luteinizing hormone-releasing hormone) neurons in suprachiasmatic-medial preoptic, medial basal hypothalamus and median eminence are involved in estrogen-negative feedback. *Endocrinology*, 107:892–901.
2. Beattie, C. W., Rodgers, C. H., and Soyka, L. F. (1972): Influence of ovariectomy and ovarian steroids on hypothalamic tyrosine hydroxylase activity in the rat. *Endocrinology*, 91:276–279.
3. Caligaris, L., Astrada, J. J., and Taleisnik, S. (1971): Release of luteinizing hormone induced by estrogen injection into ovariectomized rats. *Endocrinology*, 88:810–815.
4. Cardinali, D. P. (1979): Models in neuroendocrinology. Neurohumoral pathways to the pineal gland. *Trends Neurosci.*, 2:250–253.
5. Cardinali, D. P. (1981): Melatonin. A mammalian pineal hormone. *Endocrine Rev.*, 2:327–346.
6. Cardinali, D. P., and Gomez, E. (1977): Changes in hypothalamic noradrenaline, dopamine and serotonin uptake after oestradiol administration to rats. *J. Endocrinol.*, 73:181–182.
7. Cardinali, D. P., Nagle, C. A., and Rosner, J. M. (1975): Norepinephrine turnover in the pineal gland. Acceleration by estradiol and testosterone. *Life Sci.*, 16:1717–1724.
8. Cardinali, D. P., Nagle, C. A., and Rosner, J. M. (1975): Control of estrogen and androgen receptors in the rat pineal gland by catecholamine transmitter. *Life Sci.*, 16:93–106.
9. Cardinali, D. P., Ritta, M. N., Fuentes, A. M., Gimeno, M. F., and Gimeno, A. L. (1980): Prostaglandin E release by rat medial basal hypothalamus *in vitro*. Inhibition by melatonin at submicromolar concentrations. *Eur. J. Pharmacol.*, 67:151–153.
10. Cardinali, D. P., Ritta, M. N., Speziale, N. S., and Gimeno, M. F. (1979): Release and specific binding of prostaglandins in bovine pineal gland. *Prostaglandins*, 18:577–589.
11. Cardinali, D. P., and Vacas, M. I. (1978): Feedback control of pineal function by reproductive hormones. A neuroendocrine paradigm. *J. Neural Transm. (Suppl.)* 13:175–204.
12. Cardinali, D. P., and Vacas, M. I. (1979): Norepinephrine turnover in pineal gland and superior cervical ganglia. Changes after gonadotrophin administration to castrated rats. *J. Neural Transm.*, 45:273–284.
13. Cardinali, D. P., Vacas, M. I., Valenti, C. E., and Solveyra, C. G. (1979): Pineal gland and sympathetic cervical ganglia as sites for steroid regulation of photosensitive neuroendocrine pathways. *J. Steroid Biochem.*, 11:951–956.
14. Carrillo, A. J., and Sheridan, P. J. (1980): Estrogen receptors in the medial basal hypothalamus of the rat following complete hypothalamic deafferentation. *Brain Res.* 186:157–164.

15. Chiodo, L. A., and Caggiula, A. R. (1980): Alterations in basal firing rate and autoreceptor sensitivity of dopamine neurons in the substantia nigra following acute and extended exposure to estrogen. *Eur. J. Pharmacol.*, 67:165–166.
16. Cianarello, R. D., Jacobowitz, D., and Axelrod, J. (1973): Effect of dexamethasone on pheny-lethanolamine-*N*-methyltransferase in chromaffin tissue of the neonatal rat. *J. Neurochem.*, 20:799–805.
17. Davis, G. A. (1978): The response of adenosine-3'5'-monophosphate to norepinephrine in the hypothalamus pineal organ of female rats in proestrus or diestrus. *Endocrinology*, 103:1048–1053.
18. Demarest, K. T., Johnston, C. A., and Moore, K. E. (1981): Biochemical indices of catecholaminergic neuronal activity in the median eminence during the estrous cycle of the rat. *Neuroendocrinology*, 32:24–27.
19. Donoso, A. O., and Cukier, J. O. (1968): Oestrogen as a depressor of noradrenaline concentration in the anterior hypothalamus. *Nature*, 218:969–970.
20. Flower, R. (1974): Drugs which inhibit prostaglandin biosynthesis. *Pharmacol. Rev.*, 26:33–67.
21. Gill, G. N., and Walton, G. M. (1975): The detection and characterization of cyclic AMP-receptor proteins in animal cells. *Methods Enzymol.*, 38:376–382.
22. Kappers, J. A., and Pévet, P. (eds) (1979): *The Pineal Gland of Vertebrates including Man.* Elsevier, Amsterdam.
23. McCann, S. M., Ojeda, S. R., Harms, P. G., Wheaton, J. E., Sundberg, D. K., and Fawcet, C. P. (1976): Control of adenohypophysial hormone secretion by prostaglandins. In: *Subcellular Mechanisms in Reproductive Neuroendocrinology*, edited by F. Naftolin, K. J. Ryan, and J. J. Davies, pp. 407–422. Elsevier, Amsterdam.
24. Mizobe, F., and Kurokawa, M. (1978): Induction of a specific protein by oestradiol in rat pineals in culture. *FEBS Lett.*, 87:45–48.
25. Moore, R. Y. (1978): The innvervation of the mammalian pineal gland. *Prog. Reprod. Biol.*, 4:1–29.
26. Neill, J. D., and Smith, M. S. (1974): Pituitary-ovarian interrelationships in the rat. *Curr. Top. Exp. Endocrinol.*, 2:73–106.
27. Nishino, H., Koizumi, K., and Brooks, C. McC. (1976): The role of suprachiasmatic nuclei of the hypothalamus in the production of circadian rhythm. *Brain Res.*, 112:45–59.
28. Øgreid, D., and Døkeland, S. O. (1980): Protein kinase II has two distinct binding sites for cyclic AMP, only one of which is detectable by the conventional membrane-filtration method. *FEBS Lett.*, 121:340–344.
29. Ojeda, S. R., Negro-Vilar, A., and McCann, S. M. (1979): Release of prostaglandin E, by hypothalamic tissue: Evidence for their involvement in catecholamine-induced luteinizing hormone-releasing hormone release. *Endocrinology*, 104:617–624.
30. Oksche, A. (1973): Circumventricular organs and pituitary functions. In: *Endocrinology*, edited by R. O. Scow, F. J. G. Ebling, and I. W. Henderson, pp. 73–79. Excerpta, Amsterdam.
31. Pelayo, F., Dubocovich, M. L., and Langer, S. Z. (1977): Regulation of noradrenaline release in the rat pineal through a negative feedback mechanism mediated by presynaptic α-adrenoceptors. *Eur. J. Pharmacol.*, 45:317–318.
32. Rainbow, T. C., Degroff, V., Luine, V. N., and McEwen, B. S. (1980): Estradiol-17β increases the number of muscarinic receptors in hypothalamic nuclei. *Brain Res.* 198:239–243.
33. Reiter, R. J. (1980): The pineal and its hormones in the control of reproduction in mammals. *Endocrine Rev.*, 1:109–131.
34. Ritta, M. N., and Cardinali, D. P. (1980): Effect of indomethacin treatment on monoamine metabolism and melatonin synthesis of rat pineal gland. *Hormone Res.*, 12:305–312.
35. Ritta, M. N., and Cardinali, D. P. (1981): Prostaglandin E$_2$ increases adenosine 3',5'-monophosphate concentration and binding site occupancy, and stimulates serotonin-*N*-acetyltransferase activity in rat pineal glands *in vitro*. *Mol. Cell. Endocrinol.*, 23:151–159.
36. Sar, M., and Stumpf, W. E. (1981): Central noradrenergic neurones concentrate ³H-oestradiol. *Nature*, 289:500–502.
37. Scardapane, L., and Cardinali, D. P. (1977): Effect of estradiol and testosterone on catechol-*O*-methyl transferase activity of rat superior cervical ganglion, pineal gland, anterior hypophysis and hypothalamus. *J. Neural Transm.*, 40:81–86.
38. Smith, T. L., Eichberg, J., and Hauser, G. (1979): Postsynaptic localization of the alpha receptor-mediated stimulation of phosphatidylinositol turnover in pineal gland. *Life Sci.*, 24:2179–2184.
39. Stith, T. D., and Weingarten, D. P. (1979): Effect of a single injection of reserpine on kinetics of ³H-dexamethasone binding to receptors of the cat hypothalamus and hippocampus. *Neuroendocrinology*, 29:363–373.

40. Stumpf, W. E., and Sar, M. (1977): Steroid hormone target cells in the periventricular brain: Relationship to peptide hormone producing cells. *Fed. Proc.*, 36:1973–1983.
41. Towle, A. C., Sze, P. Y., and Lander, J. M. (1979): Cytosol glucocorticoid receptors in monoaminergic cell groups. *Trans. Am. Soc. Neurochem.*, 10:119.
42. Tsuruhara, T., Dufau, M. L. Cigorraga, S., and Catt, K. J. (1977): Hormonal regulation of testicular luteinizing hormone receptors. Effects of cyclic AMP and testosterone responses in isolated Leydig cells. *J. Biol. Chem.*, 252:9002–9009.
43. Vacas, M. I., and Cardinali, D. P. (1979): Effects of castration and reproductive hormones on pineal serotonin metabolism in rats. *Neuroendocrinology*, 28:187–195.
44. Vacas, M. I., and Cardinali, D. P. (1980): Binding sites for melatonin in bovine pineal gland. *Hormone Res.*, 13:121–131.
45. Vacas, M. I., and Cardinali, D. P. (1980): Effect of estradiol on α and β-adrenoceptor density in medial basal hypothalamus cerebral cortex and pineal gland of ovariectomized rats. *Neurosci. Lett.*, 17:73–77.
46. Vacas, M. I., Lowenstein, P. R., and Cardinali, D. P. (1979): Characterization of a cytosol progesterone receptor in bovine pineal gland. *Neuroendocrinology*, 24:84–89.
47. Vacas, M. I., Lowenstein, P. R., and Cardinali, D. P. (1980): Dihydroergocryptine binding sites in bovine and rat pineal glands. *J. Auton. Nerv. Syst.*, 2:305–313.
48. Vacas, M. I., Sarmiento, M. I. K., and Cardinali, D. P. (1981): Melatonin increases cAMP and decreases cAMP levels in rat medial basal hypothalamus *in vitro*. *Brain Res.*, 225:207–211.
49. Weiner, R. J., and Ganong, W. F. (1978): Role of brain monoamines and histamine in regulation of anterior pituitary secretion. *Physiol. Rev.*, 58:905–976.
50. Wilkinson, M., and Arendt, J. (1978): Effects of oestrogen and progesterone on rat pineal *N*-acetyltransferase activity and melatonin production. *Experientia*, 34:667–669.
51. Zatz, M. (1978): Sensitivity and cyclic nucleotides in the rat pineal gland. *J. Neural Transm. (Suppl.)*, 13:97–114.

Neural Transmission, Learning and Memory,
edited by R. Caputto and C. Ajmone Marsan.
Raven Press, New York © 1983.

Toward a Biochemistry of Memory Formation

S. P. R. Rose

Brain Research Group, The Open University, Milton Keynes, M.V.7. 6.A.A.
United Kingdom

CRITERIA FOR A BIOCHEMISTRY OF MEMORY FORMATION

When memory formation occurs, it is registered in the form of cell biological change in various neurons of the brain. It is in general believed that the change that occurs involves synaptic remodeling to reorganize pathways and connectivity (21). There is a multitude of experiments showing that, as a consequence of training, in many species and tasks, detectable biochemical changes occur in several brain regions (12,34). If we wish to discuss the relevance of these changes to the processes of information storage it is necessary to define the biochemical events that are *necessarily, sufficiently,* and *exclusively* associated with that storage. These I call the biochemical *correspondents* of memory formation, and they are to be distinguished from various necessary predispositions and concomitants of learning (32,33). For example, for learning to occur in a form which can be measured experimentally, it is generally necessary for the subject to receive sensory input, be stressed, show motor activity and so forth. While these events must occur if learning is to take place, they need to be distinguished from memory storage itself. I wish to propose six criteria which any biochemical process to be regarded as a correspondent of memory formation (or engram) must meet. I shall illustrate these criteria from the literature, including our own experiments on two forms of early learning in the chick, which we have been studying since the 1960s. The first is imprinting, in which the newly hatched chick learns to recognize and follow a prominent moving object ("mother" or "surrogate mother") and thereafter will prefer it to other more-or-less similar objects. The second is passive avoidance learning (PAL) when, following a single spontaneous peck at a small brightly colored object (generally a bead) coated with an aversive-tasting substance (methylanthranilate), the chick will thereafter avoid pecking at a similar, though uncoated object. The criteria are designed to provide a rational framework for further experimentation in this area.

Criterion 1. *The Process or Metabolite Must Show Neuroanatomically Localized Changes in Level or Rate During Memory Formation.*

This criterion is the most general; to meet it is at best to have achieved necessity but not sufficiency or exclusivity. The most important issue it raises is that of localization. It is true that memory could be represented by diffuse changes in many cells rather than in specific ones, as was the basis for holographic analogies for information storage which had a certain vogue in the 1960s. But even these would not imply that *all* regions of the brain, from cerebellum through cortex to the midbrain, were involved. There must be some specificity of localization of main effects even on the most delocalized model.

The danger of biochemical artefacts further reduces the power of this criterion (34) but it becomes the starting point for all subsequent analysis. Several laboratories including our own have made observations on particular biochemical events relevant to the criterion. Some of our own observations on changes occurring in a particular region of the chick brain, the anterior forebrain roof, are grouped below, arranged in temporal order following training:

(a) Depressed cAMP levels and elevated nuclear RNA polymerase activity within 15 to 30 min following onset of the imprinting stimulus (19,20).

(b) Transient increases of the muscarinic cholinergic receptor 30 min after training on the passive avoidance task (36) and decreases in the nicotinic (α-bungarotoxin) receptor at the same time (2).

(c) Increased incorporation of uracil into RNA within 1 to 2 hr following onset of imprinting (23,24).

(d) Elevated incorporation of [^{3}H]lysine and [^{14}C]leucine into protein 1 to 2 hr after onset of imprinting (17); increased [^{3}H]fucose incorporation into synaptic membrane glycoproteins, and [^{14}C]leucine incorporation into a tubulin fraction and amount of tubulin as measured by colchicine binding following PAL (29,37).

Such changes are compatible with a cell biological sequence involving the *de novo* synthesis of particular proteins, their post-translational modification and involvement in synaptic membrane phenomena. Their interpretation, however, is contingent on how far the observations satisfy the remaining criteria.

Criterion 2. *The Time Course of the Change in Biochemistry Must Match the Time Course of the Specific Phase of Memory Formation of Which It Is the Correspondent.*

The necessity of this criterion is plain, yet it is hard to meet—not least because of the ambiguities which surround the phenomenology of memory formation at the psychological level. If an animal is trained on a task and a biochemical measure made some hours or even days later, and a change compared to control is found, the implications are obscure unless a detailed time course of the change has been made.

A change that persists at 24 hr may have arisen during long-term memory formation and be a correspondent of that process; it can scarcely be a correspondent of the early phase(s) of memory formation, but unless it is known how long it persists subsequent to the training experience its relation to long-term memory may also be problematic. A change which occurs within minutes of the start of training may be one of two things: a correspondent of short-term memory (if such exists!) or part of the biochemical mobilization involved in "fixing" long-term memory. We have argued that changes in the cholinergic receptors (2,36) are classifiable under the first category; changes in RNA polymerase, RNA, and protein incorporation under the second. Many of the attempts in the literature to show the mobilization of *de novo* protein synthetic mechanisms: hydridization, base ratio changes, nuclear phosphorylation or changes in polysome/monosome ratio, come into the second, "mobilization" category. It may be argued that if the cell *is* to make new protein, such events are necessary preliminaries and of relatively little interest compared to the question of the cell biological role of the "end products" of all this activity, the changed proteins and other macromolecules that are part of the modulation of cell structure.

Another class of events that may be germane to this temporal question derives from the argument by Gold and McGaugh (16) and Agranoff (1) that certain of the biochemical changes detected, which may originate distant from the site of the ultimate engram itself, are some type of "fix" or "now print" signal that instructs the cell to make a transient change more lasting, to move from short to long-term memory formation. The timing of the production of these signals will be critical to their interpretation, of course; in the strict sense, they are not correspondents but concomitants of memory, as may, indeed, be many of the small peptide fragments, the presence of which seems to affect the rate and strength of memory formation and which have been investigated by the Utrecht group (11).

It will be observed that to meet criterion 2 requires a resolution of the phenomenology of memory formation. As many of the experiments germane to this phenomenology are derived from the biochemical interaction and inhibition studies described below, under criterion 4, the two issues are likely to be resolved together, if at all. Indeed much of what is known or argued about by learning neuropsychologists is a consequence, rather than a presumption, of biochemical experimentation. At any event, it is clear that the duration of distinct phases of memory formation differs with the species, task and the exact experimental design. The search for biochemical correspondents must take cognizance of this and work within the constraints given by a task the behavioural phenomenology of which has been thoroughly explored. Parenthetically, this is one of the advantages of working with imprinting or passive avoidance in the chick (3,15).

Criterion 3. *Stress, Motor Activity, or Other Necessary but not Sufficient Predispositions or Concomitants of Learning Must not in Themselves and in the Absence of the Memory Formation Result in the Changes of Criterion 1.*

This may be one of the most difficult of the criteria to meet. Note that it does not imply that memory formation is possible without the concomitants, but that the concomitants *may* occur independently of learning. One problem is the uncertainty at the behavioural level about the stages involved in memory formation, already discussed; partly devising "non-learning" controls depends on the assumption that unless the experimenter observes a measure of learning on the specific test under consideration, then the animal has learned nothing. But this implies that the organism is a sort of *tabula rasa* on which the only meaningful experience is the one imposed by the experimenter. In some experiments, "yoke controls" have been used in which the control animal experiences the cues and receives identical stimuli, for example, footshocks, to those received by the experimental, but cannot learn an escape route. But perhaps in such procedures the "controls" learn that there is no escape, and may hence be *more* stressed than the experimental (4)? In some procedures, animals are divided into two populations on the basis of success or failure to achieve a criterion of learning, which are then compared for a particular biochemical measure. Yet one only has, by definition, post-hoc knowledge of whether an animal will or will not be successful in the training, and biochemical differences may relate to endogenous behavioural differences between the populations which cannot be assessed; one can only assay an animal biochemically once!

Behind these problems, however, there lies another deeper one. Devising controls for concomitants of learning implies: (a) that we have a clear inventory of what these concomitants are; (b) that we can in fact place an animal in a situation in which the concomitants occur without the learning; and (c) that we have a clear model of the process of learning and memory formation itself in terms of initial registration and short and long-term consolidation processes so that the correspondents of these stages in memory formation can be distinguished.

Despite this formidable set of difficulties, we may reasonably adopt an experimental strategy which attempts to show that in a large number of controls in which experimenter-defined learning is absent, the biochemical change does not occur. A parsimonious interpretation would then be favourable to regarding the biochemical event as a correspondent of the memory formation. Perhaps the control of most general applicability is to compare undertrained and overtrained animals on a particular task; both groups may be performing the task, but whilst one group is learning as it performs, the other, presumably, no longer has anything (or much, at least) left to learn about it. We have used this type of control for uracil incorporation into anterior forebrain roof RNA during imprinting in the chick, and shown that the increased incorporation does not occur in the overtrained animals (6,24). Another powerful control is one in which the assumption is made that there is normally bilateral representation of the engram. Appropriate procedures may then enable learning to occur only in a particular region of a single hemisphere which can then be compared with the nonlearning side of the brain. We have used a split-brain preparation in the chick to show that increased uracil incorporation into RNA is confined to the forebrain roof of the learning compared with the naive hemisphere (23).

Such designs will control for brain effects which may be expected to be symmetrically distributed (for example, generalized circulation-borne hormones) and the sequelae of motor activity; they will not control for changes at the microcirculation level—for which there is increasing evidence (35) or for changes consequent on input into the trained compared with the untrained hemisphere—for example, sensory stimulation.

A series of separate control experiments in the imprinting model has been able to show that the increase of uracil incorporation into RNA in the chick anterior forebrain roof which occurs over the period of exposure to the imprinting stimulus was not a consequence of motor activity, stress, sensory stimulation, attention, or arousal (30,31). But there still remain problems with the use of serial control experiments of this sort. For example, the elevation in incorporation could still be a correspondent of some interaction between these several processes, none of which is sufficient individually to generate it. Further, devising a series of controls for a *particular* biochemical correspondent does not formally allow one to conclude that other related biochemical changes are themselves correspondents; for instance, in the imprinting experiments the controls were made exhaustively with uracil incorporation as the correspondent; controls for the elevated incorporation into protein which follows the uracil incorporation were much less thorough. We can make certain assumptions based on biochemical logic that the observations are interrelated parts of a single phenomenon, but these are *only* assumptions, however reasonable they may appear.

Criterion 4. *If the Cellular/Biochemical Changes of Criterion 1 Are Inhibited During the Period over Which Memory Formation Should Occur, the Memory Formation Should Be Inhibited, and Vice Versa.*

If biochemical correspondents are one-for-one (or even one-for-many) it is logically necessary that inhibition of the correspondents should inhibit memory formation, and there is a substantial body of literature which has been based on this experimental design (1,15). It is also logically necessary that the reverse should hold; inhibiting memory formation while holding the other conditions constant should inhibit the correspondent. Problems of interpretation of the experiments in the literature revolve around both behavioural and biochemical issues. If the inhibiting agent (drug, antibiotic, ECS or whatever) interferes with a concomitant of memory formation—for example, attention or arousal—a spurious correspondence may be generated with the biochemistry. Administration of the inhibitor may also affect the criteria of acquisition, so that what the animal achieves is actually a state-dependent memory for the expression of which readministration of the agent is required.

There is an analogous concern with the interpretation of the biochemistry. Few inhibitors or antibiotics have single-site effects. In early studies on protein synthesis inhibition, the antibiotic puromycin was used; later its injection was shown to result in mitochondrial swelling (14). There have been reports that cycloheximide and acetoxycycloheximide, more recently used inhibitors, interact with the catecholamine system (13).

More serious, perhaps, is that inhibition of a process so fundamental to the cell as, say, protein synthesis, has inevitable biochemical sequelae; changes in energy metabolism, amino acid uptake, etc. Recently it has been shown, scarcely surprisingly, that intracerebral injection of cycloheximide in the chick results in an intracellular accumulation of amino acids, and that some of the behavioural consequences of cycloheximide injection can be mimicked by administration of amino acids such as glutamate (18). As a strategic tool for exploring the correspondents of memory the use of inhibitors is thus limited. They have added to our information on the time course of memory formation (15,28) but the light they cast on the exact nature of the biochemical correspondents is limited to a confirmation of involvement of a correspondent demonstrated using other criteria. Every necessary and sufficient correspondent must fit criterion 4; not all phenomena that fit criterion 4 are necessary and sufficient correspondents.

There remains scope for using the reverse form of this criterion. If a biochemical process is suspected of being a correspondent, inhibition of memory formation should inhibit the process. This has been the basis of some of the experiments on the muscarinic cholinergic receptors and passive avoidance learning in the chick (36) and further work along these lines is undoubtedly possible. More specific biochemical inhibitors, for example colchicine, which disrupts microtubules and blocks axonal flow, or inhibitors of specific transmitters, may also assist in meeting this criterion. It is of interest that increases in tubulin synthesis and concentration have been found following passive avoidance learning in the chicken (29) and injection of cholchicine prevents long-term memory formation for the passive avoidance response (10).

Criterion 5. *Removal of the Anatomical Locus (or Loci) at Which the Changes of Criterion 1 Occur, should Interfere with the Process of Memory Formation and/or Recall, Depending on When, in Relation to the Training, the Region Is Removed.*

If the changes in connectivity which, it is surmised, constitute the engram, are anatomically localized rather than diffusely spread in a redundant network across entire regions of the brain, then removal of the locus subsequent to training should eliminate the memory. The regions at which the biochemical changes are observed should correspond to those whose anatomical deletion obliterates the memory. Despite the well-known objection to the interpretation of ablation studies, that what they reveal is not the function of the missing region, but of the rest of the brain in the absence of that region, the localization criterion is logically necessary, granted an otherwise identified potential correspondent. However, the reverse of this criterion does *not* apply. If ablation of a region disrupts memory formation, it does not follow that biochemical analysis must reveal changes occurring there. The same caveat about the interpretation of anatomical ablation studies must apply to the interpretation of the biochemical inhibition studies referred to in criterion 4.

There are of course many studies of the effects of ablation on memory formation and recall but most are not coupled to biochemical data; the only studies germane to this criterion of which I am aware are those of my collaborator Gabriel Horn and his colleagues in the chick imprinting system. Having localized the site of elevated uracil incorporation during imprinting to a specific region of the anterior roof, the medial hyperstriatum ventrale (MHV) (24), they have been able to show that ablation of the region following training prevents the expression of the imprinting response while ablation prior to training prevents acquisition of the response (22). The effect may be lateralised (26). There is some evidence of morphological change in the region including length of synaptic apposition, by comparison with dark-maintained controls (9). It is relevant that on the basis of independent experiments, Benowitz had earlier predicted that the MHV should be an important locus of memory storage in the chick (8). However, it remains arguable that both the biochemical change and the anatomical locus are involved in some necessary organizing responses of recognition, of the stimulus or of the following responses to it, rather than as the site of the engram itself.

Criterion 6. *Neurophysiological Recording from the Locus (or Loci) of the Changes of Criteria 1 and 5 Should Detect Altered Cellular Responses During and/or as a Consequence of Memory Formation.*

If engram formation results in changed connectivity of specific cells at a particular locus, it follows that recordings made from these cells during learning should show changes by comparison with the patterns prior to learning or following memory formation. When the animal is involved in recall, these cells should again show alteration in firing patterns. That is, there should be a coincidence of anatomical, biochemical, and physiological correspondents to engram formation and engram utilisation. There are of course reports in the literature of changes in firing responses of cells during memory formation but the triple mapping of correspondents that criterion 6 demands is still a task for future experimentation.

FURTHER QUESTIONS

If these are the set of necessary and sufficient criteria for memory formation, nonetheless, understanding the biochemistry of memory raises some further questions.

1. What is the relationship of the extent and strength of the memory to the extent of the biochemical change? Might it be that the more "powerful" the memory, the greater the extent of the modification to the connectivity which may be involved? For instance, in the chick imprinting system, we have found correlations between the preference score of the trained birds (a measure of learning) and uracil incorporation into RNA and leucine incorporation into a tubulin-enriched fraction in the anterior forebrain roof (7,27).

However, despite the tidiness of the correlation in our own imprinting studies, we must be careful of the generalization, because there is a problem about measuring the "strength" of a memory. Although a chick's preference score following imprinting can be plotted on a linear scale (5), it is not necessarily the case that all forms of learning can be so easily quantitated. Indeed even a linear preference score need not imply a linear set of internal events. Setting an arbitrary criterion for learning, and ranking performance to criterion as in maze-learning or shuttlebox tasks, may give the appearance of being metric to what is actually an ordinal scale. The biochemical and behavioural metrics are constructed in different languages and on different assumptions, and cannot automatically be assumed to be superposable in all details.

2. Do the changes involve synaptic connectivity? On the basis of the evidence reviewed in the context of the above criteria and in the case of the chick, where we have from several different sources perhaps the most complete inventory of potential correspondents, it is possible to conclude that there is reasonable, though not absolute, evidence for a sequence of events which involves transient ionic and amino acid movements across neuronal membranes (15) and changes in the activity of cholinergic receptor (2,36) in the anterior forebrain roof region in the early and short-term phases of memory fixation (minutes to an hour). Over a period of several hours (at least up to 24 hr) following training there are changes in RNA and protein turnover including soluble tubulin and synaptic membrane glycoproteins. All these changes are compatible with a model in which synaptic connectivity is being altered by changes in the communication between pre- and postsynaptic neurons and in synaptic apposition, and consequent remodelling. The morphological evidence concerning dendritic spine formation and some suggestive evidence from other experimental situations, not reviewed here, that synaptic dimensions can change as a result of experience, is also germane. The point however is not at this stage to present an elaborate model for a possible change in connectivity or a series of biochemical processes corresponding to memory formation. The semitheoretical literature and the reviews of the field of the last 2 decades are replete with such models. There is a multitude of potential ways in which we can envisage synaptic connectivity being altered, and until there are experiments which can distinguish between these possibilities, further speculation is simply burdensome; vacuous for the theoretician, useless to the experimenter. It is enough to argue that the mechanisms of connectivity change involved in memory formation (if so they be) are likely to conform to general cell-biological and neurochemical principles and not to involve fundamentally new mechanisms. The credibility of potential correspondents must be judged against this background.

3. Finally, it still seems reasonable, at least as a heuristic, to argue that the biochemical correspondents of engram formation will be found to be similar in form whatever the engram concerned; engram specificity seems more likely to be conferred by the spatial coordinates of the biochemical correspondents — that is, the addresses and connectivity of the cells concerned — rather than molecular differences between the correspondents of different memories. Despite the flurry of enthusiasm for it in the 1960s, there seems no reason to postulate molecular, rather than cellular engram formation. However, granted the degree of molecular specificity that is known to exist amongst different systems of neurons, we may in due course discover that there are differences in detail amongst the correspondents of different classes of memory. At any event a clarification of the questions involved

in the study of the biochemistry of memory formation may help to set our experimental programme onto a sound footing.

ACKNOWLEDGMENTS

The criteria proposed in this paper are discussed more fully in refs. 32 and 33, and have benefitted from discussion with many colleagues; I would like in particular to thank Martin Barker, Steve Chorover, Ruth Hubbard, Margaret Kossut, Sean Murphy and Hilary Rose, as well as colleagues and collaborators with the imprinting experiments: Pat Bateson, Gabriel Horn, Jeff Haywood, John Hambley and Alan Longstaff; and the PAL experiments: Marie Gibbs, Radmila Mileusnic, Bob Sukumar, Bob Burgoyne and Penny Tillson.

The interpretations however, remain my own, and I do not wish to commit my colleagues necessarily to them!

REFERENCES

1. Agranoff, B. W., Burrell, H. R., Dokas, L. A., and Springer, A. D. (1976): Progress in biochemical approaches to learning and memory. In: *Psychopharmacology*, edited by M. Lipton, A. De Mascio, and K. Killam, pp. 623–635. Raven Press, New York.
2. Aleksidze, N., Potempska, A., Murphy, S., and Rose, S. P. R. (1981): Passive avoidance in the young chick affects forebrain α-bungarotoxin and serotonin binding. *Abstr. 8th ISN*, p. 382.
3. Bateson, P. P. G. (1966): The characteristics and context of imprinting. *Biol. Rev.*, 177–220.
4. Bateson, P. P. G. (1970): Are they really the products of learning? In: *Short Term Changes in Neural Activity and Behaviour*, edited by G. Horn and R. A. Hinde, pp. 553–564. Cambridge University Press.
5. Bateson, P. P. G. (1976): Neural consequences of early experience in birds. In: *Perspectives in Experimental Biology, Vol. 1*, edited by P. Spencer-Davies, pp. 411–415. Pergamon Press, Oxford.
6. Bateson, P. P. G., Horn, G., and Rose, S. P. R. (1972): Effects of early experience on regional incorporation of precursors into RNA and protein in the chick brain. *Brain Res.*, 39:449–465.
7. Bateson, P. P. G., Horn, G., and Rose, S. P. R. (1975): Imprinting: Correlations between behaviour and incorporation of ^{14}C-uracil into chick brain. *Brain Res.*, 84:207–220.
8. Benowitz, L. (1980): Functional anatomy of the avian telencephalon. In: *Comparative Neurology of the Telencephalon*, edited by S. Ebbesson, pp. 389–421. Plenum, New York.
9. Bradley, P., Horn, G., and Bateson, P. P. G. (1979): Psychological correlates of imprinting in the chick brain. *Neurosci. Lett. (Suppl. 3)*, 584.
10. Cherfas, J. J., and Bateson, P. P. G. (1978): Colchicine impairs performance after learning a one-trial passive avoidance task in day old chicks. *Behav. Biol.*, 23:27–37.
11. De Wied, D., and Bohus, B. (1979): Modulation of memory processes by neuropeptides of hypothalamic hypophyseal origin. In: *Brain Mechanisms in Memory and Learning*, edited by M. A. Brazier, pp. 139–149. Raven Press, New York.
12. Dunn, A. (1980): Neurochemistry of learning and memory: An evaluation of recent data. *Annu. Rev. Psychol.*, 31:343–390.
13. Flexner, L. B., Serota, R. G., and Goodman, R. H. (1973): Cycloheximide and acetoxycycloheximide: Inhibition of tyrosine hydroxylase. *Proc. Natl. Acad. Sci. USA*, 70:354–356.
14. Gambetti, P., Gonatas, N. K., and Flexner, L. B. (1978): Puromycin: Action on neuronal mitochondria. *Science*, 161:700–902.
15. Gibbs, M. E., and Ng, K. T. (1977): Psychobiology of memory: Towards a model of memory formation. *Biobehav. Rev.*, 1:113–136.
16. Gold, P. E., and McGaugh, J. L. (1975): A single trace, two process view of memory storage processes. In: *Short Term Memory*, edited by D. Deutsch and J. A. Deutsch, pp. 355–378. Academic Press, New York.
17. Hambley, J., Haywood, J., Rose, S. P. R., and Bateson, P. P. G. (1976): Effects of imprinting on lysine uptake and incorporation into protein in chick brain. *J. Neurobiol.*, 8:1109–1118.

18. Hambley, J. A., and Rogers, L. J. (1979): Retarded learning induced by amino acids in the neonatal chick. *Neuroscience*, 4:677–684.
19. Hambley, J. W., and Rose, S. P. R. (1977): Effects of an imprinting stimulus on adenylate cyclase and adenosine 3′ 5′ phosphate in neonatal chick brain. *Neuroscience*, 2:1115–1120.
20. Haywood, J., Rose, S. P. R., and Bateson, P. P. G. (1970): Effects of an imprinting procedure on RNA polymerase activity in the chick brain. *Nature*, 228:373–374.
21. Hebb, D. O. (1949): *The Organization of Behaviour*. Wiley, New York.
22. Horn, G. (1981): Neural mechanisms of learning: An analysis of imprint in the chick. *Proc. R. Soc. Lond. (B)*, 213:101–137.
23. Horn, G., Bateson, P. P. G., and Rose, S. P. R. (1973): Monocular imprinting and reginal incorporation of tritiated uracil into the brains on intact and "split brain" chicks. *Brain Res.*, 56:227–237.
24. Horn, G., McCabe, B. J., and Bateson, P. P. G. (1979): Imprinting: An autoradiographic analysis of changes in uracil incorporation into chick brain. *Brain Res.*, 168:361–379.
25. Horn, G., Rose, S. P. R., and Bateson, P. P. G. (1973): Experience and plasticity in the nervous system. *Science*, 181:506–514.
26. Howard, K. J., Rogers, L. J., and Boura, A. L. A. (1980): Functional lateralisation of the chicken forebrain revealed by the use of intracranial glutamate. *Brain Res.*, 188:369–382.
28. Longstaff, A. and Rose, S. P. R. (1981): Ontogenetic and imprinting-induced changes in chick brain protein metabolism and muscarinic receptor binding activity. *J. Neurochem.*, 37:1089–1098.
29. McGaugh, J. L. (1966): Time dependent processes in memory storage. *Science*, 153:1351–1358.
30. Mileusnic, R., Rose, S. P. R., and Tillson, (1980): Passive avoidance learning results in region-specific changes in concentration of and incorporation into colchicine binding proteins in the chick brain. *J. Neurochem.* 34:1007–1015.
31. Rose, S. P. R. (1977): Early visual experience, learning and neurochemical plasticity in the rat and the chick. *Philos. Trans. R. Society (B)*, 278:307–318.
32. Rose, S. P. R. (1979): Neurochemical correlates of early learning in the chick. In: *Neurobiological Bases of Learning and Memory*, edited by Y. Nagata and B. W. Agranoff, pp. 179–191. Plenum Press, New York.
33. Rose, S. P. R. (1980): From causations to translations: What biochemists can contribute to the study of behaviour. In: *Perspectives in Ethology, Vol. IV*, edited by P. Klopfer and P. P. G. Bateson. Plenum Press, New York.
34. Rose, S. P. R. (1981): What should a biochemistry of learning and memory be about? *Neuroscience*, 6:811–821.
35. Rose, S. P. R., Gibbs, M. E., and Hambley, J. (1980): Transient increases in forebrain muscarinic cholinergic receptors following passive avoidance learning. *Neuroscience*, 5:169–172.
36. Rose, S. P. R., and Haywood, J. (1976): Experience, learning and brain metabolism. In: *Biochemical Correlates of Brain Structure and Function*, edited by A. N. Davison, pp. 249–292. Academic Press, London.
37. Schwartz, W. J., and Sharp, F. R. (1978): Autoradiographic maps of regional brain glucose consumption in resting awake rats using ^{14}C-2-deoxyglucose. *J. Comp. Neurol.*, 177:353–360.
38. Sukumar, R., Rose, S. P. R., and Burgoyne, R. (1980): Increased incorporation of ^{3}H-fucose into chick brain glycoproteins following training on a passive avoidance task. *J. Neurochem.*, 34:1000–1006.

Neural Transmission, Learning and Memory,
edited by R. Caputto and C. Ajmone Marsan.
Raven Press, New York © 1983.

Some Neurochemical Effects of Behavioral Training and Their Relevance to Learning and Memory Modulation

I. Izquierdo, D. A. Vendite, D. O. Souza, R. D. Dias,
M. A. Carrasco, and M. L. S. Perry

*Departamento de Bioquímica, Instituto de Biociências, U.F.R.G.S. (Centro),
90.000 Pôrto Alegre, RS, Brasil*

During training, animals associate elements such as stimuli, responses, stimuli and responses, stimuli and consequences of stimulation, etc., so that when exposed again to a similar or a related experience their behavior will be changed: the phenomenon known as learning. However, many nonassociative events also take place during training: arousal; stress; perceptual, motor, and motivational changes, etc. Even though it is possible to distinguish between some associative and some nonassociative components in at least some training paradigms (25,29,55), probably no learning can occur without concomitant nonassociative events, and perhaps it is simply not possible to design a task in which associative factors can be examined in total isolation (57).

The nonassociative events that accompany learning induce major neurochemical changes that persist after training into the so-called memory consolidation period (11,18,19,28,33,44,49). These changes include alterations in neurotransmitter release and in hormonal secretion (4,17–19,23,27,31,33,35,44,49,59). Neurotransmitters and hormones in turn affect other biochemical variables both in the brain and in the periphery: synthesis and/or release of other neurotransmitters or hormones (4,18,19,59), RNA and protein synthesis (11,12,42), etc. In addition, the neurohumoral and hormonal changes that occur during training may have modulatory influences on acquisition and memory consolidation (18,21,28,35,44,63). The secondary biochemical changes and the effects on learning and memory are not necessarily causally related (11,33). This chapter reviews recent data on the effect of training upon adrenal epinephrine secretion and central β-endorphin release, and on the influence of these substances upon brain protein synthesis and learning and memory. As will be seen, the effects on protein synthesis are probably not related to the behavioral effects.

PERIPHERAL EPINEPHRINE RELEASE DURING TRAINING, AND EFFECTS OF PERIPHERAL EPINEPHRINE ADMINISTRATION ON LEARNING AND MEMORY

It has been known for many years that the adrenal medulla secretes epinephrine in emergency situations as part of a general preparation of the body for "fight or flight" (5). So, it has been usually taken for granted that the arousal or stress associated with learning, particularly aversive learning, releases epinephrine from the adrenal glands. However, this release has actually been measured only very recently. A 5-min train of footshocks increases plasma epinephrine and norepinephrine levels in the rat (43). A single session of inhibitory avoidance training using a single 3.0-mA footshock has a similar effect (16,17). Since the major source of plasma epinephrine is the adrenal medulla (16), the increase of plasma epinephrine probably reflects an increased adrenal medullary secretion. Clearly, the effect is not specific to learning and results from a nonassociative influence of footshock stimulation.

Systemic administrations of epinephrine affect both acquisition and memory consolidation. At high doses (e.g., 100 or 500 μg/kg, i.p.) epinephrine disrupts acquisition of one- (44) and two-way active avoidance in rats (36). When given after training at similar doses it facilitates extinction of one-way active avoidance (44) and impairs retention both of shuttle (36) and of inhibitory avoidance (19). However, depending on footshock intensity (19) or on the number of footshocks (34,36), posttraining epinephrine administrations may enhance inhibitory avoidance retention (19) or have no effect in one-way avoidance situations (34). Studies using tyramine and guanethidine, a releaser and an inhibitor of the release of sympathetic nerve norepinephrine, respectively, suggested that there is a bell-shaped dose–response curve for the effect of norepinephrine on learning and memory and that the curve is displaced to the left or to the right depending on the degree of sympathoadrenal activation associated with each task; in other words, each task would require an "optimum" level of sympathoadrenal activity for learning and consolidation (34,36,50). The same may be true for peripherally injected epinephrine (19), and certainly is true for all treatments known so far which affect learning and/or memory through changes in endogenous catecholamine metabolism (18,33,63).

Among these treatments, amphetamine and nicotine have been repeatedly shown to enhance acquisition and consolidation of a variety of aversive tasks (18,29,63). Their effect is attenuated by adrenal medullectomy (44,47) or by prevention of the blood pressure increase that they produce (48). In addition, very high doses of amphetamine given i.c.v. do not enhance inhibitory avoidance consolidation whereas 4-OH-amphetamine, which does not readily cross the blood–brain barrier, causes memory facilitation when given systemically (44). The depressant effect of met-enkephalin on active avoidance acquisition (24,40), and the amnestic effect of posttraining amygdala stimulation (44) are attenuated by adrenal medullectomy. Thus, it seems that adrenal medullary secretion is important for the effects on learning and memory of a variety of treatments. Whether the adrenal glands are a target organ for those treatments (40,44), or whether epinephrine secretion has a permissive or cooperative effect (24), remains to be seen.

Epinephrine and norepinephrine, given systemically, do not readily cross the blood–brain barrier (61); therefore, it is presumable that their effect on learning and memory is mediated by peripheral receptors. Peripherally acting compounds may influence central processes such as learning and memory in a variety of ways: (a) through reflex influences of blood pressure changes on the reticular formation: the arousal produced by systemic epinephrine administration is secondary to its hypertensive effect (2), and reticular stimulation is known to facilitate memory consolidation (7); (b) through reflex influences originating in other peripheral end organs; (c) through regional changes in cerebral blood flow (34,36,50). Gold and his associates have presented convincing evidence that peripheral injections of epinephrine and other compounds may modulate consolidation through changes in brain norepinephrine levels (19,23). A moderate, but not a too large or too small, depletion of central norepinephrine seems optimum for consolidation. Clearly, the changes in central norepinephrine may result from any of the reflex influences listed above, and would readily explain the bell-shaped dose–response curves for the effects on learning and memory of peripherally injected catecholamines or of drugs that affect catecholamine metabolism.

PERIPHERAL EPINEPHRINE AND BRAIN AND LIVER PROTEIN SYNTHESIS

Many authors have reported that various forms of training are followed by an increased rate of brain protein synthesis (see 1,10,11 for reviews). Typically, this phenomenon has been related to memory consolidation. Indeed, a strong inhibition of brain protein synthesis in the posttraining period disrupts consolidation (1,10,11); however, this does not necessarily lead to the corollary that *increased* protein synthesis is essential for consolidation.

The most detailed studies on posttraining protein synthesis are those of Matthies and his group (38,42) in the rat hippocampus. After a brief session of Y-maze avoidance discrimination there are two peaks of RNA, protein, and glycoprotein labelling in this structure, one immediately after, and the other 4 to 8 hr after training (42). The first peak is not observed when protein labelling is carried out *in vitro* (38). Souza and co-workers, in this laboratory, were able to confirm Matthies's findings on protein synthesis and detected both peaks not only in the hippocampus but also in the caudate nucleus and the liver; the early peak, however, was inconstant: it was observed in some experiments (56) and not in others (57). The absence or inconstancy of the early protein synthesis peak in *in vitro* experiments may be due to the fact that the protein species whose synthesis is enhanced are different in the two peaks, at least in the hippocampus (42); it is possible that in homogenates some endogenous factor (neurohumoral or other) necessary for the first peak is either absent or inconstantly present.

Hormonal mediation of the early peak was studied by Dunn and his co-workers (10–12,52). Thirty minutes after a 15-min session of one-way active avoidance, or of buzzers alone, or of footshocks alone, there was an increased *in vivo* incorporation of [³H]lysine to protein in rat brain and liver (12,52). The fact that the phenomenon occurred after buzzer or footshock stimulation as well as after avoidance training suggests that it was a consequence of nonassociative rather than of true learning variables. The fact that the labelling changes occurred also in the liver (as was later confirmed by Souza et al., 56,57) suggested generalized hormonal mediation rather than tissue specificity. The labelling peak was not abolished by adrenalectomy, which rules out corticosterone and epinephrine, but not ACTH, as causative factors; in fact, the administration of 0.1 or 1.0 IU of ACTH caused an increase of brain and liver protein labelling similar to that caused by training (12). These findings are consistent both with the observation that hypophysectomy reduced RNA and ribosomes in brain tissue (15) and with the presumable hypersecretion of ACTH caused by the stress of the training procedures (12). The effect of ACTH appears to be due to its 4–10 segment, since $ACTH_{4-10}$, which has no actions on the adrenal gland, increases the incorporation of [¹⁴C]leucine into brain protein (51) and prevents the effect of hypophysectomy (14). Thus, there is evidence suggesting that the first peak of protein synthesis that occurs after training may be mediated by a release of pituitary ACTH caused by nonassociative factors present in the training situation (arousal, stress, etc.). The phenomenon is interesting in view of the known stimulant effects of ACTH and particularly of $ACTH_{4-10}$ on learning and memory (4,11).

Hormonal mediation of the second protein synthesis peak was studied in our laboratory. Adult female Wistar rats (120–180 g) were submitted to a 25-min session of 50 tones (1 kHz, 5 sec, 70 db) or 50 footshocks (60 Hz, 2 sec, 1.0 mA) in a 50 × 25 × 25 xm acrylic box. Interstimulus intervals varied at random between 10 and 50 sec. Animals were sacrificed by decapitation 2 or 4 hr after training. The hippocampus, caudate nucleus, and liver were dissected on an iced Petri dish, weighed, and homogenized at 4°C in 10 volumes of preboiled Ringer solution; 0.5-ml aliquots were incubated 60 min at 37°C with 2 μl of 0.01 N HCl plus 0.2 μCi of [¹⁴C](U)-leucine. Incubation was stopped with 0.375 ml of water plus 0.625 ml of 1 mM unlabelled leucine in 10% trichloroacetic acid at 4°C. The precipitate was filtered through filter paper, washed three times with 5% trichloroacetic acid at 0°C, three times with 1:1 ethanol:ether, three more times with ether alone, dried at room temperature, and taken to a scintillation mixture. Parallel samples were processed as above but incubated at 0°C ("blanks"). Data are shown in Table 1 expressed as c.p.m. mg protein minus "blank" in the precipitates/c.p.m. in total homogenates.

Table 1 shows that the two training procedures were followed by an increased protein labelling at 4 hr in the caudate nucleus and hippocampus and at 2 and 4 hr in the liver, both in intact and in sham-operated animals. The effect was not seen in animals submitted to bilateral adrenal medullectomy 30 days before; in fact, there was an actual decrease of protein labelling 2 and 4 hr after training in the demedullectomized animals.

TABLE 1. *Incorporation of [^{14}C]leucine into protein in homogenates of rat caudate nucleus, hippocampus, and liver of intact, sham-operated, and adrenal medullectomized animals*

| | | Caudate nucleus | | | |
| | | Tones | | Footshocks | |
	Control	2 hr	4 hr	2 hr	4 hr
Intact	33 ± 2 (19)	32 ± 3 (9)	42 ± 5[b] (9)	31 ± 5 (9)	40 ± 5[b] (10)
Sham-operated	34 ± 2 (11)	28 ± 2 (9)	41 ± 2[c] (15)	30 ± 2 (9)	41 ± 3[c] (15)
Medullectomized	35 ± 3 (12)	27 ± 1[a] (9)	24 ± 2[c] (10)	28 ± 2[a] (9)	24 ± 2[c] (10)

| | | Hippocampus | | | |
| | | Tones | | Footshocks | |
	Control	2 hr	4 hr	2 hr	4 hr
Intact	27 ± 1 (16)	28 ± 2 (12)	41 ± 2[c] (21)	30 ± 2 (12)	38 ± 2[b] (19)
Sham-operated	28 ± 1 (11)	30 ± 2 (9)	36 ± 2[c] (12)	29 ± 3 (10)	37 ± 2[c] (9)
Medullectomized	28 ± 2 (10)	30 ± 2 (10)	24 ± 1 (9)	31 ± 2 (9)	26 ± 2 (10)

| | | Liver | | | |
| | | Tones | | Footshocks | |
	Control	2 hr	4 hr	2 hr	4 hr
Intact	22 ± 1 (15)	33 ± 4[c] (11)	33 ± 3[c] (23)	29 ± 2[b] (12)	33 ± 2[c] (19)
Sham-operated	23 ± 1 (15)	36 ± 2[c] (9)	29 ± 3[a] (13)	33 ± 2[c] (8)	29 ± 3[a] (12)
Medullectomized	24 ± 1 (11)	27 ± 2 (6)	21 ± 2 (9)	21 ± 1 (8)	24 ± 3 (10)

Incorporation of [^{14}C]leucine expressed as (c.p.m. mg protein − blank) × 100/c.p.m in total homogenate; means ± S.E.M. Animals were sacrificed 2 or 4 hr after tones or footshock training during 25 min.

Significant differences from control in a Duncan multiple range test: [a]at 0.05 level; [b]at 0.01 level; [c]at 0.005 level. In this and following tables the number of animals per group is given in parentheses.

These findings suggest that the protein synthesis increase caused by training may be mediated by the adrenal medulla. Table 2 shows the effect of intraperitoneal injections of saline or of 12 μg/kg of epinephrine HCl on protein synthesis in the caudate, hippocampus, and liver. Saline caused an increased protein labelling in the liver at 2 hr from injection, and epinephrine caused a similar increase in both the caudate nucleus and the liver. The effect of saline might be mediated by the release of endogenous epinephrine, since it causes also a transient hyperglycemia which is abolished by adrenal medullectomy (60). Therefore, it seems that the second protein labelling peak which occurs after training requires the presence of intact adrenal medullary glands, either as mediators of the effect, or as a permissive or cooperative factor (which makes it different from the first or early peak, which is not abolished by adrenalectomy, 12). If the adrenal glands had merely a permissive or cooperative effect, the second peak would nevertheless be mediated by some other agent with a generalized action, such as a hormone (the peak occurs simultaneously in the brain and the liver).

It is unlikely that the second post-training protein synthesis peak is directly related to memory consolidation processes. First, in our laboratory, rats with bilateral adrenal medullectomy show no impairment of shuttle avoidance acquisition or retention (24; see also 44,47), and they lack the second protein synthesis peak. Second, this peak occurs not only after tones or footshock training but also after shuttle avoidance or pseudoconditioning training (56); pseudoconditioning (random tones and footshocks) leaves no detectable memory (29), and footshock training corresponds to a very different form of learning than habituation (tones alone) or shuttle avoidance, if any (58). Third, the peak occurs simultaneously in brain and liver, whereas memory consolidation probably takes place only in the former.

Therefore, the second peak of protein synthesis that occurs after training may be regarded as a byproduct of nonassociative factors present during training; it requires the presence of intact adrenal medullary glands, but it is not related to either learning or memory processes, or to the influence of the adrenal medullary glands on learning and memory.

RELEASE OF β-ENDORPHIN IN THE BRAIN CAUSED BY DIFFERENT FORMS OF TRAINING

Training in any of the four behavioral situations mentioned above (50 tones alone, 50 footshocks alone, 50 tone-footshock shuttle avoidance trials, or 50 tones and

TABLE 2. *Effect of saline (1 ml/kg, i. p.) and epinephrine HC1 μg/kg, i. p.) on the incorporation of [^{14}C]leucine into protein in homogenates of rat caudate nucleus, hippocampus, and liver*

Treatment	Caudate	Hippocampus	Liver
Saline: 2 hr	30 ± 3 (11)	32 ± 4 (12)	41 ± 4[c] (10)
Saline: 4 hr	30 ± 4 (11)	24 ± 2 (15)	30 ± 3[b] (10)
Epinephrine: 2 hr	41 ± 3[a,b] (13)	30 ± 2 (13)	42 ± 3[c] (17)
Epinephrine: 4 hr	32 ± 3 (12)	29 ± 2 (9)	32 ± 4[b] (16)

Incorporation of [^{14}C]leucine expressed as (c.p.m. mg protein − blank) × 100/ c.p.m. in total homogenate; means ± S.E.M. Animals were sacrificed 2 or 4 hr after injection.

[a]Significant difference from saline groups in Duncan multiple range test at 0.005 level; [b,c]significant difference from intact control groups of Table 1 at 0.01 and 0.005 levels, respectively.

25 footshocks in random sequence) causes a reduction of β-endorphin immuno-reactivity in the rest of the brain but not in the hypothalamus of rats (32,35). Footshock stimulation, but not the other forms of training, causes in addition a release of β-endorphin immunoreactive material from the pituitary gland into the general circulation (33,54). When the animals are submitted for a second time to the same behavioral procedure in which they had been trained, there is no change of brain β-endorphin immunoreactivity after the second session (32,33,35). If, however, there is a change of task between the training and the test session (for example, if animals trained with tones alone are tested in the avoidance situation or vice versa), there is again a reduction of brain β-endorphin immunoreactivity in the test session (32). The decrease of β-endorphin immunoreactivity observed during training is of 20 to 50 ng of β-endorphin ($\sim$30 to 70 ng of β-endorphin immu-noreactive material, 32,33,35) per brain over 25 min $\cong$ 1.0 to 1.5 ng/brain/min (28,35).

Clearly, the β-endorphin changes result from nonassociative, rather than from learning, factors in the training sessions, and appear to be related to novelty of the task (28,32,33,35).

β-endorphin (β-lipotropin$_{61-91}$) is synthetized very slowly (3) and brain levels of β-endorphin immunoreactive substances would not be expected to change in 25 min even if protein synthesis were completely arrested, which is certainly not the case with any of the behavioral paradigms mentioned above (see preceding section). In addition, with the exception of footshock stimulation, there was no release of β-endorphin immunoreactive substances into the blood (and in that case they came from the pituitary gland, 33). Therefore, it must be concluded that the decrease of β-endorphin immunoreactivity that occurs in the brain during training is due to local release and subsequent metabolization of the substance(s) (24,27,28,32,33,35).

Electroconvulsive shock, a well-known amnestic treatment (9,18), causes a much larger depletion of brain β-endorphin immunoreactivity than the one observed after any of the four behavioral treatments mentioned above; in the case of electrocon-vulsive shock, the depletion occurs also in the hypothalamus and there is no change of pituitary or plasma β-endorphin immunoreactivity levels (9). Electroconvulsive shock also releases Met-enkephalin from the rat brain amygdala and hypothalamus (6). Twenty-five-min training with tones alone or shuttle avoidance does not alter brain Met-enkephalin levels (6).

ROLE OF THE β-ENDORPHIN THAT IS RELEASED IN THE BRAIN DURING TRAINING ON LEARNING AND MEMORY

Experiments carried out in 1978–1979 in three different laboratories showed that the immediate posttraining administration of low doses of the opiate receptor an-tagonist, naloxone (0.2–5.0 mg/kg i.p., or 0.156–2.5 nmoles into the amygdaloid nucleus), causes memory facilitation of a wide variety of tasks in the rat: inhibitory avoidance (13,37,46), one-way active avoidance (46), two variants of shuttle avoid-ance, classic conditioning in the shuttle-box, classic training-avoidance testing and vice versa in the shuttle-box (20), and habituation of a rearing response to a tone

(20,30). The memory facilitating action of naloxone was independent of the response requirements of the tasks (activity, response suppression), of the presence of pain during the training session (no pain in the habituation task), and, when footshocks were present, of the number of footshocks (20). In all cases, the administration of similarly low doses of morphine or levorphanol had an opposite effect and counteracted the effect of naloxone (13,20,37,46). These findings suggested that endogenous opioid substances may normally be inhibitory modulators of memory consolidation (13,20,30,37,46). In view of the finding that β-endorphin is released during training in the rat brain, β-endorphin appeared as a very likely candidate for such a physiological role (28,35).

Indeed, it was shown shortly thereafter that the posttraining intraperitoneal administration of β-endorphin (0.4–10.0 μg/kg ≅ 55–1,400 ng/rat) causes retrograde amnesia for the same tasks in which naloxone caused retrograde memory facilitation (21,24,35,41), and that its effect is shared by other opioid peptides, such as Met-, Leu-, and des-Tyr-Met-enkephalin (21,23,24,26). The ED_{50} of these substances is very low: ~1.0 μg/kg ≅ 140 ng/rat for β-endorphin (35) and ~0.4 μg/kg ≅ 60 ng/rat for the enkephalins (26). In all cases, the effect of the peptides was antagonized competitively by low doses of naloxone which on their own had no influence on memory (24,26). The pretraining administration of β-endorphin (22) or of Met-Leu-, or des-Tyr-Met-enkephalin (24) also causes amnesia, in this case anterograde amnesia, which is reverted by the posttraining adminstration of naloxone (22). The amnestic effect of the peptides appears to be central, since it can be obtained with doses as low as 5.0 to 25.0 ng/rat given i.c.v. (39). It requires, however, the presence of intact adrenal medullary glands, which suggests again a permissive or cooperative role of the epinephrine secreted by these glands (24).

Since approximately 20% of a systemically injected dose of β-endorphin reaches the brain within 120 min from injection (see references in 33,35), the amnestic ED_{50} of this drug at the brain level may be estimated to be of about 30 ng when it is given systemically (35), and has been shown to be lower than that when given by the i.c.v. route (39). Therefore, since memory is normally not perfect and it can be improved by naloxone, and since the amount of β-endorphin released in the brain is compatible with partially amnestic doses of this substance *(see above)*, it may be concluded that there is a physiological amnestic mechanism mediated by β-endorphin, and possibly by other opioid peptides as well, which prevents memory from being as good as it could be (27,28,32,33,35). In addition, the amnestic effect of electroconvulsive shock might be explained by a massive release of β-endorphin in the brain (9,33).

It should be noted that the amnestic doses of morphine or of the peptides mentioned above are in all cases subanalgesic doses (see 8,24,33), which favors the idea that the primary physiological role of the opioids may be to modulate behavior, rather than to produce analgesia (28,33).

At higher doses, morphine (33), β-endorphin (24,41), and the enkephalins (24) do not cause amnesia. Table 3 shows the effect of three different dose levels of β-endorphin, Met-, Leu-, and des-Tyr-Met-enkephalin on retention of a shuttle avoid-

TABLE 3. *Training-test difference in performance of shuttle avoidance responses over 50 trials in rats receiving either saline or three different dose levels of β-endorphin, Met-, Leu-, and des-Tyr-Met-enkephalin i.p. within 1 min from termination of the training session*

Treatment	Dose (μg/kg)	n	Training-test difference (avoidance responses)
Saline	—	12	14.9 ± 1.9
β-Endorphin	1.0	8	8.5 ± 2.9[a]
β-Endorphin	10.0	8	−0.7 ± 2.9[c]
β-Endorphin	20.0	8	13.3 ± 1.9
Saline	—	9	17.3 ± 1.8
Met-enkephalin	0.8	10	3.0 ± 4.8[b]
Met-enkephalin	10.0	7	−3.7 ± 1.7[c]
Met-enkephalin	20.0	6	17.3 ± 3.5
Leu-enkephalin	0.8	10	3.1 ± 2.0[b]
Leu-enkephalin	10.0	7	−0.6 ± 3.7[c]
Leu-enkephalin	20.0	6	13.7 ± 3.2
Des-Tyr-Met-enkephalin	0.8	10	3.4 ± 5.4[b]
Des-Tyr-Met-enkephalin	10.0	6	−0.7 ± 2.3[c]
Des-Tyr-Met-enkephalin	20.0	6	18.0 ± 1.9

Training session performances not different among groups, range 19.6 to 21.2, f (13,101) = 0.20, $p > 0.2$. Training-test interval, 24 hr.
Data expressed as means ± S.E.M.
[a]Significant difference from saline group in Duncan multiple range test at 0.05 level; [b]same, at 0.01 level; [c]same, at 0.005 level.

ance response (50 tone-footshock trials on training and test session; training-test interval, 1 day; drugs injected intraperitoneally 1 min after training). Note that at the highest dose level (20.0 μg/kg) the four drugs are not amnestic. Therefore, as occurs with many other compounds active on memory and learning, opioids also have a bell-shaped dose–response curve. Motivational or other secondary effects at the higher dose levels may explain this peculiarity (see 33 and preceding sections).

The fact that β-endorphin is released during training raises the question of whether it might not also have an influence on acquisition. Indeed, Met-, Leu- (24,40), and des-Tyr-Met-enkephalin (24) depress acquisition at low doses, an effect that is naloxone-reversible (40); in the shuttle avoidance task, the doses of these substances that depress acquisition are lower than those necessary to cause anterograde amnesia (24). This puts them in a separate category from β-endorphin, which depresses acquisition of the shuttle avoidance and the habituation task only at doses that are no longer amnestic (20 μg/kg, i.p.) (22,24). In fact, there is evidence that the endogenous release of β-endorphin might be necessary for acquisition and that avoidance and habituation may normally be dependent on a state caused by that substance. A sufficiently large dose of naloxone given prior to training in these two tasks (0.8–1.6 mg/kg, i.p.) depresses their acquisition; 2.0 μg/kg of β-endorphin have no effect (which suggests that the amount released endogenously is sufficient for this purpose) (21). When given prior to the test session, in which, as shown above, there is no β-endorphin release (32,35), naloxone has no effect, but

2.0 μg/kg of β-endorphin markedly improve retrieval of these two tasks (21). The result is consonant with previous data by DeWied and his group (8) and by Rigter (53) who had observed that the administration of opioids prior to a test session enhances retrieval of other avoidance behaviors. It is not known whether the effects of opioids on acquisition, consolidation, and retrieval refer to different actions or to different mechanisms, or whether, at least in the case of β-endorphin, they are all reflections of a common basic process (21). At any rate, it is clear that β-endorphin and the enkephalins affect learned behavior at various stages, and that this is independent both of pain perception and of the response requirements of the tasks.

EFFECTS OF OPIOID PEPTIDES ON BRAIN REGIONAL PROTEIN SYNTHESIS

Rats were injected intraperitoneally with 10.0 or 20.0 μg/kg of Met- or Leu-enkephalin or β-endorphin, or with 10.0, 20.0, or 50.0 μg/kg of des-Tyr-Met-enkephalin, and sacrificed 2 hr later by decapitation. Incorporation of $[^{14}C](U)$-leucine to protein was measured in homogenates of brain regions by the methods described in a preceding section. Lower doses and shorter times after injection were found to be ineffective in a pilot study, not shown here. Results are shown in Table 4. They varied with the drug. At the low dose, Leu-enkephalin reduced protein synthesis in all structures, Met-enkephalin reduced it in the rest of the brain and increased it in the caudate nucleus, and des-Tyr-Met-enkephalin reduced it in both caudate nucleus and rest of the brain, whereas β-endorphin caused a slight increase of amygdala protein synthesis. At a dose of 20.0 μg/kg, Leu-enkephalin increased protein labelling in amygdala and caudate nucleus, Met-enkephalin increased it in amygdala, hippocampus, and rest of the brain, and des-Tyr-Met-enkephalin increased protein synthesis in amygdala, caudate, and hippocampus; the effect of the latter on the amygdala was higher at a dose of 50.0 μg/kg, which, however, had no effect on the hippocampus.

Obviously no correlation is possible between these findings and the effect of these same drugs on learning and memory *(see above)*. The reductions of protein labelling obtained with the enkephalins at the lower dose are probably unrelated to the amnestic effect obtained with this same dose (Table 3): first, the protein synthesis effect varied with the drug, whereas the amnestic effect does not; second, much larger reductions of brain protein synthesis obtained with specific inhibitors have no effect on learning or memory (1,10,11); third, β-endorphin causes as much amnesia as the enkephalins at that dose, and it did not decrease brain protein synthesis. In addition, the increases of protein labelling obtained in one or other structure with different doses of the various compounds occurred at an amnestic dose in the case of β-endorphin (10.0 μg/kg), and at doses that are no longer amnestic in the case of the other compounds (see Table 3).

Thus, opioid peptides affect brain synthesis; the regions affected are different for each compound, and the nature of the effect is also different. These effects may

TABLE 4. Effect of Leu-, Met-, des-Tyr-Met-enkephalin, and β-endorphin on the incorporation of [¹⁴C]leucine to protein in homogenates of rat brain structures

Treatment	Dose (μg/kg)	Protein labelling (1) in			
		Amygdala	Caudate	Hippocampus	Rest of brain
Saline	—	39 ± 2 (26)	33 ± 1 (28)	34 ± 2 (33)	42 ± 2 (32)
Leu-enkephalin	10.0	32 ± 4[a] (12)	28 ± 2[b] (12)	22 ± 1[b] (12)	32 ± 4[c] (13)
Leu-enkephalin	20.0	68 ± 14[c] (12)	42 ± 5[c] (11)	38 ± 6 (12)	42 ± 5 (11)
Met-enkephalin	10.0	37 ± 3 (11)	38 ± 3[b] (12)	29 ± 3 (12)	29 ± 2[c] (12)
Met-enkephalin	20.0	82 ± 11[c] (16)	35 ± 2 (12)	45 ± 5[a] (16)	49 ± 6[a] (14)
Des-Tyr-Met-enkephalin	10.0	35 ± 3 (13)	28 ± 2[b] (12)	30 ± 3 (12)	35 ± 4[a] (11)
Des-Tyr-Met-enkephalin	20.0	47 ± 7[a] (12)	42 ± 3[c] (13)	44 ± 4[a] (11)	45 ± 3 (11)
Des-Tyr-Met-enkephalin	50.0	54 ± 7[c] (15)	40 ± 3[b] (14)	36 ± 4 (14)	45 ± 4 (14)
Des-Tyr-Met-endorphin	10.0	48 ± 14[a] (10)	31 ± 4 (10)	33 ± 7 (10)	40 ± 7 (11)
Des-Tyr-Met-endorphin	20.0	42 ± 9 (10)	32 ± 7 (10)	28 ± 4 (9)	41 ± 9 (10)

Injections were i.p. and the animals were sacrificed 2 hr later.
Data expressed as means ± S.E.M. (1). See Tables I and 2 for units of measure.
[a]Significant difference from saline group in Ducan multiple range test at 0.05 level; [b]same, at 0.01 level; [c]same, at 0.005 level.

be regarded as neuropharmacological actions which are separate from, and unrelated to, the known influences of these compounds on learning and memory consolidation.

SUMMARY AND CONCLUSIONS

Hypersecretion of epinephrine by the adrenal medulla and β-endorphin release in the brain are two consequences of training triggered by nonassociative events that occur during training. Both have important influences on learning and memory consolidation. Peripheral epinephrine administration affects learning and memory, and the influence of various drugs and other agents on memory requires the presence of intact adrenal medullary glands. β-Endorphin appears to be the mediator of a physiological amnesic mechanism, and, perhaps together with other opioid peptides, is an important regulator of acquisition and retrieval.

In addition, the adrenal medulla is necessary for the occurrence of a late post-training peak of protein synthesis in the brain and liver, and β-endorphin and other opioids have diverse effects on brain protein synthesis. However, these biochemical effects appear to be entirely unrelated to the influence of peripheral epinephrine and central β-endorphin on learning and memory.

These findings point to the need of distinguishing between neurochemical correlates and concomitants of learning and memory, and to the fact that neurochemical consequences of training may be very prominent but not necessarily very important for acquisition and retention (11,33).

ACKNOWLEDGMENTS

This work was supported by FAPERGS, PROPESP-UFRGS, PROPLAN-UFRGS and CNPq, Brasil. The technical assistance of Susana V. Hampe and Paulo P. Branco, Jr. in the protein labelling experiments is gratefully acknowledged.

REFERENCES

1. Agranoff, B. W., Burrell, H. R., Dokas, L. A., and Springer, A. D. (1978): Progress in biochemical approaches to learning and memory. In: *Psychopharmacology: A Generation of Progress*, edited by M. A. Lipton, A. DiMascio, and K. F. Killam, pp. 623–636. Raven Press, New York.
2. Baust, W., Niemczyk, H., and Vieth, J. (1963): The action of blood pressure on the ascending reticular activating system with special reference to adrenaline-induced EEG arousal. *Electroencephalogr. Clin. Neurophysiol.*, 15:63–72.
3. Beaumont, A., and Hughes, J. (1979): Biology of opioid peptides. *Annu. Rev. Pharmacol. Toxicol.*, 19:245–267.
4. Bohus, B., *unpublished material*.
5. Cannon, W. B. (1929): *Bodily Changes in Pain, Hunger, Fear and Rage*. Appleton-Century-Crofts, New York.
6. Carrasco, M. A., Dias, R. D., Perry, M. L., and Izquierdo, I. (1982): Effect of training and of electroconvulsive shock on brain Met-enkephalin levels. *Behav. Neural Biol.*, 34:1–4.
7. Denti, A., McGaugh, J. L., Landfield, P. W., and Shinkman, P. (1970): Effects of post-trial electrical stimulation of the mesencephalic reticular formation on avoidance learning in rats. *Physiol. Behav.*, 5:659–662.
8. DeWied, D., Bohus, B., van Ree, J. M., and Urban, I. (1978): Behavioral and electrophysiological effects of peptides related to lipotropin (β-LPH). *J. Pharmacol. Exp. Ther.*, 204:570–580.
9. Dias, R. D., Perry, M. L. S., Carrasco, M. A., and Izquierdo, I. (1981): Effect of electroconvulsive shock on β-endorphin immunoreactivity of rat brain, pituitary gland, and plasma. *Behav. Neural Biol.*, 33 *(in press)*.
10. Dunn, A. J. (1976): Biochemical correlates of training experiences: A discussion of the evidence. In: *Neural Mechanisms of Learning and Memory*, edited by M. R. Rosenzweig and E. L. Bennett, pp. 311–320. MIT Press, Cambridge (Mass.).
11. Dunn, A. J. (1980): Neurochemistry of learning and memory: An evaluation of recent data. *Annu. Rev. Psychol.*, 31:343–390.
12. Dunn, A. J., and Rees, H. D. (1977): Brain RNA and protein synthesis during training: The interpretation of changes of precursor incorporation. In: *Neurobiology of Sleep and Memory*, edited by R. R. Drucker-Colín and J. L. McGaugh, pp. 33–54. Academic Press, New York.
13. Gallagher, M., and Kapp, B. S. (1978): Opiate administration into the amygdala: Effects on memory processes. *Life Sci.*, 23:1973–1978.
14. Gispen, W. H., DeWied, D., Schotman, P., and Jansz, H. S. (1970): Effects of hypophysectomy on RNA metabolism in rat brain stem. *J. Neurochem.*, 17:751–761.
15. Gispen, W. H., and Schotman, P. (1970): Effect of hypophysectomy and conditioned avoidance behavior on macromolecule metabolism in the brain stem of the rat. *Prog. Brain Res.*, 32:236–244.
16. Gold, P. E., and McCarty, R. (1981): Plasma catecholamines: Changes after footshock and seizure-producing frontal cortex stimulation. *Behav. Neural Biol.*, 31:247–260.
17. Gold, P. E., and McGaugh, J. L. (1975): A single-trace, two-process view of memory storage processes. In: *Short-term Memory*, edited by D. and J. A. Deutsch, pp. 355–378. Academic Press, New York.
18. Gold, P. E., and van Buskirk, R. (1976): Effect of posttrial hormone injections on memory processes. *Hormones Behav.*, 7:509–517.

19. Gold, P. E., and van Buskirk, R. (1978): Post-training brain norepinephrine concentrations: Correlation with retention performance of avoidance training and with peripheral epinephrine modulation of memory processing. *Behav. Biol.*, 23:509–520.
20. Izquierdo, I. (1979): Effect of naloxone and morphine on various forms of memory in the rat: Possible role of endogenous opiate mechanisms in memory consolidation. *Psychopharmacology*, 66:199–203.
21. Izquierdo, I. (1980): Effect of β-endorphin and naloxone on acquisition, memory and retrieval of shuttle avoidance and habituation learning in rats. *Psychopharmacology*, 69:111–115.
22. Izquierdo, I. (1980): Effects of a low and a high dose of β-endorphin on acquisition and retention in the rat. *Behav. Neural Biol.*, 30:460–464.
23. Izquierdo, I., Beamish, D. G., and Anisman, H. (1979): Effect of an inhibitor of dopamine-beta-hydroxylase on the acquisition and retention of four different avoidance tasks in mice. *Psychopharmacology*, 63:173–178.
24. Izquierdo, I., Carrasco, M. A., Dias, R. D., Perry, M. L. S., Netto, C. A., and Souza, D. O. (1982): Effect of opioid peptides on learning and memory: Single or dual effect? In: *Pharmacology of Learning and Memory*, edited by S. Saito and J. L. McGaugh. Excerpta Medica, Amsterdam.
25. Izquierdo, I., and Cavalheiro, E. A. (1976): Three main factors in rat shuttle behavior: Their pharmacology and sequential entry in operation during a two-way avoidance session. *Psychopharmacology*, 49:145–157.
26. Izquierdo, I., and Dias, R. D. (1981): Retrograde amnesia caused by Met-, Leu- and des-Tyr-Met-enkephalin in the rat and its reversal by naloxone. *Neurosci. Lett.*, 22:189–193.
27. Izquierdo, I., Dias, D. O., Perry, M. L., Souza, D. O., Elisabetsky, E., and Carrasco, M. A. (1981): A physiological amnesic mechanism mediated by endogenous opioid peptides and its possible role in learning. In: *International Neurobiological Symposium on Learning and Memory*, edited by H. Matthies, pp. 89–111. Raven Press, New York.
28. Izquierdo, I., Dias, R. D., Souza, D. O., Carrasco, M. A., Elisabetsky, E., and Perry, M. L. (1980): The role of opioid peptides in memory and learning. *Behav. Brain Res.*, 1:451–468.
29. Izquierdo, I., and Elisabetsky, E. (1979): Physiological and pharmacological dissection of the main factors in the acquisition and retention of shuttle behaviour. In: *Brain Mechanisms in Memory and Learning: From the Single Neuron to Man*, edited by M. A. B. Brazier, pp. 227–248. Raven Press, New York.
30. Izquierdo, I., and Graudenz, M. (1980): Memory facilitation by naloxone is due to release of dopaminergic and beta-adrenergic systems from tonic inhibition. *Psychopharmacology*, 67:265–268.
31. Izquierdo, I., Paiva, A. C. M., and Elisabetsky, E. (1980): Post-training intraperitoneal administration of Leu-enkephalin and Beta-endorphin causes retrograde amnesia for two different tasks in rats. *Behav. Neural Biol.*, 28:246–250.
32. Izquierdo, I., Perry, M. L. S., Dias, R. D., Orsingher, O. A., and Carrasco, M. A. (1981): Effect of training and testing rats in two different behavioral paradigms on brain beta-endorphin immunoreactivity. *Arq. Biol. Tecnol.*, 24:327–331.
33. Izquierdo, I., Perry, M. L., Dias, R. D., Souza, D. O., Elisabetsky, E., Carrasco, M. A., Orsingher, O. A., and Netto, C. A. (1981): Endogenous opioids, memory modulation and state-dependency. In: *Endogenous Peptides and Learning and Memory Processes*, edited by J. L. Martinez, Jr., R. A. Jensen, R. B. Messing, H. Rigter, and J. L. McGaugh, pp. 269–290. Academic Press, San Diego.
34. Izquierdo, I., Salzano, F., and Thomé, F. (1976): The effect of adrenaline, tyramine and guanethidine on one-way step-up avoidance. *Acta Physiol. Latin Am.*, 26:218–219.
35. Izquierdo, I., Souza, D. O., Carrasco, M. A., Dias, R. D., Perry, M. L., Eisinger, S., and Vendite, D. A. (1980): Beta-endorphin causes retrograde amnesia and is released from the rat brain by various forms of training and stimulation. *Psychopharmacology*, 70:173–177.
36. Izquierdo, I., and Thaddeu, R. C. (1975): The effect of adrenaline, tyramine and guanethidine on two-way avoidance conditioning and pseudoconditioning. *Psychopharmacologia*, 43:85–87.
37. Jensen, R. A., Martinez, J. L., Jr., Messing, R. B., Spiehler, V., Vasquez, B. J., Soumireu-Mourat, B., Liang, K. C., and McGaugh, J. L. (1978): Morphine and naloxone alter memory in the rat. *Neurosci. Soc. Abstr.*, 4:260.
38. Jork, R., and Matthies, H. (1982): *In vitro* protein synthesis in hippocampus after training. In: *International Neurobiological Symposium on Learning and Memory*, edited by H. Matthies. Raven Press, New York.

39. Lucion, A. B., Rosito, G., Sapper, D., Palmini, A. L., and Izquierdo, I. (1982): Intracerebro-ventricular administration of nanogram amounts of β-endorphin and Met-ekephalin causes retrograde amnesia in rats. *Behav. Brain Res.*, 4:111–115.
40. Martinez, J. L., Jr., and Rigter, H. (1980): Endorphins alter acquisition and consolidation of an inhibitory avoidance response in rats. *Neurosci. Lett.*, 19:197–201.
41. Martinez, J. L., Jr., Rigter, H., and van der Gugten, J. (1981): Enkephalin effects on avoidance conditioning are dependent on the adrenal glands. In: *Advances in Physiological Sciences, Vol. 13. Endocrinology, Neuroendocrinology, Neruopeptides-I*, edited by E. Stark, G. B. Makara, Zs. Acs, and E. Endröczi, pp. 273–277. Pergamon Press and Akadémiai Kiadó, Budapest.
42. Matthies, H. (1979): Biochemical, electrophysiological and morphological correlates of brightness discrimination in rats. In: *Brain Mechanisms in Memory and Learning: From the Single Neuron to Man*, edited by M. A. B. Brazier, pp. 197–215. Raven Press, New York.
43. McCarty, R., and Kopin, I. J. (1979): Stress-induced alterations in plasma catecholamines and behavior in rats: Effects of chlorisondamine and bretylium. *Behav. Neural Biol.*, 27:249–265.
44. McGaugh, J. L., Martinez, J. L., Jr., Liang, K. C., Brewton, C., Jensen, R. A., Vasquez, B. J., Messing, R. B., and Ishikawa, K. (1982): Learning modulating hormones. In: *Pharmacology of Learning and Memory*, edited by S. Saito and J. L. McGaugh. Excerpta Medica, Amsterdam.
45. Marlo, A. B., and Izquierdo, I. (1967): The effect of catecholamines on learning. *Med. Pharmacol. Exp.*, 16:343–349.
46. Messing, R. B., Jensen, R. A., Martinez, J. L., Jr., Spiehler, V. R., Vasquez, B. J., Soumireu-Mourat, B., Liang, K. C., and McGaugh, J. L. (1979): Naloxone enhancement of memory. *Behav. Neural. Biol.*, 27:266–275.
47. Orsingher, O. A., and Fulginiti, S. (1971): Effects of α-methyltyrosine and adrenergic blocking agents on the facilitating action of amphetamine and nicotine on learning in rats. *Psychopharmacologia*, 19:231–240.
48. Orsingher, O. A., and Fulginiti, S. (1973): Influence of peripheral mechanisms on the facilitatory learning action of amphetamine and nicotine in rats. *Pharmacology*, 9:138–144.
49. Peters, D. A. V., Anisman, H., and Pappas, B. A. (1978): Monoamines and aversively motivated behaviors. In: *Psychopharmacology of Aversively Motivated Behaviors*, edited by H. Anisman and G. Bignami, pp. 257–343. Plenum Press, New York.
50. Rachid, C., de Souza, A. S., and Izquierdo, I. (1977): Effect of pre- and post-trial tyramine and guanethidine injections on an appetitive task in rats. *Behav. Biol.*, 21:294–299.
51. Reading, H. W. (1972): Effects of some adrenocorticotrophin analogues on protein synthesis in brain. *Biochem. J.*, 127:12P.
52. Rees, H. D., Brogan, L. L., Entingh, D. J., Dunn, A., Shinkman, P. G., DamstraEntingh, T., Wilson, J. E., and Glassman, E. (1974): Effect of sensory stimulation on the uptake and incorporation of radioactive lysine into protein of mouse brain and liver. *Brain Res.*, 68:143–156.
53. Rigter, H. (1978): Attenuation of amnesia in rats by systemically administered enkephalins. *Science*, 200:83–85.
54. Rossier, J., French, E. D., Rivier, C., Ling, N., Guillemin, R., and Bloom, F. (1977): Foot shock induced stress increases β-endorphin levels in blood but not brain. *Nature*, 270:618–620.
55. Schütz, R. A., and Izquierdo, I. (1979): Effect of brain lesions on rat shuttle behavior in four different tests. *Physiol. Behav.*, 23:97–105.
56. Souza, D. O. (1980): Estudo Neuroquímico do Aprendizado Aversivo em Ratos. Doctor's Thesis, Universidade Federal do Rio de Janeiro.
57. Souza, D. O., Elisabetsky, E., Dias R. D., and Izquierdo, I. (1979): Neurochemical effects of aversive learning in rats. *Neurosci. Soc. Abstracts*, 5:323.
58. Souza, D. O., Elisabetsky, E., and Izquierdo, I. (1980): Effect of various forms of training and stimulation on the incorporation of ^{32}P into nuclear phosphoproteins of the rat brain. *Pharmacol. Biochem. Behav.*, 12:481–485.
59. Teledgy, G., and Kovács, G. L. (1979): Role of monoamines in mediating the action of hormones in learning and memory. In: *Brain Mechanisms in Memory and Learning: From the Single Neuron to Man*, edited by M. A. B. Brazier, pp. 249–268. Raven Press, New York.
60. Vendite, D. A. (1981): Efeitos neuroquímicos do treinamento: papel da medula adrenal. Master's Thesis, Universidade Federal do Rio Grande do Sul.
61. Weil-Malherbe, H., Whitby, L. G., and Axelrod, J. (1961): The uptake of circulating [^{3}H]norepinephrine by the pituitary gland and various areas of the brain. *J. Neurochem.*, 8:55–64.

62. Yang, H.-Y. T., Hong, J. S., Fratta, W., and Costa, E. (1978): Rat brain enkephalins: Distribution and biosynthesis. In: *Advances in Biochemical Pharmacology. Vol. 18. The Endorphins*, edited by E. Costa and M. Trabucchi, pp. 149–159. Raven Press, New York.
63. Zornetzer, S. F. (1978): Neurotransmitter modulation and memory: A new neuropharmacological phrenology? In: *Psychopharmacology: A Generation of Progress*, edited by M. A. Lipton, A. DiMascio and K. F. Killam, pp. 637–649. Raven Press, New York.

Neural Transmission, Learning and Memory,
edited by R. Caputto and C. Ajmone Marsan.
Raven Press, New York © 1983.

Neurobiology of Central Monoamine Neurotransmission: Functional Neuroanatomy and Noradrenaline and 5-Hydroxytryptamine Involvement in Learning and Memory

*K. Fuxe, †L. F. Agnati, ‡S.-O. Ögren, *K. Andersson, and †F. Benfenati

*Department of Histology, Karolinska Institutet, Stockholm, Sweden;
†Department of Human Physiology, University of Modena, Modena, Italy;
and ‡Astra Pharmaceuticals, Södertälje, Sweden

In the exact science of physics the importance of mathematics is universally accepted, but in the "softer" sciences of biology and medicine the value and indeed the feasibility of a mathematical treatment are widely and frequently questioned (10). It should be admitted that in these fields mathematics does not allow to reach, through formal deductions, "new" statements as it does, e.g., in theoretical physics. However, it can be used to describe in an exact, i.e., a nonambiguous, way biological structures. In particular, stereology and morphometry enable us to describe and then to demonstrate changes in cell populations and tissues that would otherwise have escaped our detection. By stereology it is possible to obtain three-dimensional information on structures from two-dimensional sections of the same structures. Morphometry can be defined as the commensurations of structures. Stereology, instead, is the rigorous extrapolation from the two- to the three-dimensional space (24).

These techniques have already been applied to the nervous system both at the structural as well as at the ultrastructural level (23,39). However, to date no application of morphometry has been carried out on transmitter-identified neurons. In the present chapter, some new morphometric approaches to this field will be presented as well as some functional correlates of this investigation and the involvement of noradrenaline (NA) and serotonin (5-hydroxytryptamine, 5-HT) neurotransmission in learning and memory. Finally, a heuristic hypothesis will be presented that arises from neuroanatomical findings and was already "in nuce" in the work of Cajal.

CHARACTERIZATION OF CELL GROUPS OF TRANSMITTER-IDENTIFIED NEURONS

The mapping of the different types of monoamine-identified cell groups in the rat brain has so far been based on subjective evaluation of various neuroanatomists. For example, the early work of the Swedish groups described the NA-containing cell groups A1–A7, the dopamine (DA)-identified cell groups A8–A14, the 5-HT-identified cell groups B1–B9, and the adrenaline-identified cell groups C1–C2 (19). Already in 1974, Fuxe and Jonsson (20) suggested the existence of subgroups within, e.g., the B7 cell group. Recently a more objective criterion has been developed to assess not only when a cluster of transmitter-identified cells forms a cell group, but also when it is possible to detect within this group subgroups. This procedure can be exemplified with the B7 cells visualized by means of indirect immunofluorescence methodology (40,41). The procedure consists of five steps (4,7):

(a) Coronal sections of the region under study are processed for immunocytochemical visualization of 5-HT-positive cells. From these sections micrographs are taken and photomontages are prepared (Fig. 1).

(b) A Cartesian representation of these micrographs is obtained. In this case the midline has been considered as the x-axis. The zero point of the x-axis has been placed in the intersection between the midline and the ventral border of the aqueductus Sylvii. The y-axis has been defined as the axis perpendicular to the midline and crossing the zero point. In this way the localization of each 5-HT nerve cell body can be determined by the coordinates obtained with these two axes (Fig. 2); the fluorescence picture of this representation is not shown.

(c) The density of nerve cell body distribution is obtained by means of considering squares that cover the Cartesian plane of Fig. 2. These squares have a side that is 10 times the mean nerve cell body diameter. The number of nerve cell bodies present in each of these squares is then counted. In this way a complete picture of the density distribution of the nerve cell bodies in the area under study is obtained. To recognize 5-HT cell clusters we have pooled (thicker marking in Fig. 3) three types of squares:

(1) squares with at least two nerve cells;

(2) squares with only one nerve cell but in continuity with at least one marked square;

(3) squares with no nerve cells but with the four sides in contact with marked squares.

By means of this procedure two big clusters can be demonstrated, which clearly correspond to the 5-HT nerve cell groups B7 and B8 + B9 of Dahlström and Fuxe, 1964 (13).

(d) It is now possible to study whether B7 can be, at this level, subdivided into at least two subgroups. For this purpose the "frequency polygon approach" developed by us in a previous theoretical paper has been used (7). Thus, two frequency polygons have been considered: one with class marks (distances from the zero point)

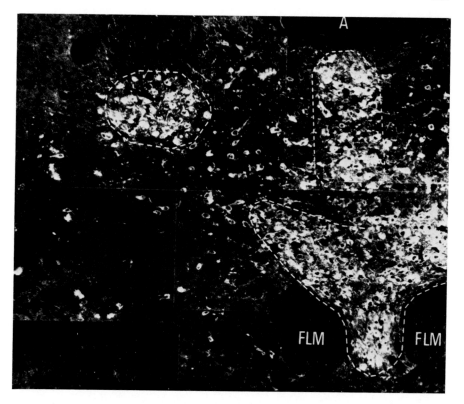

FIG. 1. Coronal section of the midbrain at the level A 200 according to König and Klippel (25a). The section has been stained by means of the indirect immunofluorescence technique using antibodies against 5-HT. ×140. A, aqueductus Sylvii; FLM, fasciculus longitudinalis medialis. The areas surrounded by *dashed lines* represent the three subgroups of group B7 as described by Fuxe and Jonsson (20).

along the x-axis and the other one with class marks along the y-axis (Fig. 4). The class interval is still equal to 10 times the mean cell body diameter. The criterion previously introduced to evaluate the frequency polygons is illustrated in Fig. 5. This criterion is based on the distance between the two modal values along the axis where the class marks are reported and on the ratio between the two modal values. As is seen in Fig. 4 the value that quantitates the degree of bimodality is equal to 0.9 for the polygon with the class marks along the midline, and it is equal to 0.4 for the other one. Thus, there exist at least two subgroups of 5-HT nerve cells within B7, which can be recognized mainly via inspecting B7 in a dorso-ventral direction.

(e) Finally, the problem of obtaining an objective criterion to assess whether a cluster of transmitter-identified nerve cells form a cell group or only scattered cells must be considered. One important parameter is obviously the mean free distance among cells. This parameter represents the uninterrupted intercell distance through the nervous tissue averaged between all the possible pairs of transmitter-identified

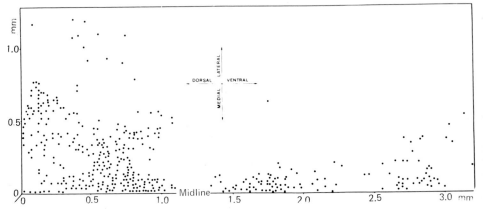

FIG. 2. Cartesian representation of 5-HT cell body distribution in a mesencephalic coronal section at the level A 160 according to König and Klippel (the morphological picture is not shown). The origin of the axes is placed in the ventral border of the aqueductus Sylvii in the midline. On the axes the true distances from the origin (in millimeters) are reported (4).

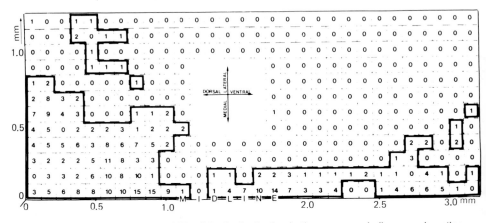

FIG. 3. The density of the 5-HT cell body distribution in the mesencephalic coronal section represented in Fig. 2 has been evaluated by counting the number of cell bodies falling within the squares of 107 μm by side. Marks have been made in those squares containing at least two cells. The squares with one cell have been marked only if they were continuous with at least one nonempty square. Squares with no 5-HT cell bodies have been marked only when they were completely bordered by nonempty squares. In this way two main cell assemblies can be seen, which correspond to the B7 and B8 + B9 groups. A much smaller one (Bx?) is seen in the dorsomedial area (4).

nerve cells. It is obvious that by increasing this distance the transmitter-identified cell group is converted into scattered transmitter-identified nerve cells. Thus, we have suggested that a cluster of transmitter-identified nerve cell bodies should be considered as a cell group when, within a 10 μm thick section, the mean free distance among cells is less than 15 times the mean cell diameter and when the number of transmitter-identified nerve cells is above 10. Thus, this procedure in particular allows us to detect a *"topological hetereogeneity"* within a cell group. However, a *"functional hetereogeneity"* and a *"biochemical hetereogeneity"* within

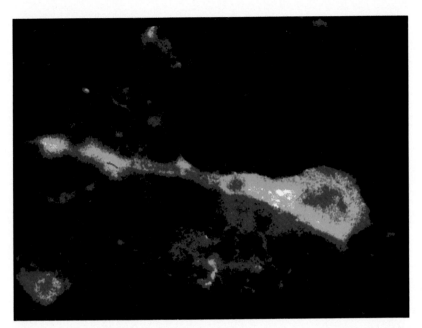

FIG. 6. Intensity evaluation of DA fluorescence in a DA nerve cell of the substantia nigra, using high-contrast Kodalith plates (1,2). Red, yellow, and white colours represent low, medium, and high intensity, respectively. ×300.

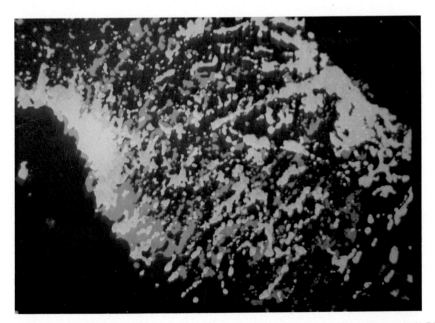

FIG. 9. The distribution pattern in adjacent sections of tyrosine hydroxylase (TH) and LH-RH (luteinizing hormone-releasing hormone) immunoreactive nerve terminals in the lateral palisade zone of the rat median eminence. Terminals with blue colour represent TH immunoreactive terminals and terminals with yellow colour represent LH-RH immunoreactive terminals. White colour represents region of overlapping LH-RH and TH immunoreactive nerve terminals. ×300.

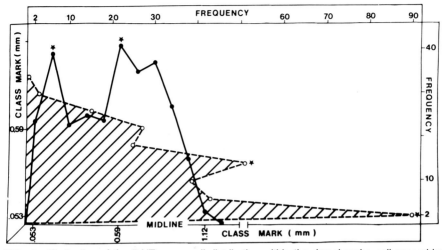

FIG. 4. Evaluation of the 5-HT nerve cell distribution within the dorsal raphe cell assembly (B7) delimited in Fig. 3. This evaluation has been carried out by means of the frequency polygon analysis (4). On the x-axis class marks are reported along the midline. For each of these classes (class interval = 107 μm) the number of cells (frequency) falling in it has been plotted (axis on the right). On the y-axis class marks are reported along the axis perpendicular to the midline (class interval = 107 μm). For each of these classes the number of cells (frequency) falling in it has been plotted (axis on the top of the plot). According to the criterion suggested (4), the population plotted in the polygon which has the class marks along the midline is clearly bimodal (degree of bimodality = 0.9). This is true also for the polygon plotted with its class marks along the y-axis (degree of bimodality = 0.4). *Asterisks* mark the values accepted as modal values of different subpopulations present in the cell assembly under study.

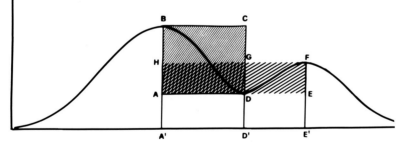

FIG. 5. Schematic representation of the criterion on which the existence of a bimodality in a frequency polygon is assessed. On the x-axis the class marks are reported; the unity of measurement is a unit of length (e.g., mm). On the y-axis the frequencies, i.e., the number of cell bodies that fall within each class, are reported. For further details, see text (7).

cell groups of transmitter-identified neurons have also been demonstrated. It is our opinion that a new important field in neuroanatomy will be the study of how these different types of hetereogeneities correlate with each other.

Functional hetereogeneity has been detected at the level of A10 group by means of a densitometric approach based on an elaboration of high-contrast Kodalith plates (1) (Fig. 6), using the Falck-Hillarp visualization of DA cell bodies in the area

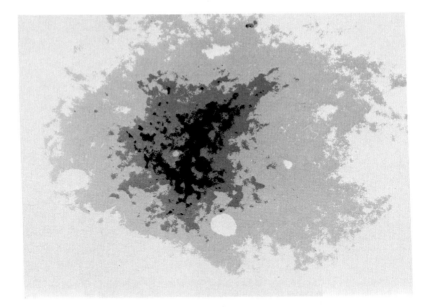

FIG. 7. Intensity evaluation of DA fluorescence in an island of DA nerve terminals of the nuc. caudatus of the rat (1,2). The black tone represents the highest intensity and the weak gray tone the lowest intensity. × 600.

surrounding the nucleus interpeduncularis. Thus, the A10 subgroup of small-sized DA cell bodies located in the midline has a very high DA turnover. On the basis of such data we have suggested that the A10 mesolimbic system can be subdivided into several subgroups (2) the midline one (nuc. interfascicularis) having a very high DA turnover in their cell bodies. Hökfelt et al. (22) have shown that there probably exists a biochemical hetereogenity within a monoamine-identified cell group. Some monoamine neurons store more than one putative transmitter. Thus, e.g., within the A10–A9 cell groups they have discovered neurons which also store cholecystokinin (CCK)-like material. It is apparent that these heterogeneities also exist at the nerve terminals. Studies with the Falck-Hillarp procedure indicated that hetereogenity exists in the DA terminals (16). Thus, dotted (or islandic) types of DA terminals can be distinguished from diffuse types of DA terminals (Fig. 7). These terminals have different DA turnover rates, suggesting a possible different functional role of these two terminal systems. Turnover studies with the DA receptor agonist, the ergolene derivative, PTR 17402, have shown that it is possible to reduce DA turnover preferentially in the dotted type of DA terminals (17). It is notable that the dotted but not the diffuse types of DA terminals may contain cholecystokinin (CCK)-like immunoreactivity (22). Functional and biochemical hetereogeneity can be a very important feature, since the complexity of the local circuit organization can be increased and the same neurotransmitter can acquire different functional roles in the local circuit. The biochemical heterogeneity may be especially relevant, since the same terminal may change its functional characteristics according to the relative release of transmitter and cotransmitter in the local circuit system.

The development of neuroanatomical methods to study the transmitter-identified terminal in the context of the local circuit is timely. An important step in this direction is the recent development by Schipper (37) of a scanning microfluorimetric method that allows determination of NA in various segments of the sympathetic nerve fibres in the rat iris.

Our group has also developed a method to study the morphofunctional role of the local circuit organization. This method is schematically illustrated in Fig. 8 (5). In short, fluorescence intensity measurements (or for PAP technique different transmittances through the section) are measured for circular fields of increasing diameters. If we consider a plot with the log of radius on the *x*-axis *(r)* and the log of fluorescence intensities *(I)* on the *y*-axis, and if we assume an even distribution of the transmitter-identified terminals in the area under study, a straight line should be obtained.

In fact intensity *(I)* is proportional to the area in the selected circular field *(A)*. Thus, $I = K' \cdot A$ and since $A = \tau r^2$ it is possible to put $K = \tau \cdot K'$ as a new constant of proportionality and then $I = K \cdot r^2$. From this expression we can get $\log I = \log K + 2 \log r$, which is the expression of a straight line in a log–log plot, that is in a plot, where $X = \log r$ and $Y = \log I$. The theoretical value of the slope of this line is equal to 2. It should be noted that the fluorescence intensity yields a good approximation of terminal transmitter density. Now if by changing

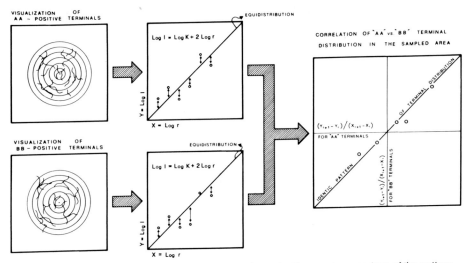

FIG. 8. Schematic illustration of the quantitative determinations and comparison of the pattern of distribution of two types of transmitter-identified nerve terminal networks in the same area of the same or adjacent section. The degree of equidistribution is evaluated from the scattering of the points around the equidistribution line. The evaluation of these points for "AA" and "BB" positive nerve terminals is shown in this example to be highly significant since an almost identical distribution pattern is obtained (5).

the radius from a certain value to a subsequent value a densely innervated area falls within the wider circular field, the fluorescence intensity will pass from Y_0 to Y_1 $>> Y_0$. Further, $(Y_1 - Y_0)/(X_1 - X_0) > 2$, that is we will observe a slope value higher than the theoretical value of equidistribution. Hence, it is possible to map the topography of the density of innervation of transmitter-identified terminals of a certain area. This procedure can be repeated on the same section using Tramu's elution technique (44), or on the subsequent section with another type of transmitter-identified terminal. It is therefore possible to test the correlation between these two patterns of innervation. If there is a highly significant correlation, the two terminal systems probably interact in this particular area and take part in the organization of the same local circuits. This method has been used in the lateral palisade zone (LPZ) level of the median eminence. Tyrosine hydroxylase (TH)-positive terminals (TH can be used as marker of DA) and luteinizing hormone-releasing hormone (LH-RH)-positive terminals were visualized to determine whether an axo–axonic interaction between these systems could be the morphological counterpart of the dopaminergic control of LH-RH release into the hypophyseal portal vessels. The visual inspection of the two systems (Fig. 9) suggested such a possibility. There was a significant ($p < 0.01$) correlation between the distribution of the TH- and LH-RH-positive terminals in the LPZ (Fig. 10). A more extensive use of these new techniques for the study of local circuits can be a key to understanding high-level integrative functions in the CNS. In fact, until now local circuits have not been explored by means of morphofunctional analysis. The interest in the local circuit is based on indirect findings that suggest that integrative functions may be linked to the local circuit organization (35,38). Already Cajal stated that "the functional superiority of the human brain is intimately linked up with the prodigious abundance and unaccustomed wealth of forms of the so called neurons with short axons." Local circuits are today defined as a set of neuronal parts (synaptic knobs, somas, and dendrites) that under given conditions function as an independent integrative unit. It now remains for the functional role of the local circuits to be defined in operative terms. In this context also heuristic hypotheses are important, even if they later on may be disproved. We have recently put forward a new hypothesis on the functional role of local circuit that takes into account not only electrical events (which have been preferentially considered up till now) but also biochemical events and suggests a possible complementarity among these two sets of phenomena. Further, if it is true that local circuits can operate as independent functional units, then the old view of the neuron theory should be revised. The neuron could have its trophic center at soma level, but the functional unit would be not the *neuron* but the *local circuit*. Thus, on functional grounds we may therefore move back again from the neuron theory to the reticular theory, where we could recognize two types of critical nodes:

(a) the integrative nodes, which are represented by the local circuits
(b) the trophic nodes, which are represented by the somas.

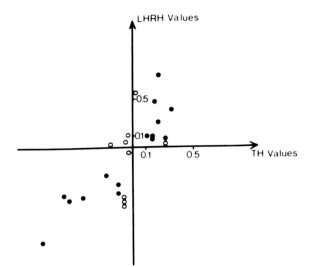

FIG. 10. Correlation between patterns of LH-RH versus TH fluorescence distribution in corresponding areas of LPZ of the median eminence. LH-RH and TH ($\Delta Y/\Delta X - b$) values obtained from corresponding regions for the same radius increase have been reported as y and x coordinates, respectively. The *open symbols* represent points for which either LH-RH ($\Delta Y/\Delta X - b$) value or TH ($\Delta Y/\Delta X - b$) value falls out of the 50% confidence limits for the respective slope, whereas the *closed symbols* represent points for which both LH-RH ($\Delta Y/\Delta X - b$) value and TH ($\Delta Y/\Delta X - b$) value fall within the 50% confidence limits for the respective slopes. Pearson's correlation coefficient was found to be highly significant when considering all the points ($r = 0.721; p << 0.01; df = 22$) and also when considering only the points marked by *closed symbols* ($r = 0.824; p << 0.01; df = 13$) (5).

POSSIBLE ROLE OF LOCAL CIRCUITS IN THE MEMORY TRACE FORMATION

On the Role of Central NA Neurons in Learning

It was early suggested by Kety (25) and by Crow (12) that central NA neurotransmission associated with reinforcement can produce persistent changes in synaptic conductivity. It could also be demonstrated that electrolytic lesion of locus coeruleus produced a marked reduction in the acquisition of a runway response for food reward (8). On the other hand, a number of recent investigations have failed to support the involvement of central NA neurons in learning. Thus, 6-hydroxydopamine (6-OHDA)-induced degenerations of the coeruleocortical NA systems have failed to counteract the acquisition of positively or negatively reinforced tasks (27,32). By the use of a new NA neurotoxin [N-(2-chloroethyl)-N-ethyl-2-bromobenzylamine] (DSP4), however, it has been possible to obtain evidence for the role of the locus coeruleus NA system in aversive learning processes (31). Thus, this neurotoxin produces a marked and selective degeneration of the locus coeruleus NA system and at the same time impairs one- and two-way avoidance acquisition in rats (Fig. 11). The specificity of the actions is demonstrated by the fact that the NA uptake blocking agent, desipramine, counteracts both the neurochemical and the behavioural effects of the neurotoxin. The major difference between the DSP4- and the 6-OHDA-induced lesions quoted above is that DSP4 treatment results in a degeneration of all the branches of the locus coeruleus NA cells whereas the intracerebral injections of 6-OHDA lesion the ascending branches. Thus, it seems as if the locus coeruleus NA system in its entire extent is involved in regulation of learning processes (31) and it is possible that the collateral innervation by the locus coeruleus of the lower brainstem may play a critical role by, e.g., being part of a filter mechanism only allowing relevant stimuli to reach the cortical hemispheres where higher brain functions are located.

On the Role of the Pituitary Adrenal Axis in Learning and Its Interaction with Central NA Neurons

It is known that the pituitary adrenal axis plays an important role in aversive learning and memory processes (45). In view of the fact that adrenalectomy and treatment with the glycocorticoids could produce changes in NA turnover in large parts of the brain (18), we early investigated a possible interaction between the locus coeruleus NA system and glycocorticoids in avoidance learning. It was dis-

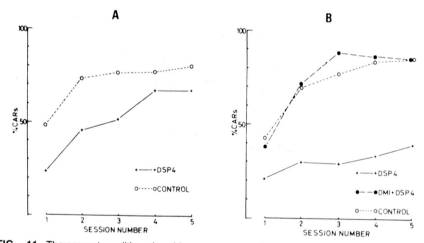

FIG. 11. The percent conditioned avoidance responses (CARs) during each session for control and DSP4-treated rats. DSP4 was injected once (50 mg/kg, i.p.) 7 days prior to the start of acquisition training. DMI + DPS4-treated rats were injected with desipramine (20 mg/kg, i.p.) 20 min prior to the DSP4 injection. Controls received i.p. injections of distilled water (1 ml/kg). **A:** Tukey's HSD test indicated a significant difference in the 1% level on the first three sessions. **B:** Tukey's HSD test indicated significant differences at the 1% level in each of the final four sessions (see text). Two-way avoidance acquisition took place in a shuttlebox as previously described. Each trial consisted of 10 sec tone (1000 Hz) presentation followed by 5 sec shock (1.0 mA). A 40 sec intertrial interval was maintained and 60 trials were presented during each daily session (31).

covered that the combination of 6-OHDA-induced lesions of the ascending dorsal NA bundle to the cerebral cortex and bilateral adrenalectomy resulted in a marked retention deficit in a two-way condition avoidance response and in a complete failure to relearn this response (32,33). On the other hand, adrenalectomy alone or 6-OHDA-induced lesions of the dorsal NA bundle alone, did not impair the acquisition of two-way avoidance learning. It could be demonstrated that the failure to learn a two-way active avoidance response following adrenalectomy and dorsal noradrenaline bundle lesion was not due to a motor deficit or to change in pain sensitivity. Moreover, it does not seem to be due to abnormalities in the cortical EEG or in the hippocampal EEG, since they appeared normal also during learning (Henriksson, Fuxe, Roberts, Ögren, and Bloom, *unpublished data*). Subsequently it could also be shown that a reacquisition of a one-way active avoidance response was significantly impaired in 6-OHDA dorsal NA bundle lesioned and adrenalectomized rats (30), which is a substantially easier task to learn compared with a two-way active avoidance response. The learning deficit in the one-way situation and to a certain degree also in the two-way situation was counteracted by treatment with corticosterone in twice daily doses of 1 mg/kg given subcutaneously. It deserves mentioning that a deficit in passive avoidance acquisition and in the 24-hr retention of step-down passive avoidance has been noted following 6-OHDA-induced lesions of the dorsal NA bundle combined with adrenalectomy (36).

These findings could be evidence for an important complementary role of glycocorticoids and cortical NA receptor activity in avoidance learning. Both these systems may be regarded as survival systems, and removal of one of them does not result in a deficit unless the other survival system also is lesioned. In view of the widespread distribution of corticosterone receptors (43) in the cerebral cortex as well as of the vast networks of the cortical NA nerve terminals it seems likely that this interaction involves large parts of the cerebral hemispheres.

A discussion of the mechanisms by which changes in pituitary adrenal activity can influence central NA neurotransmission is of substantial interest. It should be noted that adrenalectomy can counteract the increase in the number of β-adrenergic binding sites in the cerebral cortex following a 6-OHDA-induced lesion of the coeruleocortical noradrenaline pathway using as radioligand the β-adrenergic receptor blocking agent [³H]dihydroalprenolol (30). These results strongly suggest that adrenal steroids are of importance for the adaptive changes occurring in the β-adrenergic receptors in the cerebral cortex following removal of the cortical NA afferent input. The blockade of supersensitivity development at β-adrenergic receptors following adrenalectomy should further enhance the deficit in cortical NA neurotransmission obtained after the lesion of the coeruleocortical NA pathway and could in this way at least partly be responsible for the learning deficit observed in animals that have been adrenalectomized and in which the dorsal NA bundle has been lesioned. Mobley and Sulser (28) have also shown that adrenal corticoids can regulate NA receptor-coupled adenylate cyclase in the brain. On the basis of these observations it seems reasonable that corticosterone receptors present in cortical nerve cells, showing β-adrenergic receptors in their nerve cell membranes, via changes in genetic transcription can influence the biochemical signals regulating biological effectors, coupling proteins and recognition sites of the receptors that are essential for the induction of especially adaptive responses occurring in, e.g., β-adrenergic receptors (6).

It should be noted that the deficit in learning in the DSP4-treated animals may not be produced via exactly the same mechanisms as in the 6-OHDA-treated and adrenalectomized rats, since in the DSP4-treated animals there exists an increase in the secretion of corticosterone (30). However, in spite of this situation corticosterone (1 mg/kg, twice daily) given to DSP4-treated animals can significantly counteract the impairment of learning produced by DSP4 shown in the experiments on two-way active acquisition (9).

It deserves mentioning, however, that corticosterone treatment does not modify the increase in the number of β-adrenergic receptors found in the cerebral cortex in the DSP4-treated rats. Under all conditions, these experiments also underline the view that glycocorticoids can increase learning ability in animals showing learning deficits due to an impairment of neurotransmission in the locus coeruleus NA systems.

ON THE ROLE OF CENTRAL 5-HT NEURONS IN AVOIDANCE LEARNING

Studies by Ögren and colleagues (29,34) have clearly demonstrated that parachloroamphetamine (PCA) produces an impairment of active avoidance learning by releasing 5-HT and increasing 5-HT receptor activity within the brain (Fig. 12). Thus, it has been shown that tryptophan hydroxylase inhibitors such as parachlorophenylalanine can antagonize the action of PCA (Fig. 13) and likewise pretreatment with 5-HT uptake blocking agents such as zimelidine also blocks the capacity of PCA to produce active avoidance learning impairment. Finally, a 5-HT receptor blocking agent such as methergoline can antagonize the behavioural effects of PCA (29,34).

As seen from the dose–effect curves very small doses of PCA are sufficient to produce an avoidance deficit in spite of the fact that these doses of PCA only produce slight effects on 5-HT concentrations (Fig. 12). These results indicate that PCA can release 5-HT from extragranular sites, especially since PCA is capable of releasing 5-HT also following reserpine treatment.

The evidence suggests that the learning deficit produced by PCA is not related to changes in nonassociative processes such as pain, sensitivity, and motor activity. Instead the studies of Ögren and colleagues (29,34) suggest that the learning deficit produced is due to an effect on the formation of the memory trace. There is little doubt that PCA has its highest activity during the early phase of acquisition. Thus, it seems as if central 5-HT systems are controllers of the acquisition and storage of acquired information. Since PCA mainly affects the ascending 5-HT pathways it seems as if these systems innervating the forebrain have an inhibitory role in the

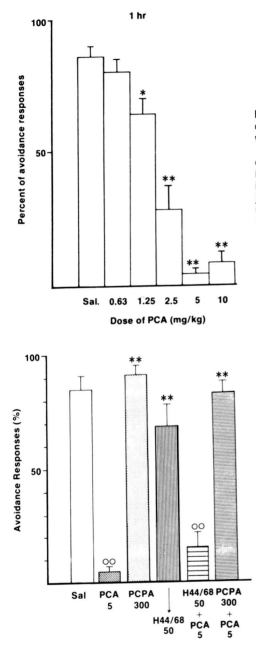

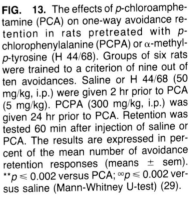

FIG. 12. The effect of PCA administration on the retention of an unsignalled active one-way avoidance response. Groups of rats (n = 5–6) were trained to a criterion of nine out of ten consecutive avoidance responses and injected with saline or PCA (0.63 – 10 mg/kg, i.p.). Retention was tested 60 min after injection of saline or PCA. *p ≤ 0.05; **p ≤ 0.01, versus the saline group (Mann-Whitney U-test) (29).

FIG. 13. The effects of p-chloroamphetamine (PCA) on one-way avoidance retention in rats pretreated with p-chlorophenylalanine (PCPA) or α-methyl-p-tyrosine (H 44/68). Groups of six rats were trained to a criterion of nine out of ten avoidances. Saline or H 44/68 (50 mg/kg, i.p.) were given 2 hr prior to PCA (5 mg/kg). PCPA (300 mg/kg, i.p.) was given 24 hr prior to PCA. Retention was tested 60 min after injection of saline or PCA. The results are expressed in percent of the mean number of avoidance retention responses (means ± sem). **p ≤ 0.002 versus PCA; ∞p ≤ 0.002 versus saline (Mann-Whitney U-test) (29).

information processing. This inhibitory role may mainly be caused by the fact that 5-HT neurotransmission can reduce the activity in the filter mechanisms for sensory inputs in the brainstem. In this way irrelevant sensory stimuli can reach the cortical regions with their local circuits where memory traces probably are formed (see *below)*. There exists clearcut behavioural and neurophysiological evidence that 5-HT terminals can participate in regulation of sensory inputs (14). In agreement with this view Ögren and colleagues have recently shown that by increasing afferent inputs of various types during the learning sessions, the behavioural potency of PCA can be considerably enhanced, provided the afferent stimuli are of no help for the discrimination in the learning process. As a matter of fact, Ögren and colleagues found that by increasing the possibility of rats to discriminate during the learning process the learning deficit produced by PCA could be almost completely attenuated.

In agreement with the view that 5-HT neurotransmission can impair avoidance learning by increasing the access of sensory stimuli to reach the local circuits of the cerebral cortex it has been found that the well-known hallucinogen, *d*-LSD, and the indoleamine hallucinogens, which also are 5-HT receptor agonists, can impair avoidance learning (42). In the lower dose range the hallucinogens instead increase avoidance learning, which probably is related to the fact that they, in this dose range, preferentially stimulate the presynaptic 5-HT receptors in this way reducing 5-HT neurotransmission (42). It is possible that 5-HT receptors in the hippocampal formation may be of particular importance in the regulation of memory storage processes, since microinjections of 5-HT into the hippocampal formation immediately after the acquisition of a passive avoidance response produces a clearcut deficit in retention tested 24 hr later (15).

Possible Role of Local Circuits in the Formation of the Memory Trace

The concept of synaptic plasticity seems to be the essence of various theories of learning and memory (21). Local circuits may be the seat of the synaptic plasticity related to memory, since they represent very important integrative elements in the brain (Fig. 14). As defined by Rakic (35), a local circuit is any portion of a neuron or neurons that can function as an independent integrative unit. Recently we have underlined the idea that local circuits not only are the seat for bioelectrical events, especially electrotonic currents, but that they could also act as biochemical units (3). As a matter of fact the bioelectrical events can produce biochemical events in the local circuits, and we hypothesize that the biochemical events generated by the bioelectrical signals can form the memory trace. The biochemical events may result in the synthesis of macromolecules related to the memory processes. This hypothesis postulates the formation of local "memory" molecules in the local circuit that is a "biochemical mirror" of the sequence for electrical events occurring in the local circuits. It is further hypothesized that this molecule has the capacity to play back the specific sequence or electrical activity in the local circuit. Thus, the local molecule formed can modulate the characteristics of the receptor complexes of the membranes of the local circuit in such a way that the electrical sequence that has just taken place can be repeated in the same order as earlier. The local molecule may in this way produce a short-term memory by changing the degree of positive or negative cooperativity to the interactions within or between channel and/or receptor macromolecules or their subunits (see 38). These changes will in turn produce graded changes in the sensitivity of the various gating mechanisms in the local circuit so that it will be preferentially activated according to a certain sequence

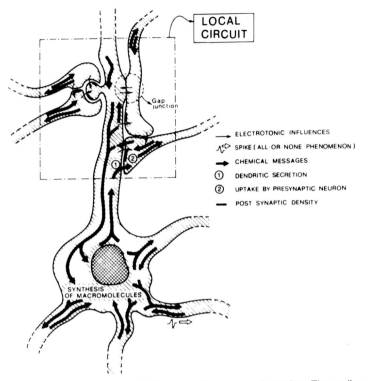

FIG. 14. Schematic representation of information flow in neural circuitry. The coding of the information by means of either electrical phenomena (graded electrotonic potentials and action potentials) or molecules (bidirectional transport within axons and dendrites and transsynaptic transport between neurons) is shown (3).

order. In the presence of a local macromolecule formed it may be sufficient to trigger one part of the electrical sequence to obtain the complete electrical sequence (short-term memory). In this way a possible feedback mechanism is also obtained that can ensure the maintained synthesis of the specific memory molecule. It must further be postulated that the local memory molecule must be resynthesized to obtain a long-term memory. Resynthesis may be obtained by postulating that some of the local molecules via the retrograde flow can reach the cell body region, where it may have the capability of entering the nucleus and initiating the synthesis of a new type of messenger RNA that leads to the formation of a precursor to the local memory molecule formed in the local circuit. These newly synthesized precursors to local memory molecules can flow to the various local circuits via the axoplasmic flow and also reach other types of nerve cells via transsynaptic transport and represent the basis of long-term memory. According to this hypothesis the engram is not a permanent trace in the neurons but rather a biochemical trigger that can induce the trace in a large number of local circuits in various parts of the brain (long-term memory).

The role of the large diffuse NA and 5-HT networks all over the cerebral cortices could partly be regulation of the causal access to the local circuits. The NA nerve terminal networks appear to be involved in selective attention and may, thus, allow relevant afferent inputs to enter into the local circuit of the cortex. The NA terminals may also erase ongoing activity in the local circuit at the same time as they enhance the responsivity of the nerve cell membranes of the local circuits to afferent inputs (11). In this way noise level can be reduced, allowing the relevant afferent inputs to dominate together with the local memory molecules formed. As already mentioned, the experimental evidence indicates that the diffuse 5-HT nerve terminal systems, on the other hand, may interfere with short-term memory formation by allowing irrelevant afferent inputs to reach into the local circuits, making it difficult to set up the correct sequences within the local circuits. Still other types of unspecific cortical afferent systems may play an active role in setting up various types of sequences of impulses in various local circuits. If then part of the sequence is correct the full sequence will be obtained (memory recall). The recall or retrieval of a memory trace may according to this hypothesis trigger the new production of the specific local molecule, further reinforcing the maintenance of the memory trace (memory consolidation). In view of the above it then appears as if memory consolidation can be greatly facilitated by the capacity of certain types of unspecific cortical afferents to set up sequences at the level of the local circuits. Memory consolidation will of course also be increased by a proper regulation of the access of sensory stimuli to the local circuits (see discussion on NA involvement above), leading in view of above to a role of NA terminals also in memory consolidation (26).

Following up this discussion, it may be speculated that the physiology of sleep and especially paradoxic sleep could be to allow the diffuse unspecific cortical afferents access to the local circuits to facilitate memory consolidation. Thus, in this state, which is characterized by a functional deafferentation of the cerebral hemispheres, afferent inputs will not disturb the memory processes.

ACKNOWLEDGMENTS

This work has been supported by a grant (04X-715) from the Swedish Medical Research Council, by a grant from Magnus Bergvall's Foundation, and by a grant from Knut and Alice Wallenberg's Foundation.

REFERENCES

1. Agnati, L. F., Benfenati, F., Cortelli, P., and D'Alessandro, R. (1978): A new method to quantify catecholamine stores visualized by means of the Falck-Hillarp technique. *Neurosci. Lett.*, 10:11–17.
2. Agnati, L. F., Fuxe, K., Andersson, K., Benfenati, F., Cortelli, P., and D'Alessandro, R. (1980): The mesolimbic dopamine system: Evidence for a high amine turnover and for a heterogeneity of the dopamine neuron population. *Neurosci. Lett.*, 18:45–51.
3. Agnati, L. F., Fuxe, K., Ferri, M., Benfenati, F., and Ögren, S.-O. (1981): A new hypothesis on memory—A possible role of local circuits in the formation of the memory trace. *Med. Biol.* 59:224–229.

4. Agnati, L. F., Fuxe, K., Hökfelt, T., Benfenati, F., Calza, L., Johansson, O., and De Mey, J. (1981): Stereological characterization and criteria for subdivision of transmitter-identified nerve cell groups in the central nervous system: Analysis of mesencephalic 5-HT nerve cell bodies. *Brain Res. Bull. (in press)*.
5. Agnati, L. F., Fuxe, K., Hökfelt, T., Goldstein, M., and Jeffcoate, S. L. (1977): A method to measure the distribution pattern of specific nerve terminals in sampled regions studies on tyrosine hydroxylase LHRH, TRH and GIH immunofluorescence. *J. Histochem. Cytochem.*, 24:1222–1236.
6. Agnati, L. F., Fuxe, K., Kuonen, D., Blake, C. A., Andersson, K., Eneroth, P., Gustafsson, J.-Å., Battistini, N., and Calza, L. (1982): Effects of estrogen and progesterone on central- and β-adrenergic receptors in ovariectomized rats: Evidence for gonadal steroid receptor regulation of brain α- and β-adrenergic receptors. In: *Steroid Hormone Regulation of the Brain*, edited by K. Fuxe, J.-Å. Gustafsson, and L. Wetterberg, Pergamon Press, Oxford.
7. Agnati, L. F., Fuxe, K., Scardovi, I., Monari, P., Calza, L., Benfenati, F., Hökfelt, T., and De Mey, J. (1982): Principles for stereological characterization of transmitter-identified cell groups. *J. Neurosci. Methods*, 6:157–167.
8. Anlezark, G. M., Crow, T. J., and Greenway, A. P. (1973): Impaired learning and decreased cortical norepinephrine after bilateral locus coeruleus lesions. *Science*, 181:682–684.
9. Archer, T., Ögren, S.-O., Fuxe, F., Agnati, L. F., and Eneroth, P. (1981): On the interactive role of noradrenaline and corticosterone in two-way active avoidance acquisition. *Neurosci. Lett.*, 27:341–346.
10. Baley, N. T. (1970): *The Mathematical Approach to Biology and Medicine*. John Wiley, London.
11. Bloom, F. E. (1978): Central noradrenergic systems: Physiology and pharmacology. In: *Psychopharmacology: A Generation of Progress*, edited by M. A. Lipton, A. DiMascio, and K. F. Killam, pp. 131–143. Raven Press, New York.
12. Crow, T. J. (1973): The coerulo-cortical norepinephrine system and learning. In: *Frontiers in Catecholamine Research*, edited by E. Usdin and S. H. Snyder, pp. 723–726. Pergamon Press, New York.
13. Dahlström, A., and Fuxe, K. (1964): Evidence for the existence of monoamine containing neurons in the central nervous system. I. Demonstration of monoamines in the cell bodies of brain stem neurons. *Acta Physiol. Scand. (Suppl. 232)*, 62:1–55.
14. Davis, M., and Sheard, M. H. (1976): *p*-Chloroamphetamine (PCA): Acute and chronic effects on habituation and sensitization of the acoustic startle response in rats. *Eur. J. Pharmacol.*, 35:261–273.
15. Essman, W. B. (1973): Neuromolecular modulation of experimentally-induced retrograde amnesia. *Confin. Neurol.*, 35:1–22.
16. Fuxe, K., Andersson, K., Schwarcz, R., Agnati, L. F., Perez de la Mora, M., Hökfelt, T., Goldstein, M., Ferland, L., Possani, L., and Tapia, R. (1979): Studies on different types of dopamine nerve terminals in the forebrain and their possible interaction with hormones and with neurons containing GABA, glutamate and opioid peptides. *Adv. Neurol.*, 24:199–215.
17. Fuxe, K., Fredholm, B. B., Agnati, L. F., and Corrodi, H. (1978): Dopamine receptors and ergot drugs. Evidence that an ergolene derivative is a differential agonist at subcortical limbic dopamine receptors. *Brain Res.*, 146:295–311.
18. Fuxe, K., Hökfelt, T., Jonsson, G., Levine, S., Lidbrink, P., and Löfström, A. (1973): Brain and pituitary-adrenal interaction studies on central monoamine neurons. In: *Brain-Pituitary-Adrenal Interrelationships*, edited by A. Brodish and E. S. Redgate, pp. 239–269. Karger, Basel.
19. Fuxe, K., Hökfelt, T., Olson, L., and Ungerstedt, U. (1977): Central monoaminergic pathways with emphasis on their relation to the so called "extrapyramidal motor system". *Pharmacol. Ther. B.*, 3:169–210.
20. Fuxe, K., and Jonsson, G. (1974): Further mapping of central 5-hydroxytryptamine neurons: Studies with the neurotoxic dihydroxytryptamine. *Adv. Biochem. Psychopharmacol.*, 10:1–12.
21. Hebb, D. O. (1949): *The Organization of Behaviour*. John Wiley, New York.
22. Hökfelt, T., Rehfeld, J. F., Skirboll, L., Ivemark, B., Goldstein, M., and Markey, K. (1980): Evidence for coexistence of dopamine and CCK in mesolimbic neurons. *Nature (Lond.)* 285:476–478.
23. Huang, H. (1979): Model cases from biological morphometry: Nervous tissue. In: *Stereological Methods, Vol. 1*, edited by E. R. Werbel, pp. 311–322. Academic Press, New York.

24. James, N. T. (1977): Stereology. In: *Analytical and Quantitative Methods in Microscopy*, edited by G. A. Meck and H. T. Elder, pp. 9–28. Cambridge University Press, Cambridge.

25. Kety, S. S. (1970): The possible role of the adrenergic system of the cortex in learning. *Res. Publ. Assoc. Res. Nerv. Ment. Dis.*, 50:376–389.

25a. König, J. F. R., and Klippel, R. A. (1963): The rat brain. In: *A Stereotaxic Atlas of the Forebrain and Lower Part of the Brain Stem*. Williams & Wilkins, Baltimore.

26. Kovacz, G. L., Bohus, B., and Versteeg, D. H. G. (1979): Facilitation of memory consolidation by vasopressin: Mediation by terminals of the dorsal noradrenergic bundle. *Brain Res.*, 172:73–85.

27. Mason, S. T., and Fibiger, H. C. (1979): Noradrenaline and avoidance learning in the rat. *Brain Res.*, 161:321–333.

28. Mobley, P. L., and Sulser, F. (1980): Adrenal corticoids regulate sensitivity of noradrenaline receptor-completed adenylate cyclase in brain. *Nature*, 286:608–609.

29. Ögren, S.-O. (1981): Acute effects of the serotonin releasing compound p-chloroamphetamine on active avoidance learning in the rat. Evidence for an involvement of forebrain serotonin pathways in avoidance learning. *Pharmacol. Biochem. Behav. (submitted)*.

30. Ögren, S.-O., Archer, T., Fuxe, K., Eneroth, P., and Agnati, L. F. (1982): Glucocorticoids, catecholamines and avoidance learning. In: *Steroid Hormone Regulation of the Brain*, edited by K. Fuxe, J.-Å. Gustafsson, and L. Wetterberg, Pergamon Press, Oxford.

31. Ögren, S.-O., Archer, T., and Ross, S. B. (1980): Evidence for a role of the locus coeruleus noradrenaline system in learning. *Neurosci. Lett.*, 20:351–356.

32. Ögren, S.-O., and Fuxe, K. (1974): Learning, brain noradrenaline and the pituitary-adrenal axis. *Med. Biol.*, 52:399–405.

33. Ögren, S.-O., and Fuxe, K. (1977): On the role of noradrenaline and the pituitary-adrenal axis in avoidance learning. Studies with corticosterone. *Neurosci. Lett.*, 5:291–296.

34. Ögren, S.-O., Fuxe, K., Archer, T., Hall, H., Holm, A. C., and Köhler, C. (1982): Studies on the role of central 5-HT neurons in avoidance learning: A behavioural and biochemical analysis. In: *Serotonin: Current Aspects of Neruochemistry and Function*, edited by B. Haber and S. Gabay. Plenum Press, New York.

35. Rakic, P. (1979): Genetic and epigenetic determinants of local neuronal circuits in the mammalian central nervous system. In: *The Neurosciences: Fourth Study Program*, edited by F. O. Schmitt and F. G. Worden, pp. 109–129. The MIT Press, Cambridge.

36. Roberts, D. C. S., and Fibiger, H. C. (1977): Evidence for interactions between central noradrenaline neurons and adrenal hormones in learning and memory. *Pharmac. Biochem. Behav.*, 7:191–194.

37. Schipper, J. (1979): A scanning microfluorimetric study on noradrenergic neurotransmission. M.D. Thesis, Amsterdam.

38. Schmitt, F. O. (1979): The role of structural, electrical and chemical circuitry in brain function. In: *The Neurosciences: Fourth Study Program*, edited by F. O. Schmitt and F. G. Worden, pp. 5–21. The MIT Press, Cambridge.

39. Schwartz, D. E. (1971): Stereology: Application to biomedical research. *Physiol. Rev.*, 51:158–200.

40. Steinbusch, H. W. N. (1981): Distribution of serotonin-immunoreactivity in the central nervous system of the rat. Cell bodies and terminals. *Neuroscience*, 6:557–618.

41. Steinbusch, H. W. N., Verhofstad, A. A. J., and Joosten, H. W. J. (1978): Localization of serotonin in the central nervous system by immunohistochemistry. Description of a specific and sensitive technique and some applications. *Neuroscience*, 3:811–819.

42. Stoff, D. M., Gorelick, D. A., Bozewicz, T., Bridger, W. H., Gillin, J. C., and Wyatt, R. J. (1978): The indole hallucinogens N,N-dimethyltryptamine (DMT) and 5-methoxy-N,N-dimethyltryptamine (5-MeO-DMT) have different effects from mescaline on rat shuttlebox avoidance. *Neuropharmacology*, 17:1035–1040.

43. Stumpf, W. E. (1979): Binding of estrogens, progestagens, androgens and corticosteroids in the central nervous system. In: *Interaction between the Nervous and the Endocrine Systems*, edited by A. A. J. Verhofstad and J. A. M. van Kermenade, pp. 103–134. University of Nijmegen, The Netherlands.

44. Tramu, G., Pillez, A., and Leonardelli, J. (1978): An efficient method of antibody elution for the successive or simultaneous location of two antigens by immunocytochemistry. *J. Histochem. Cytochem.*, 26:322–324.
45. Wied, D. de (1974): Pituitary-adrenal system hormones and behavior. In: *The Neurosciences: Third Study Program*, edited by F. Schmitt and F. Warden, pp. 653–666. The MIT Press, Cambridge.

Neural Transmission, Learning and Memory,
edited by R. Caputto and C. Ajmone Marsan.
Raven Press, New York © 1983.

Role of Learning and Memory in Maternal Behavior

J. Prilusky

*Laboratorio de Reproducción y Lactancia (LARLAC), Consejo Nacional de
Investigaciones Científicas y Técnicas (CONICET), Mendoza, Argentina*

In general, the influence that learning and experience may have on the performance of a particular task can be determined in experimental situations in which naive subjects are unable to perform what their experienced counterparts do.

This is not true in the case of maternal behavior, since it is always present after parturition, even in primiparous animals, enabling the new mother to take care of the litter in a way difficult to distinguish from the manner of the multiparous one (33). The principal activities that comprise maternal behavior: nest building, retrieving, cleaning and nursing of the pups, are performed in a functionally adequate form, few minutes after the first pup is raised, even by primiparous rats (1).

Although the mother-pups relationship is generally considered as instinctive, "the fact that a behavioral pattern occurs effectively the first time the animal is in the biologically appropriate situation does not necessarily indicate that learning has played no role in its genesis" (29).

Three phases can be distinguished in the rat maternal behavior: the initiation phase, from the 1st to the 3rd postpartum day; the maintenance phase (4th to 14th day); and the declination phase, which extends until the 21st to 28th postpartum day (45,47). We believe that memory, learning, and previous experience play an important role in each of these phases, interacting with pups' stimuli and endocrine changes to allow the full expression of maternal behavior.

SENSORY AND HORMONAL INFLUENCES

The initiation of maternal behavior presumably depends both on the presence of pups (44) and on the endogenously determined variation in circulating hormone levels (see 16,45 for review). It seems that estrogen, progesterone, and prolactin are implicated, but none of them is individually sufficient for the initiation of maternal behavior (25). Studies done on ovariectomized pregnant rats (9), on hysterectomized pregnant females, and on hysterectomized-ovariectomized rats treated with estrogen (48–50) have shown that estrogen facilitates the initiation of maternal behavior. Progesterone, on the other hand, has an inhibitory effect on the onset of this behavior (7,8,36,51). Prolactin by itself, however, does not seem to have a direct effect on maternal responsiveness (6,41). Instead, it seems to act through the adrenal gland by "buffering" the stress responses (31,54) that could interfere with the expression of maternal behavior.

The optimal hormonal balance seems to be present only around the time of parturition. The injection of blood plasma taken from mothers within 48 hr after parturition (58) reduces the latency for the onset of maternal behavior in virgin recipients from 4–6 days to 2 days. The cross-transfusion of blood taken from newly parturient rats can induce maternal behavior in virgin female rats in a shorter time (45 hr), when the experimental procedure is initiated just after parturition (59).

Parturition itself is not crucial for the initiation of maternal behavior, since females after cesarean section before term develop maternal behavior toward foster pups (15,29,61). In fact, maternal behavior is present shortly before term (48,53) in the intact pregnant female.

In any case, the presence of pups provides the stimuli for the initiation of maternal behavior. Among these stimuli, the olfactory ones seem to play an important role. Studies in which virgin rats were exposed to pups have shown that the young are first actively avoided by nonmaternal animals. Only after several days, naive rats will tolerate a close and continuous contact with pups and initiate maternal behavior (11).

Deafferentation of the olfactory and vomeronasal system prior to pups' exposure, either by intranasal infusion of zinc sulfate, by bulbectomy or by lesions of the olfactory and vomeronasal tracts, reduced the aversive responses to pups in non-pregnant animals, leads to a short latency initiation of maternal behavior (12,13,23,24).

These evidences suggest that one of the differences between a naive and an experienced rat may be the knowledge the latter has of pup odors. The long latencies for initiation of maternal behavior may be related to the time the rat needs to overcome the aversive impact of chemical stimuli from the pups.

Any experimental procedure able to minimize the "odor-impact" should be conducive to shorter latencies in the appearance of maternal behavior in naive non-pregnant rats. Noirot (32) found that the "priming" of nonmaternal subjects by exposure to pup odors, greatly increases the maternal responses (retrieving and nest building). The retention of maternal behavior on subjects kept in a room with other mothers and their pups, but without pups of their own (Deis, *unpublished results*), may be related to the same mechanism, since the continuous exposure to odors from pups in other cages may reduce the aversive impact of odors from pups introduced later in their same cages.

The maintenance phase of maternal behavior, on the other hand, seems to depend mainly on pups' stimulation (46). Once maternal behavior is established, either in postpartum or virgin pup-induced rats, it can be maintained as long as fresh pups are provided. Such a maternally behaving rat will stay in the maintenance phase for as long as her pups are periodically replaced by younger pups. The declination of maternal behavior is not associated with internal changes in the mother, but seems to be a consequence of the growing independence of the young (45). Prolactin may effectively help to maintain the mother-pup relationship by contributing to the emission of the maternal pheromone, which plays an important role from the 14th postpartum day onward (19–21,27).

With regard to the endocrine control of maternal behavior it should be emphasized, finally, that the only feature of this behavior that is clearly affected by hormones is the latency of its initiation. In fact, maternal behavior has been elicited in intact and castrated rats of both sexes, as well as in hypophysectomized females (44) and immature intact rats (22,26,45).

THE NEURAL BASIS

Certain brain structures must be present for the expression of maternal behavior. Radiofrequency lesions in the ventral mesencephalic tegmentum disrupt maternal behavior (14). The multiparous rats studied did not build nests either before or after parturition, cannibalized their pups, and did not nurse a foster litter.

Beach (1,2) and Davis (10) also showed that extensive cortical ablations interfered with the efficiency of various aspects of maternal behavior of the rat. Beach (2) found that lesions performed during infancy had far less effect than similar lesions performed in adulthood, implying that removal of cortex in adults interfered with learned patterns that did not yet exist in infants. More recently, Stamm (55) and Slotnick (52) confirmed and extended these results. They found that the sole removal of the cingulate cortex is effective to disrupt maternal behavior and they suggested that this may be the consequence of a more general role of the cingulate cortex in the organization of complex activities.

Besides the cingulate cortex, other limbic structures are also involved in maternal behavior, and they may be acting through modulating the activity of the preoptic area (34,35,37,54). Transection of dorsal limbic afferents to the preoptic area abolish maternal behavior (60), and this effect may be exerted through changes in brain norepinephrine (42,43,56). Cuts made laterally (36,37,57) but not posteriorly to the preoptic area (60) produce deficits in maternal behavior.

ROLE OF EXPERIENCE

Some evidence substantiates the view that the previous experience of simple tasks such as carrying objects or self-licking the genitalia are indispensable for the expression of maternal behavior. In fact, this might be questioning the "naiveness" of the primiparous mother when she is first confronted with a pup.

Riess (40) raised rats in isolation, preventing them from manipulating or carrying objects. The floor of the cage consisted of netting to draw the feces out of reach. All food was powdered, so that the rat never carried food pellets. When mature, placed in a regular breeding cage, these rats failed to build a nest before or during pregnancy, and failed to retrieve their pups normally. They scattered the nesting material all over the cage and moved the litter from place to place without grouping them in the nest.

Birch (3) showed that rats that had no opportunity to perform genital self-licking during pregnancy, generally eat their young, and do not take care of the surviving ones. Apparently, a rat must learn that something that smells and tastes like her genitalia must be licked, not bitten.

These are just two examples of behaviors that might be considered unrelated to maternal behavior, but that affect the normal development of maternal responses in the rat. We believe that we must not diminish the importance of previous experiences when considering the performance of a new response. In this sense, maternal behavior appears as a recombination of previously learned tasks, which is fully developed under appropriate environmental and endocrine conditions.

Even the basic level of maternal responsiveness (44) seems not to be innate, but gradually acquired as a result of animal-environment interactions (20,21).

RETENTION OF MATERNAL BEHAVIOR

After the onset of maternal behavior, maternal responsiveness continues for some time, since this behavior is exhibited by nonlactating primiparous rats upon presentation of foster pups, weeks after the cessation of lactation (4). Reinduction of maternal behavior in a previously sensitized virgin female occurred with a shorter latency than did in the first induction (11). Cesarean operated animals on day 22 of gestation, exposed to pups for 70 hr and then housed singly for 25 days, exhibited a rapid onset of maternal behavior upon reintroduction of 2- to 5-day-old pups, showing that the act of parturition is not essential for the establishment of the long-term retention of maternal behavior (5).

When the hormonal balance of the peripartum period is altered, either by ovariectomy (30) or by progesterone administration (28), only multiparous females show normal maternal behavior, indicating that experience can also overcome the adverse effects of hormone unbalance.

It is clear, therefore, that maternal responsiveness should be stored in some way in the rat. A possible explanation may be a change in excitability of nervous circuits involved in these responses (30). Another possibility is the accumulation of a brain substance or substances that might modulate the excitability of those neurons. Recent studies conducted with two brain peptides, oxytocin and vasopressin, have shown that they may serve an important role in the induction of maternal behavior (38). Oxytocin was clearly superior to Arg-vasopressin in producing full maternal responses, this effect being estrogen dependent. Brain extracts obtained from primiparous mothers on day 16 of lactation cause a rapid maternal response to foster pups (39). Neither blood nor kidney extracts from mothers on day 16 of lactation influenced maternal responsiveness. These results suggest the development, within the brain of the lactating mother, of a factor capable of inducing maternal behavior in a nonlactating rat. The factor is present in the microsomal and soluble fractions of the brain homogenate, and has a molecular weight of less than 12,000.

They further suggest that the accumulation of this putative factor is related to experience, since brain extracts prepared from virgin rats or from primiparous rats killed on the 1st postpartum day were ineffective in inducing maternal behavior (39).

CONCLUSIONS

The considerations made above point to the role that learning and memory play in maternal behavior. The presence of the young triggers a maternal mechanism that is affected by the hormonal background and that involves several brain structures, neurotransmitters, and, probably, peptides. In such a mechanism, previous experience has certainly a role of its own, providing at least some of the elementary behaviors which are incorporated, at the time of parturition, into a broader and more specialized behavioral frame. Moreover, experience may consolidate maternal responsiveness in a way that the full behavior can be expressed even in adverse hormonal conditions.

ACKNOWLEDGMENTS

The author is a Career Scientist of the Consejo Nacional de Investigaciones Científicas y Técnicas of Argentina. The assistance of Dr. A. Castro-Vázquez for criticism during the preparation of the manuscript and Dr. A. M. Fages for editing the manuscript is gratefully acknowledged.

REFERENCES

 1. Beach, F. R. (1937): The neural basis of innate behavior. I. Effects of cortical lesions upon the maternal behaviour pattern in the rat. *J. Comp. Physiol. Psychol.*, 24:393–439.
 2. Beach, F. R. (1938): The neural basis of innate behavior. II. Relative effects of partial decortication in adulthood and infancy upon the maternal behavior of the primiparous rat. *J. Gen. Psychol.*, 53:109–148.
 3. Birch, H. G. (1956): Sources of order in maternal behavior of animals. *Am. J. Orthopsychiatry*, 26:279–284.
 4. Bridges, R. S. (1975): Long-term effects of pregnancy and parturition upon maternal responsiveness in rat. *Physiol. Behav.*, 14:245–249.
 5. Bridges, R. S. (1977): Parturition: Its role in the long term retention of maternal behavior in the rat. *Physiol. Behav.*, 18:487–490.
 6. Bridges, R. S., Goldman, B. D., and Bryant, L. P. (1974): Serum prolactin concentrations and the initiation of maternal behavior in the rat. *Horm. Behav.*, 5:219–226.
 7. Bridges, R. S., Rosenblatt, R. S., and Feder, H. H. (1978): Serum progesterone concentrations and maternal behavior in rats after pregnancy termination: Behavioral stimulation after progesterone withdrawal and inhibition by progesterone maintenance. *Endocrinology*, 102:258–267.
 8. Bridges, R. S., Rosenblatt, J. S., and Feder, H. H. (1978): Stimulation of maternal responsiveness after pregnancy termination in rats: Effects of the time of onset of behavioral testing. *Horm. Behav.*, 10:235–245.
 9. Catala, S. and Deis, R. P. (1973): Effect of oestrogen upon parturition, maternal behaviour and lactation in ovariectomized pregnant rats. *J. Endocrinol.*, 56:219–225.
10. Davis, C. D. (1939): The effect of ablations of neocortex on mating, maternal behavior and the production of pseudopregnancy in the female rat and on copulatory activity in the male. *Am. J. Physiol.*, 127:374–380.
11. Fleming, R. S., and Rosenblatt, J. S. (1974): Maternal behavior in the virgin and lactating rat. *J. Comp. Physiol. Psychol.*, 86:957–972.
12. Fleming, R. S., and Rosenblatt, J. S. (1974) : Olfactory regulation of maternal behavior in rats: I. Effects of olfactory bulb removal in experienced and inexperienced lactating and cycling females. *J. Comp. Physiol. Psychol.*, 86:221–232.
13. Fleming, R. S., and Rosenblatt, J. S. (1974): Olfactory regulation of maternal behavior in rats. II. Effects of peripherally induced anosmia and lesions of the lateral olfactory tract in pup-induced virgins. *J. Comp. Physiol. Psychol.*, 86:233–246.

14. Gaffori, O., and Le Moal, M. (1979): Disruption of maternal behavior and appearance of cannibalism after ventral mesencephalic tegmentum lesions. *Physiol. Behav.*, 23:317–323.
15. Labriola, J. (1953): Effects of cesarean delivery upon maternal behavior in rats. *Proc. Soc. Exp. Biol.*, 83:556–567.
16. Lamb, M. E. (1975): Physiological mechanism in the control of maternal behavior in rats: A review. *Psychol. Bull.*, 82:104–119.
17. Lehrman, D. S. (1953): A critique of Konrad Lorenz's theory of instinctive behavior. *Q. Rev. Biol.*, 28:337–363.
18. Lehrman, D. S. (1956): On the organization of maternal behavior and the problem of instinct. In: *L'instinct dans le Comportement des Animaux et des l'Homme.* Masson et Cie, Paris, pp. 425–520.
19. Leidahl, L. C., and Moltz, M. (1975): Emission of the maternal pheromone in the nulliparous female and failure of emission in the adult male. *Physiol. Behav.*, 14:421–424.
20. Leon, M., and Moltz, M. (1971): Maternal pheromone: Discrimination by pre-weanling albino rats. *Physiol. Behav.*, 7:265–267.
21. Leon, M., and Moltz, M. (1972): The development of the pheromonal bond in the albino rat. *Physiol. Behav.*, 8:683–686.
22. Mayer, A. D., Freeman, N. C. G., and Rosenblatt, J. S. (1979): Ontogeny of maternal behavior in the laboratory rat: Factors underlying changes in responsiveness from 30 to 90 days. *Dev. Psychol.*, 12:425–439.
23. Mayer, A. D., and Rosenblatt, J. S. (1975): Olfactory basis for the delayed onset of maternal behavior in virgin female rats. Experiential effects. *J. Comp. Physiol. Psychol.*, 89:701–710.
24. Mayer, A. D., and Rosenblatt, J. S. (1977):Effects of intranasal zinc sulfate on open field and maternal behavior in female rats. *Physiol. Behav.*, 18:101–109.
25. Mayer, A. D., and Rosenblatt, J. S. (1979): Hormonal influences during the ontogeny of maternal behavior in female rats. *J. Comp. Physiol. Psychol.*, 93:879–898.
26. Mayer, A. D., and Rosenblatt, J. S. (1979): Ontogeny of maternal behavior in the laboratory rat: Early origins in 18- to 27-day-old young. *Dev. Psychol.*, 12:407–424.
27. Moltz, M., and Leidahl, L. C. (1977): Bile, prolactin and the maternal pheromone. *Science*, 196:81–83.
28. Moltz, M., Levin, R., and Leon, M. (1969): Differential effects of progesterone on the maternal behavior of primiparous and multiparous rats. *J. Comp. Physiol. Psychol.*, 67:36–40.
29. Moltz, H., Robbins, D., and Parks, M. (1966): Cesarean delivery and maternal behavior of primiparous and multiparous rats. *J. Comp. Physiol. Psychol.*, 61:455–460.
30. Moltz, M., and Wiener, E. (1966): Effects of ovariectomy on maternal behavior of primiparous and multiparous rats. *J. Comp. Physiol. Psychol.*, 62:382–387.
31. Myers, M. M., Denemberg, V. H., Thoman, E., Holloway, W. R., and Bowerman, D. R. (1975): The effects of litter size on plasma corticoesterone and prolactin response to ether stress in the lactating rat. *Neuroendocrinology*, 19:54–58.
32. Noirot, E. (1969): Changes in responsiveness to young in the adult mouse. V. Priming. *Anim. Behav.*, 17:542–546.
33. Noirot, E. (1972): The onset of maternal behavior in rats, hamsters and mice. A selective review. In: *Advances in the Study of Behavior, Vol. 4*, pp. 107–145. Academic Press, New York and London.
34. Noonan, M., and Dristal, M. B. (1979): Effects of medial preoptic lesions on placentophagia and the onset of maternal behavior in the rat. *Physiol. Behav.*, 22:1197–1202.
35. Numan, M. (1974): Medial preoptic area and maternal behavior in the female rat. *J. Comp. Physiol. Psychol.*, 87:746–759.
36. Numan, M. (1978): Progesterone inhibition of maternal behavior in the rat. *Horm. Behav.*, 11:209–231.
37. Numan, M., Rosenblatt, J. S., and Komisaruk, B. R. (1977): Medial preoptic area and onset of maternal behavior in the rat. *J. Comp. Physiol. Psychol.*, 91:146–164.
38. Pendersen, C. R., and Prange, J. (1979): Induction of maternal behavior in virgin rats after intracerebroventricular administration of oxytocin. *Proc. Natl. Acad. Sci. USA*, 76:6661–6665.
39. Prilusky, J. (1981): Induction of maternal behavior in the virgin rat by lactating-rat brain extracts. *Physiol. Behav.*, 26:149–152.
40. Riess, B. F. (1950): The isolation of factors of learning and native behavior in field and laboratory studies. *Ann. NY Acad. Sci.*, 51:1093–1102.

41. Rodriquez-Sierra, J. F., and Rosenblatt, J. S. (1977): Does prolactin play a role in estrogen-induced maternal behavior in rats: apomorphine reduction of prolactin release. *Horm. Behav.*, 9:1–7.
42. Rosenberg, P., Halaris, A., and Moltz, M. (1977): Effects of central norepinephrine depletion on the initiation and maintenance of maternal behavior in the rat. *Pharmacol. Biochem. Behav.*, 6:21–24.
43. Rosenberg, P., Leidahl, L., Halaris, A., and Moltz, M. (1976): Changes in the metabolism of hypothalamic norepinephrine associated with the onset of maternal behavior in the nulliparous rat. *Pharmacol. Biochem. Behav.*, 4:647–649.
44. Rosenblatt, J. S. (1967): Nonhormonal basis of maternal behavior in the rat. *Science*, 156:1512–1514.
45. Rosenblatt, J. S. (1969): The development of maternal responsiveness in the rat. *Am. J. Orthopsychiatry*, 39:36–56.
46. Rosenblatt, J. S. (1970): Views on the onset and maintenance of maternal behavior in the rat. In: *Development and Evolution of Behavior*, edited by L. R. Aronson, E. Tobach, J. S. Rosenblatt, and D. S. Lehrman, pp. 489–518. Freeman, San Francisco, California.
47. Rosenblatt, J. S., and Lehrman, D. S. (1963): Maternal behavior of the laboratory rat. In: *Maternal Behavior in Mammals*, edited by H. L. Rheingold, p. 8. John Wiley & Sons, New York.
48. Rosenblatt, J. S., and Siegel, H. I. (1975): Hysterectomy-induced maternal behavior during pregnancy in the rat. *J. Comp. Physiol. Psychol.*, 89:685–700.
49. Siegel, H. I., and Rosenblatt, J. S. (1975): Estrogen-induced maternal behavior in hysterectomized-ovariectomized virgin rats. *Physiol. Behav.*, 14:465–471.
50. Siegel, H. I., and Rosenblatt, J. S. (1975) : Hormonal basis of hysterectomy-induced maternal behavior in the rat. *Horm. Behav.*, 6:211–222.
51. Siegel, H. I., and Rosenblatt, J. S. (1978): Duration of estrogen stimulation and progesterone inhibition of maternal behavior in pregnancy-terminated rats. *Horm. Behav.*, 11:12–19.
52. Slotnick, B. M. (1967): Disturbance of maternal behavior in the rat following lesions of the cingulate cortex. *Behaviour*, 24:204–236.
53. Slotnick, B. M., Carpenter, M. L., and Fusco, R. (1973): Initiation of maternal behavior in pregnant nulliparous rats. *Horm. Behav.*, 4:53–59.
54. Smotherman, W. P., Hennessy, J. W., and Levine, S. (1977): Medial preoptic area cuts in the lactating female rat: Effects on maternal behavior and pituitary-adrenal activity. *Physiol. Psychol.*, 5:243–246.
55. Stamm, J. S. (1955): The function of the median cerebral cortex in maternal behavior of rats. *J. Comp. Physiol. Psychol.*, 48:347–356.
56. Steele, M. K., Rowland, D., and Moltz, H. (1979): Initiation of maternal behavior in the rat: Possible involvement of limbic norepinephrine. *Pharmacol. Biochem. Behav.*, 11:123–130.
57. Terkel, J., Bridges, R. S., and Sawyer, C. H. (1979): Effects of transecting lateral neural connections of the medial preoptic area on maternal behavior in the rat: Nest building, pup retrieval and prolactin secretion. *Brain Res.*, 169:369–380.
58. Terkel, J., and Rosenblatt, J. S. (1968): Maternal behavior induced by maternal blood plasma injected into virgin rats. *J. Comp. Physiol. Psychol.*, 65:479–482.
59. Terkel, J., and Rosenblatt, J. S. (1972): Humoral factors underlying maternal behavior at parturition: Cross transfusion between freely moving rats. *J. Comp. Physiol. Psychol.*, 80:365–371.
60. Velasco, M. E., Castro-Vazquez, A., and Rotchild, I. (1974): Effects of hypothalamic deafferentation on criteria of prolactin secretion during pregnancy and lactation in the rat. *J. Rep. Fert.*, 41:385–395.
61. Wiesner, B. P., and Sheard, N. M. (1933): *Maternal Behaviour in the Rat*. Oliver and Boyd, London.

Author Index

Numbers in parentheses before page of citation are reference numbers; italicized numbers represent the page on which the reference appears.

Subject Index